Perinatal Medicine

Perinatal Medicine

Edited by

J. Clinch
and
T. Matthews

*Proceedings of the IX European Congress of
Perinatal Medicine held in Dublin, Ireland
September 3rd–5th 1984*

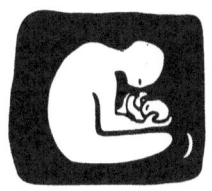

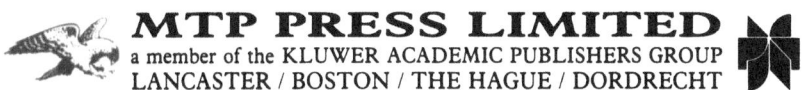

MTP PRESS LIMITED
a member of the KLUWER ACADEMIC PUBLISHERS GROUP
LANCASTER / BOSTON / THE HAGUE / DORDRECHT

Published in the UK and Europe by
MTP Press Limited
Falcon House
Lancaster, England

British Library Cataloguing in Publication Data

European Congress of Perinatal Medicine (*9th:*
  1984: Dublin)
  Perinatal medicine: proceedings of the IX
  European Congress of Perinatal Medicine held in
  Dublin, Ireland, September 3rd–5th 1984.
  1. Obstetrics 2. Pediatrics
  I. Title   II. Clinch, J.   III. Matthews, T.
  618.3'2   RG524
  ISBN-13: 978-94-010-8679-0   e-ISBN-13: 978-94-009-4918-8
  DOI: 10.1007/978-94-009-4918-8

Published in the USA by
MTP Press
A division of Kluwer Boston Inc
190 Old Derby Street
Hingham, MA 02043, USA

Contents

Committee Members

Scientific Committee:

J. Alvey, Ireland
K. Jaehrig, German Democratic Republic
M. Thiery, Belgium
L.-E. Bratteby, Sweden
M. Orzalesi, Italy
G. McClure, Northern Ireland
A. Van Assche, Belgium
E. Papiernik, France

Local Organizing Committee:

Chairman: J. Clinch
Secretary: T. Matthews

J. O'Sullivan
R. Harrison
R. Counahan
K. Ritchie

List of Contributors

L. AERTS
The Unit for the Study of Reproduction
U.Z. Gasthuisberg
3000 Leuven
BELGIUM

C. AMIEL-TISON
Clinique Universitaire Baudelocque
123, Boulevard de Port-Royal
75674 Paris Cedex 14
FRANCE

P. BERGSJØ
Department of Obstetrics &
Gynaecology
Kvinneklinikken N-5016
Haukeland Sykehus
Bergen
NORWAY

J. BONNAR
T.C.D. Medical School
St. James's Hospital
Dublin 8
IRELAND

J. BOYD
8409–112th Street
Edmonton T6G IK6
CANADA

G. BREART
Epidemiological Research Unit on
    Mother and Child
INSERM U149
123, Boulevard de Port-Royal
75014 Paris
FRANCE

P. BUEKENS
Universite Libre de Bruxelles
Laboratorie d'Epidemiologie
    et de Medicine Sociale
Route de Lennik 808
1070 Bruxelles
BELGIUM

L. J. BUTTERFIELD
Department of Perinatology
The Children's Hospital
1056 East 19th Avenue
Denver
Colorado 80218
USA

I. CHALMERS
National Perinatal Epidemiology Unit
Radcliffe Infirmary
Oxford OX2 6HE
UK

P. CHAMBERLAIN
Department of Obstetrics and
    Gynecology
Regional Hospital
Galway
Ireland

J. CLINCH
Coombe Lying-In Hospital
Dublin 8
IRELAND

J. CONNOLLY
24, Dornden Park
Booterstown
Co. Dublin
IRELAND

R. COOKE
Liverpool Maternity Hospital
Oxford Street
Liverpool L7 7BN
UK

G. DAWES
University of Oxford
The Nuffield Institute for Medical
    Research
Headley Way
Headington
Oxford OX3 9DS
UK

R. DEROM
Department of Obstetrics
University Hospital
De Pintelaan 185
B-9000 Gent
BELGIUM

M. I. DRURY
Department of Endocrinology
Mater Hospital
Eccles Street
Dublin 7
IRELAND

G. DUC
University Department of Neonatology
Frauenklinikstrasse 10
CH-8091 Zurich
SWITZERLAND

P. DUNN
University of Bristol
Department of Child Health
Southmead Hospital
Bristol BS10 5NB
UK

J. FALCK-LARSEN
Department of Obstetrics and
    Gynaecology
Herlev University Hospital
2730 Herlev Copenhagen
DENMARK

K. FUHRMANN
Zentralinstitut fur Diabetes
2201 Karlsburg
GERMAN DEMOCRATIC
REPUBLIC

E. GRAUEL
Kinderklinik
20, Schumannstrasse
104 Berlin
GERMAN DEMOCRATIC
REPUBLIC

H. HALLIDAY
Department of Neonatal Medicine
Royal Maternity Hospital
Grosvenor Road,
Belfast BT12 6BJ
NORTHERN IRELAND

D. HARVEY
Institute of Obstetrics and Gynaecology
Queen Charlotte's Maternity Hospital
Goldhawk Road
London W6 0XG
UK

M. J. N. C. KEIRSE
Department of Obstetrics and
    Gynecology
University Hospital
Rijnsburgerweg 10
2333 AA Leiden
THE NETHERLANDS

G. L. KLOOSTERMAN
University of Amsterdam
Wildenborch 8
1082 KD Amsterdam
THE NETHERLANDS

F. KUBLI
Universität Frauenklinik
Voss Strasse 9
D-6900 Heidelberg
FEDERAL REPUBLIC OF
GERMANY

M. I. LEVENE
Department of Child Health
Clinical Sciences Building
Leicester Royal Infirmary
Leicester LE2 7LX
UK

G. McLURE
Nuffield Department of Child Health
Queens University of Belfast Institute of
   Clinical Science
Grosvenor Rd
Belfast BT12 6BJ
NORTHERN IRELAND

D. MACDONALD
National Maternity Hospital
Holles Street
Dublin 2
IRELAND

J. A. McGARRY
Division of Obstetrics and Gynaecology
Southern General Hospital
Glasgow G51 4TF
SCOTLAND

T. MATTHEWS
Department of Paediatrics
Rotunda Hospital
Dublin I
IRELAND

C. MORLEY
University Department of Paediatrics
Addenbrooke's Hospital
Cambridge CB2 2QQ
UK

J. N. OATS
University Department of Obstetrics and
   Gynaecology
Mercy Maternity Hospital
Clarendon Street
East Melbourne 3002
AUSTRALIA

P. O'CONNELL
Coombe Lying-In Hospital
Dublin 8
IRELAND

M. ODENT
Maternité
Centre Hospitalier General de
   Pithiviers
Boulevard Beauvallet
45300 Pithiviers
FRANCE

K. O'DRISCOLL
National Maternity Hospital
Holles Street
Dublin 2
IRELAND

N. R. C. ROBERTON
University Department of Paediatrics
The Rosie Maternity Hospital
Robinson Way
Cambridge CB2 2QQ
UK

B. ROBERTSON
Department of Pediatric Pathology
St. Gorans Hospital
Box 12506
S112 81 Stockholm
SWEDEN

G. ROOTH
Perinatal Research Unit
University Hospital
S-750 14 Uppsala
SWEDEN

H. RYDHSTROM
Department of Obstetrics and Gynecology
University Hospital
221 85, Lund
SWEDEN

E. SALING
Unit of Perinatal Medicine
Free University of Berlin
Mariendorfer Weg 28
D-1000 Berlin 44
FEDERAL REPUBLIC OF
GERMANY

B. L. SHEPPARD
University Department of Obstetrics &
  Gynaecology
Sir Patrick Dun Research Centre
St. James's Hospital
Dublin 8
IRELAND

N. SVENNINGSEN
Neonatal Intensive Care Unit
Department of Pediatrics
University Hospital
S-221 85 Lund
SWEDEN

M. THIERY
Verloskundige Kliniek
De Pintelaan 135
B-9000 Gent
BELGIUM

B. C. L. TOUWEN
Department of Developmental
  Neurology
University Hospital Groningen
Oostersingel 59
9713 EZ Groningen
THE NETHERLANDS

P. E. TREFFERS
Department of Obstetrics and
Gynaecology,
Academisch Medisch Centrum
Meibergdreef 9
1105 AZ Amsterdam
THE NETHERLANDS

R. USHER
Royal Victoria Hospital
687 Avenue des Pins Ouest
Montreal
Quebec H3A 1A1
CANADA

A. VAN ASSCHE
Universitair Ziekenhuis
Sint-Rafael
Gasthuisberg
3000 Leuven
BELGIUM

H. P. VAN GEIJN
Department of Obstetrics and
  Gynecology
Academisch Ziekenhuis der Vrije
  Universiteit
De Boelelaan 1117
1007 MB Amsterdam
THE NETHERLANDS

D. V. WALTERS
Department of Paediatrics
University College Hospital Medical
  School
Rayne Institute
University Street
London WC1E 6JJ
UK

M. WESTGREN
Department of Obstetrics and
  Gynecology
Karolinska Institutet
Danderyd Hospital
S–182–88 Danderyd
SWEDEN

A. WHITELAW
Department of Paediatrics and Neonatal
  Medicine
Royal Postgraduate Medical School
Hammersmith Hospital
Du Cane Road
London W12 0HS
UK

C. R. WHITFIELD
Department of Midwifery
University of Glasgow
Queen Mother's Hospital
Yorkhill
Glasgow G3 8SH
SCOTLAND

J. S. WIGGLESWORTH
Department of Paediatrics and Neonatal
  Medicine
Royal Postgraduate Medical School
Hammersmith Hospital
Du Cane Road
London W12 0HS
UK

A. WILKINSON
Neonatal Unit
University of Oxford
John Radcliffe Maternity Hospital
Oxford OX3 9DU
UK

Y. Y. H. Yu
Department of Neonatal
 Intensive Care
Queen Victoria Medical Centre
Monash University
172, Lonsdale Street
Melbourne
Victoria 3000
AUSTRALIA

Preface

Perinatal Medicine is a relatively new specialty, sited between the mechanistic approach of traditional obstetrics and the anticipatory and preventative outlook expressed in the study of fetal growth which extends into monitoring neonatal progress and development. It is of primary importance that obstetricians and neonatologists should think alike and should not allow their interests to develop along separate lines. Frequent clinical consultations with neonatologists cooperating in prenatal care and obstetricians visiting the special nursery on a regular basis are essential if every fetus is to reach its full potential. Such aims have been advanced by previous European Congresses and it was our privilege in Dublin to host the IXth Congress held at the Royal Dublin Society from September 3rd to 5th 1984. Over nine hundred delegates representing thirty-nine countries attended the scientific and social programme.

The theme of the congress was the mature baby. The organizers felt that while major advances had been made in the management of prematurity there were still far too many mature fetuses dying and too many deaths in the normally formed appropriate weight for gestational age neonate. Hence antenatal fetal assessment, the management of labour including electronic monitoring in normal women and asphyxial brain damage were major topics. Pregnancy hypertension, caesarean section, breech presentation, diabetes and unexplained mature stillbirth were workshop topics. The subject of perinatal training was awarded a session and we feel that this will become more prominent in future congresses. In order that advances should be scientifically audited, workshop five dealt with means of assessing perinatal statistics. The premature baby was not ignored: workshops on persistent fetal circulation and surfactant examined the major problems associated with immaturity.

The overall conclusion from the congress was that while many advances had been made, much work remains to be done in the vital area of presenting every

xix

mother at the end of pregnancy with a fit healthy baby and giving that baby the best possible start in life.

Contributions from fifty-five of the fifty-eight speakers are included in this book of proceedings. It differs from the congress programme in that rather than being laid out on a daily basis, it starts with the three main presentations, goes on to the major symposia and then continues with the nine workshops. At most of the sessions, the chairman delivered a formal introduction. In some there was a concluding discussion and in others, where the chairman was a speaker, these were amalgamated into the chairman's paper. The text follows these variations.

A pleasant aspect of the congress was the quality of papers submitted as free communications. Many of these were from younger doctors and the standard displayed indicates that the future of perinatal medicine should be in good hands. These contributions are summarized in the book of abstracts which was made available to participants at the congress and should be read in conjunction with these proceedings. Together they form a synopsis of modern clinical practice and recent research in perinatal medicine.

Publication was greatly assisted by a generous donation from the Ireland Fund made possible by a grant to it from the H. J. Heinz Company Foundation. The editors acknowledge this with gratitude and trust that readers will remember the support which was given to the congress by this and other business firms.

J. Clinch
T. Matthews

Presentation of the Maternité Prize to Albert and Renate Huch

E. Saling

As the founder president of this society I have the honour and pleasure to present the Maternité Prize of the European Society of Perinatal Medicine for the 5th time. The prize is donated by Humana Milchwerke of Herford, and consists of a sum of 5000 German Marks and a bronze statue made by Madame Guastalla from Paris.

Professor Ewerbeck in Cologne aptly described the bronze statue as symbolizing perinatal medicine. The mother is medicine, her two children are obstetrics and paediatrics and jointly they go forwards. The European prize has been awarded four times before. To Geoffrey Dawes in Oxford, to Mont Liggins in New Zealand, to Gösta Rooth in Uppsala and to me.

The committee members for the present prize-giving were: our president, Dr Joseph Alvey, Dublin, Dr K. Jaehrig, Greifswald (GDR), Professor von Muralt, Bern and Dr J. Koppe, Amsterdam. We are happy that the small number of international prize winners will increase by leaps and bounds today. For the first time the prize is awarded to two, a pair of Maternité twins. The European Maternité prize was awarded by the committee to Renate and Albert Huch. Working together the Huchs have had a spectacular career, acknowledged by a number of reputed scientists not least from abroad.

The fact that the prize is awarded in this pleasant country, with its particular charm, adds to this festive and solemn occasion.

Renate Huch studied medicine in Göttingen. Between 1967 and 1979 she worked in the Department of Obstetrics and Gynaecology of the University of Marburg, many of these 12 years as assistant to Professor Lübbers in clinical physiology. In 1978 she was appointed Professor of Perinatal Physiology. Five years ago she became Director of the Perinatal Physiological Unit in the Department of Obstetrics in Zürich.

Albert Huch also did his medical studies in Göttingen and then spent two years in respiratory research at the Max Planck Institute. In 1973 he was appointed Professor of Obstetrics and Gynaecology in Marburg and in 1978 he became chairman of the Department of Obstetrics in Zürich.

The Huchs have become world famous for the introduction of the transcutaneous technique of monitoring blood gases. This non-invasive approach is of outstanding clinical importance in neonatal medicine and of particular scientific value during labour.

Transcutaneous Po_2 is today an integrated part of neonatal medicine and the use of transcutaneous Pco_2 is spreading rapidly at present. By this technique small neonates are saved from repeated harmful punctures with their risk of fall in pH and circulatory disturbances. The transcutaneous technique very rapidly attracted a lot of interest and drew numerous research workers to Marburg first and then later to Zürich. Thereby they have also made many friends in the research community.

The crowning peak of their academic careers was of course their appointment to the prestigious and well endowed University of Zürich.

The Huchs early considered their research a joint family undertaking and hobby. Thus their work and their private lives have largely merged.

Albert Huch is always soberly dressed with bow tie. If you see someone whom you think is Albert, but wears an ordinary tie, it is not Albert. Renate is the rather unusual combination of a productive, effective and constructive research worker and a beautiful lady full of charm. Both of them love to meet their friends in cultured surroundings and offer them delicious food and wines. The 'secret' of the success of the Huchs very much lies in their complementary skills. Albert has the technical and inventive ability. Renate the systematic testing and analysing capacity.

Albert's technical knowledge is not limited to electronics and medical equipment. He also loves to restore old houses and is his own master builder. The jewel of his crown is their house in Marburg overlooking the city and with foundations which include part of the still intact old city wall and also including two towers dating about 1150.

Outside Renate's door in the laboratory in Zürich is a collection of addresses from which we may perhaps be allowed to draw some conclusions.

Mr Professor Dr Renate Huch. Is *she* the boss?

Dr Renate Huch's University is of course an appropriate but perhaps somewhat premature honour.

Laboratory-Professor Huch and Huch-Electrode Dept. of Electronic Development are both obviously correct.

It is definitely more difficult to understand Laboratory of Perminatology.

To a frightened or insecure person it might be nice to go to Perinatal Psychiatry.

The modern trend in childbirth is apparent in Peri Natural Physiology Laboratory.

The Huchs and their collaborators are active in several fields. Let me list eight of them: inhibition of labour, prostaglandins, skin blood flow measurements with the Laser Doppler technique, flying and pregnancy, smoking and pregnancy, pregnancy and work at high altitude, hyperventilation in pregnancy and cardiopulmonary reactions during pregnancy in relation to posture.

By themselves or together with collaborators the Huchs have written or edited eight books, published 251 scientific papers and read 277 papers at meetings at home or abroad. To sum up: The Huchs have made lasting scientific and clinical contributions.

The transcutaneous technique is a milestone in perinatal medicine. I must now ask you both to accept the prize. The official text as written on the scroll is:

For their contributions to one of the most outstanding advances in perinatal medicine, namely the transcutaneous measurements of oxygen tension and carbon dioxide tension for the intensive care of prematures and other neonates.

Winners awarded the Maternité Prize presented by The European Association of Perinatal Medicine

1976   Professor Geoffrey Dawes F.R.S.
University of Oxford
Nuffield Institute for Medical Research
Headley Way
Headington
Oxford OX3 9DS
England

1978   Professor Dr Graeme Collingwood Liggins
Postgraduate School of Obstetrics & Gynaecology
National Women's Hospital
Claude Road
Auckland 3
New Zealand

1980   Professor Dr Gösta Rooth
Perinatal Research Unit
University Hospital
S–750 14 Uppsala
Sweden

1982   Professor Dr Erich Saling
Chief of the Department of Obstetrics of the Women's Hospital
Neukölln and of The Unit of Perinatal Medicine of the Free
University of Berlin
Mariendorfer Weg 28
D–1000 Berlin 44
Germany

1984   Professor Dr Albert Huch and Dr Renate Huch,
Universitäts–Frauenklinik Zurich,
Frauenklinikstrasse 10,
Ch–8006 Zürich
Switzerland

Section 1
Main Lectures

1

Randomized trial of fetal monitoring

D. MacDonald

INTRODUCTION

During the past two decades there have been marked advances in the methods available for assessing the condition and wellbeing of the fetus during labour. Improvements in the quality of continuous electronic monitoring equipment have led to such equipment being employed routinely in many centres. In some, the technique has been backed up by the use of scalp blood sampling to measure the fetal pH. Others rely solely on fetal heart rate patterns to decide whether the baby is in a healthy condition or whether immediate delivery, often by caesarean section, is necessary. Another alternative, often employed because of financial stringency, is to use clinical methods of assessing the fetus and, should these be abnormal, to perform scalp sampling directly.

Controversy continues to exist about the relative merits of these different methods. Although there is some evidence of a consensus that the use of the more intensive means of intrapartum monitoring is appropriate when the fetus is deemed to be at high risk, there is no such agreement concerning the application of these methods for fetuses at average or low risk of adverse outcome [1-3]. These uncertainties reflect difficulties in the interpretation of information derived from randomized trials which have been designed to compare alternative methods of intrapartum monitoring.

To date, five such randomized trials have been reported [4-8]. The only benefit that these have suggested might result from more intensive monitoring is the possibility that neonatal convulsions may be reduced by using continuous electronic methods in conjunction with fetal acid–base estimations. Set against this possible benefit, however, is the evidence from the same trials that continuous fetal heart monitoring may lead to a substantial increase in the incidence of caesarean section, particularly if no attempt is made to support this with fetal scalp sampling [9].

Because of these controversial findings a randomized trial was organized at the National Maternity Hospital, Dublin, Ireland. Selection of cases for continuous electronic monitoring had hitherto been based on examination of the liquor once a diagnosis of labour had been made. In the 5% of cases in which liquor had either been absent or significantly meconium-stained, a fetal blood sample would be taken immediately. If the results were reassuring, the fetal heart was electronically monitored until delivery. In the remaining 95% of patients the fetus was assessed at regular intervals by auscultation of the fetal heart, and by scalp blood sampling if this was indicated[10]. The trial reported here was designed to compare this latter policy, used in the vast majority of patients, with the most promising alternative practice, i.e. continuous fetal heart rate monitoring using a scalp electrode and supported by scalp blood sampling when indicated by the finding of an abnormal heart trace.

Full details of the prior hypotheses, methods and findings of the trial have been reported elsewhere[11]. This brief presentation concentrates on comparing the two policies in respect of the most serious adverse outcomes in normally formed babies: intrapartum or neonatal death, as well as the presence or absence of convulsions in the neonatal period.

PATIENTS AND METHODS

Patients were considered eligible for inclusion in the trial if they had a live fetus of at least 28 weeks gestation, if a diagnosis of labour had been made and provided liquor without significant meconium staining had been demonstrated on admission to the hospital or at early amniotomy. A total of 13 025 women met these entry requirements; 99.5% of these eligible patients (12 960) were then allocated randomly (by opening a sealed envelope) to either continuous electronic monitoring (EFM) or intermittent auscultation (IA) of the fetal heart. Six thousand four hundred and seventy-four patients were entered in the first group and 6486 in the second. Table 1 compares the two groups for age, marital status, race, parity, gestational age, the incidence of induction of labour, and baby birth weight. There were no significant differences for any of these parameters and all subsequent analyses are based on the unbiased comparisons between the two randomized groups.

RESULTS

Table 2 demonstrates that 10% of those allocated to the EFM group delivered too rapidly for the method to be set up. A further 6% refused the technique and a small proportion could not be monitored for technical or other reasons; 81.3% of those originally chosen were successfully monitored. Virtually all (97.7%) of those allocated to the IA group were supervised in this fashion until delivery.

The differences occurring during labour between the two groups are illustrated in Table 3. The incidence of scalp blood sampling prompted by abnormalities of the fetal heart rate was 2.7% among those allocated to electronic monitoring, and only 1% in patients in whom the fetal heart was auscultated intermittently. This difference is highly significant. Mothers who were moni-

Table 1 Comparison of the two groups

	EFM	IA
Mean maternal age (years)	27.1	27.3
Married (%)	90	90
Non-Caucasian (%)	0.3	0.3
Parity (%) 0	41	40
1–3	51	52
4+	8	8
Mean gestational age (weeks)	39.9	39.9
Induction of labour (%)	6.9	7.7
Mean birthweight (g)	3543	3558
Total mothers entered	6474	6486

EFM = electronic fetal monitoring; IA = intermittent auscultation

Table 2 Actual method of intrapartum assessment (%)

Allocated to EFM		Allocated to IA	
		EFM indicated for the following reasons:	
Delivered too rapidly	10.5	Prolonged labour	1.3
Refused EFM	6.5	Meconium or no liquor	0.2
Machine failure	0.7	FHR abnormality	0.4
No machine available	0.4	Other	0.4
Other	0.6		
Actually monitored by EFM	81.3	Actually monitored by IA	97.7

tored electronically were less likely to require pethidine for analgesia and had significantly shorter labours. However, more of them required delivery by forceps, a variation caused entirely by an increased number of cases with abnormalities of the fetal heart rate. There was no difference between the two groups in the incidence of caesarean section.

Table 4 demonstrates that the number of babies with an Apgar score of less than four at 1 minute after delivery was the same in both groups of patients. Post-delivery admission to the special care nursery was also identical. The combined intrapartum and neonatal death rate for normally formed infants was identical in the two groups at 1.9 per thousand. The timing of death in relation to labour was also similar. Trauma accounted for three deaths, all occurring in the electronically monitored group. These were associated with forceps delivery undertaken because of failure to advance in the second stage of labour.

The outstanding difference between the two groups was the significantly reduced incidence of neonatal convulsions amongst infants who had been electronically monitored during labour. This difference was reflected both

Table 3 Intrapartum variations between the two groups (total mothers 12 960)

	EFM	IA	Significance
FBS for FHR abnormality	2.7%	1.0%	$p < 0.001$
Pethidine	46%	49%	$p < 0.05$
Mean duration of labour	3.9 (h)	4.2 (h)	$p < 0.05$
Forceps delivery	8.2%	6.2%	$p < 0.05$
Caesarean section	2.4%	2.2%	NS

Table 4 Gross perinatal outcome (total babies 13 077)

	EFM	IA
Apgar <4 at 1 minute (%)	1.1	1.1
SCBU admission (%)	8.0	8.0
Intrapartum stillbirths	3	2
Neonatal deaths	9	10

Table 5 Number of infants demonstrating seizures in the newborn period (total babies 13 077)

	EFM	IA	Significance
Convulsions followed by neonatal death	3	6	$p < 0.01$
Convulsions followed by survival	9	21	$p < 0.05$
Total babies with convulsions	12	27	$p < 0.025$

amongst those babies who survived the neonatal period and those in whom convulsions were followed by neonatal death (Table 5).

Follow-up examination at 1 year of age of the 30 survivors showed that three babies in each group suffered serious sequelae after their seizures. Of those electronically monitored, two infants were affected by cerebral palsy associated with microcephaly and another baby had spasticity of the lower limbs. In the IA group there was one case with gross cerebral palsy and two infants with developmental delay, one severe and one moderate (Table 6).

DISCUSSION

The results presented here suggest that the frequency of convulsions in the

Table 6 Follow-up at 1 year of the 30 babies who survived neonatal seizures

	EFM	IA
Spasticity with microcephaly	2	
Spasticity of lower limbs	1	
Cerebral palsy		1
Developmental delay		2
Development normal	6	18

neonatal period is reduced by 56% when continuous fetal heart monitoring and fetal acid–base assessment is used in place of intermittent auscultation, even if the latter is backed up by fetal scalp sampling. However, this variation is compatible with a real reduction of as little as 10% or as great as 78%. This means that while on average to prevent one case of neonatal convulsion it would be necessary to monitor 433 fetuses electronically, this number might be as low as 240 or as high as 2167.

One aspect of our work that should be emphasized is the importance of using scalp blood sampling as an adjunct to continuous electronic monitoring. It is our view that there can be little justification for employing the latter without the facilities to assess the acid–base status of the fetus before proceeding to caesarean section when the baby is thought to be compromised. The similar incidence in caesarean section between our two groups of patients demonstrates that intensive monitoring during labour need not lead to an increase in abdominal delivery.

Neonatal convulsions often have serious sequelae. A recent review of the literature[12] has suggested that between one-quarter and one-third of all cases die in early infancy, and that a similar proportion go on to survive with severe disabilities. Our work confirms this finding with nine deaths out of 39 babies who suffered from seizures. Of the 30 survivors, three babies in each group were found to be handicapped at follow-up examination when 1 year old.

References

1. Gillmer, M. D. G. and Combe, D. (1979). Intrapartum fetal monitoring practice in the United Kingdom. *Br. J. Obstet. Gynaecol.*, **86**, 753–758
2. National Institutes of Health (1979). Report of a Task Force on Predictors of Fetal Distress. In *Antenatal Diagnosis*, Washington: US Department of Health, Education and Welfare, p. 166
3. Social Services Committee (1980). *Report on Perinatal and Neonatal Mortality.* (London: HMSO)
4. Haverkamp, A. D., Thomson, H. E., McFee, J. and Cetrulo, C. (1976). The evaluation of continuous fetal heart rate monitoring in high risk pregnancy. *Am. J. Obstet. Gynecol.*, **125**, 310–320
5. Renou, P., Chang, A., Anderson, I. and Wood, C. (1976). Controlled trial of fetal intensive care. *Am. J. Obstet. Gynecol*, **126**, 470–476

6. Kelso, I. M., Parsons, R. J., Lawrence, G. F., Arora, S. S., Edmonds, D. K. and Cooke, I. D. (1978). An assessment of continuous fetal heart rate monitoring in labour. A randomised trial. *Am. J. Obstet. Gynecol.*, **131**, 526–532

7. Haverkamp, A. D., Orleans, M., Langendoerfer, S., McFee J. G. and Murphy, J. (1979). A controlled trial of the differential effects of intrapartum fetal monitoring. *Am. J. Obstet. Gynecol.*, **134**, 399–412

8. Wood, C., Renou, P., Oats, J., Farrell, E., Beischer, N. and Anderson, I. (1981). A controlled trial of fetal heart rate monitoring in a low risk obstetric population. *Am. J. Obstet. Gynecol.*, **141**, 527–534

9. Chalmers, I. (1979). Randomised controlled trials of fetal monitoring 1973–1977. In: Thalhammer, O., Baumgarten, K. and Pollak, A. (eds), *Perinatal Medicine*, pp. 260–265. (Stuttgart: George Thieme)

10. O'Driscoll, K., Coughlan, M., Fenton, V. and Skelly, M. (1977). Active management of labour: care of the fetus. *Br. Med. J.*, **2**, 1451–1453

11. MacDonald, D., Grant, A., Pereira, M., Boylan, P. and Chalmers, I. (1985). The Dublin randomised controlled trial of intrapartum electronic fetal heart rate monitoring. (In press)

12. Dennis J. and Chalmers I. (1982). Very early neonatal seizure rate: a possible epidemiological indicator of the quality of perinatal care. *Br. J. Obstet. Gynaecol.*, **89**, 418–426

2

The contribution of perinatal physiology to clinical practice

G. S. Dawes

Twelve years ago, at the Third European Congress of Perinatal Medicine in Lausanne in 1972, you were kind enough to ask me to give a main lecture on animal physiology and perinatal medicine[1]. This is the Ninth European Congress and much has happened since the Third Congress. But I am now being asked a different question: to discuss the contribution not of animal physiology to perinatal medicine, but of perinatal physiology to clinical practice. Twelve years ago I summarized the recent experiments which had shown that, in the fetal lamb, parturition is preceded and determined by fetal secretion of corticosteroids followed by a fall in plasma progesterone and a rapid rise in estrogen, associated with a rise in prostaglandin $F_{2\alpha}$ in the maternal placenta and myometrium. The missing link had been found between the steroids and myometrial activity, it seemed.

I gave an account of the animal experiments which laid the basis for the discovery of pulmonary surfactant, an amazing story to which so many had contributed. By that time Liggins had also found the association between steroid secretion and lung surfactant synthesis as a result of animal experiments. Finally, breathing movements coinciding with rapid eye movement sleep during the last few weeks of gestation had been identified, and the net outward flow of fetal pulmonary fluid secretion had been measured. New developments in neurobiology were evident, particularly in relation to critical periods of development as exemplified by the experiments of Huebel and Wiesel, for which they received a Nobel Prize last year.

On this occasion I have decided to take a wide view and to tell some stories of discovery and the painstaking application to clinical practice. Julius Comroe, a long-time friend and teacher, died last month. He spent some years of his very active life identifying the source of discoveries in cardiovascular and respiratory medicine. A series of reviews[2] were collected into the *Retrospectoscope: Insights into Medical Discovery* (1977), where he identified the sources of the major experimental advances in these fields, ranging from the treatment of heart diseases with simple remedies to replacement by transplantation. The conclusion was that about 60% of practical discoveries in adult medicine in these fields was derived from basic research.

I commend the *Retrospectoscope* to your attention. The last three chapters, on 'Premature science and immature lungs' are required (and light-hearted) reading for every student of perinatal medicine. These chapters tell the story of the elucidation of the physical forces which determine lung expansion; it was animal research on chemical warfare which led to the discovery of pulmonary surfactant. This also gives the best account I have read of the discovery of the effectiveness of CPAP (continuous positive airways pressure) in the treatment of the respiratory distress syndrome. In a fascinating footnote (to p. 171) Comroe refers to the preceding unsuccessful efforts by several other groups of investigators. For this was not a discovery in isolation; the idea was around. Dr Gregory, who has rightly received much credit, was working in an institution where the principles of perinatal physiology were constantly reviewed and discussed. Comroe asks the question (p. 173) why did we have to wait until 1970 for this discovery? Why not 1960? I will refer you to his own explanation which, as usual, is perceptive and informed; in a word the time was not ripe. He adds 'physicians engaged in clinical trials on the human fetus and newborn have special tribulations in addition to the usual ones... they are damned by some if they *don't* do research and damned by others if they *do*'.

I too have had a painful experience as to the unripeness of time. In 1958 my colleagues and I found that the arterial pH in asphyxia was an important factor in fetal or neonatal survival in sheep. If you corrected the pH by infusion of alkali, then anaerobic metabolism could continue to supply energy and prevent death. So I asked the pediatrician in charge of the newborn ward at the Radcliffe Infirmary, Oxford, if she would like me to install a pH meter and help with clinical studies. I was told that there was no room for the machine. Meanwhile Stan James at Columbia Presbyterian, New York, had begun to work on this problem, and was able to set the scene by getting good basic data on normal babies. We were able to combine forces in Puerto Rico, thanks to Bill Windle, and to prove that in acute asphyxia in rhesus monkeys maintenance of the arterial pH prevented or attenuated cerebral damage[3].

So transfer of the products of perinatal physiology, whether based on research in man or animals, to clinical practice has to await the right time, the talent and the opportunity. The practitioner wants to see good clear results, and indeed the results of introducing CPAP were so dramatic that they hardly required a formal clinical trial.

NIFEDIPINE: A CALCIUM CHANNEL BLOCKER

There are clinical experiments and animal experiments, and everyone would agree that it is much easier to organize, and sometimes easier to interpret, animal experiments than clinical observations.

About a year ago, at Alec Turnbull's suggestion, Margaret Roebuck and Bruce Castle started to investigate the effects of the calcium channel blocker nifedipine on the fetal lamb. Their results[4] are interesting, and illustrate an important principle. They found that nifedipine given to the mother in doses which attenuate or abolish spontaneous uterine contractions in sheep within the last fifth of gestation cause a small fall in fetal arterial pressure, as well as a fall in maternal arterial pressure. This is not surprising; drugs which cause falls of arterial pressure by a peripheral mechanism in adults should do the same in the fetus. There was a small increase in fetal heart rate, but no effect on PaO_2, on fetal breathing or electrocortical activity. Administration of propranolol alone also does not affect fetal PaO_2; but given together nifedipine and propranolol cause a fall in fetal arterial PaO_2. That too is not altogether surprising; the two drugs block different arms of the mechanisms of fetal cardiovascular homeostasis. So a drug may have no obvious deleterious effect upon a normal fetus; but if a fetus has something wrong with it, insufficient of itself to cause a departure from normal values, the sum of the two effects may be quite evident. Hence even if a manufacturer has tested a drug upon normal fetal animals, and states that it has no effect, that statement should not be accepted without critical assessment. It is an inadequate guarantee of safety. A couple of weeks ago I happened to tell this story to one of my clinical colleagues, who said with astonishment, 'but we have just had two fetuses like that'. Well, on review they were not quite like that. The mothers in question had been given labetalol rather than propranolol; but when nifedipine was added there were gross changes in fetal heart rate which led to withdrawal of the drug in one instance and caesarean section in the other. The principle is clear.

EXERCISE IN PREGNANCY

Another example of what may be a practical guide in relation to clinical practice concerns exercise in pregnancy. In the past few years jogging or more strenuous exercise has become more common, and young women wish to know whether this may affect the outcome of pregnancy. It is difficult to design satisfactory trials because of the many factors which affect pregnancy. It was reassuring to read the excellent review by Lotgering et al.[5], which covered both animal and clinical observations. Evidence is presented that exhaustive exercise in pregnant sheep, for 40 minutes at 70% of maximal O_2 consumption, causes a small fall in mean uterine blood flow whose effect on the fetus is almost wholly offset by the rise in haematocrit and in gas transfer across the placenta. There was no evidence of a decline in fetal oxygen supply with this brief but exhaustive exercise. It would be difficult to obtain comparable evidence in human pregnancy. How one interprets the evidence is another matter.

Of course one should not expect a close correlation between observations on fetal sheep and human infants. There are, we know, quantitative differences, but the general principles which control physiological mechanisms, and hence the response to perturbations of normal health, are similar. Since 1972 a few differences have emerged. Thus umbilical blood flow appears to be higher in lambs (about 210 ml (kg^{-1} fetal body weight) min^{-1}) compared with many estimates using Doppler ultrasound in man (about 115–130 ml kg^{-1} min^{-1}). Breathing movements in the human fetus respond to changes in maternal (and hence fetal) blood glucose concentrations, increasing in incidence after each meal; this phenomenon is not seen in sheep, though hypoglycaemia arrests fetal breathing movements. However there seems no doubt that the general principles which control cardiac output and its distribution and ante-natal breathing movements are similar in both species.

FETAL BREATHING

The main problem as to the clinical application of observations on fetal breath-ing is its episodic character. In sheep we record it continuously, but in man this has so far proved impractical. Near term the episodes of apnoea are long (e.g. Patrick et al.[6]). This is a pity, for in sheep it is a good guide to fetal health; it is a useful addition to measurements of blood gases, for example; for it should be appreciated that neither blood pressure nor heart rate nor blood gases alone or together tell the whole story, as every good neonatologist knows. I cannot see why the same should not be true of the human fetus. Only Frank Manning and his colleagues in California and Winnipeg have incorporated the observation of fetal breathing movements (and amniotic fluid volume) into a biophysical profile which helps in the assessment of fetal health.

I do not propose to discuss the advantages or otherwise of this method of fetal assessment as compared with others, but to direct your attention to another issue. Some years ago it was found that breathing movements declined or were arrested shortly before or at the onset of labour in sheep[7] and in man using A-scan ultrasound[8]. Castle and Turnbull[9] have explored the possibility of detecting the group of women (about half) presenting in preterm labour who do not deliver within the next few days, by looking for fetal breath-ing. At the gestational age (28–34 weeks) where this distinction is most import-ant the interval between episodes of breathing is less than at term. So the idea proved practicable, and a preliminary analysis looked promising. With larger numbers and the recognition that rupture of the membranes and infection also are important factors, the results still look promising in singleton preg-nancies[10].

THE RESPONSE OF THE FETUS TO SOUND AND SHAKING

The quality of the sound environment of the fetus in utero is a matter of dis-pute. Observations in humans have been made at term by inserting a micro-phone to lie at or just inside the cervix before or after rupture of the membranes. On physical grounds this is unsatisfactory and may explain the odd conclusion that the acoustic environment is dominated by maternal card-iovascular sounds, for turbulent blood flow, sufficient to cause sound produc-tion, occurs very rarely in peripheral blood vessels, and then only with partial obstruction to generate streams which exceed the Reynolds number. This seems most unlikely unless the blood vessels are kinked. Clearly the micro-phone must be introduced into the amniotic cavity, whose volume should be within normal limits.

Margaret Vince and her colleagues in Cambridge, using a microphone implanted chronically into the amniotic cavity of fetal lambs, has reported that sounds from the maternal blood flow were picked up rarely and at very low frequencies and amplitude. There were other intermittent low-frequency sounds associated with the ewe's feeding and digestion. There were louder sounds of vocalization from the ewe, from the flock and human voices 'whose attenuation was rarely more than 30 dB and, especially at low frequencies, usually much less'[11]. The sound of the mother's voice was transmitted effectively through the diaphragm, and there were long, loud low-frequency sounds associated with uterine contractions in labour.

Before we consider whether or how the fetus reacts to acoustic stimuli we must have regard to the changes which have taken place in our appreciation of fetal development in the past 12 years. In the early 1970s evidence became available to show that the lamb fetus changes episodically from high-voltage electrocortical activity (characteristic of quiet sleep postnatally) and low voltage associated with rapid eye movements. Henrique Rigatto and his colleagues in Winnipeg[12], who have succeeded in implanting a transparent plastic window into the wall of the uterus and the maternal adbomen, reported that they could not identify episodes of fetal wakefulness. In the human fetus too there is good evidence in normal human fetuses *in utero* that, as in sheep, behavioural states related to sleep are established by 34–36 weeks[13]; the first changes are perceptible (as aggregation of fetal movements in association with episodes of high heart rate variation) as early as 28 weeks gestation[14]. It should be noted that it has proved difficult to record electrocortical activity from the human fetus *in utero*, but that eye movements can be observed. It has been suggested by many observers that the episodes of low heart rate variation in human fetuses, first described by Timor-Tritsch *et al.* in 1978[15], correspond to quiet sleep postnatally.

Now newborn infants in quiet sleep are difficult to arouse, as is well known to parents and pediatricians. Attempts to arouse lambs during high-voltage electrocortical activity also have met with singular failure. So Gerry Visser *et al.* recently re-examined the hypothesis that human fetuses respond to tactile stimuli in episodes of low heart rate variation[16]. This was also a practical problem, since for many years it had become the practice of some midwives in England, Holland and elsewhere to shake the fetus in such episodes. They expected a normal fetus to respond by one or more cardiac accelerations. The design of this experiment required some care, because episodes of quiet sleep last for different lengths of time. It is all too easy for a midwife to conclude that a fetus has responded to shaking when the episode of quiet sleep has come to its natural end. In fact, when proper controls are made on the same infant *in utero*, it is evident that it does *not* respond to shaking in episodes of low heart rate variation. So we may draw two conclusions: first this is consistent with such episodes coinciding with quiet sleep; and secondly it would seem that shaking human fetuses *in utero* during low heart rate variation, to test responsiveness and hence normal health, is pointless.

During 1984 papers have appeared, both from Scandinavia and North America, in which it is stated that human fetuses *in utero* respond by cardiac accelerations to acoustic stimuli. These papers repeat statements made in the obstetric literature during the past 14 years. The question arises whether these statements are true. Will a fetus respond to a sound stimulus applied in a period of low heart rate variation analogous to quiet sleep postnatally? We need properly designed experiments to test this hypothesis. It is worrying that the implications of sleep states have been so wholly disregarded in the clinical literature, although the phenomenon has become well known.

Let us turn to another aspect of the same problem, i.e. responsivenes to tactile or acoustic stimuli during episodes of high heart rate variation. The difficulty is that the period of time between successive cardiac accelerations is, normally, small and variable. At 36–38 weeks gestation the modal (i.e. most common) value is < 0.5 minute; so once again we have a difficult problem in experimental design. Only Patrick and his colleagues[5] have yet taken account of this in experiments on human infants *in utero* near term using tactile stimuli. They concluded that there was *no consistent response*. It is easy to choose illustrative figures which show a stimulus closely followed by an acceleration. What must be proven is that the incidence of accelerations following the stimulus is greater than that which would occur by chance in that type of episode in that fetus.

It is possible that the views of previous investigators may have been influenced by the statement so commonly made that fetal cardiac accelerations result from fetal movements. It is true that they are closely associated in time, in sheep as in man. However when the sheep fetus is paralysed by a neuromuscular blocking agent (gallamine) there is no significant decrease in heart rate variation or the incidence of accelerations.

Perhaps we should also consider what may happen in fetal lambs or human infants before the differentiation of electrocortical activity and associated sleep states, i.e. before 110 days gestation or 28 weeks respectively. Do they fail to respond to stimuli, episodically? It might be worth consideration, since work on fetal lambs between 110 and 125 days shows that there are progressive complex changes in the behavioural patterns and the same may be true of man. Perhaps the sensory input before 110 days gestation in sheep or 28 weeks in man is too small. The development of these states may be determined independently of sensory input. So far we have not been able to identify any developmental anomalies, in man or sheep, which might help answer these questions.

We also have to consider whether the presence of normal episodic behaviour, characteristic of sleep states, could be a useful indicator of health. It has been known for some years that episodes of high and low heart rate variation persist into and probably throughout normal labour. Six years ago Chris Redman and I began to collaborate in measuring human fetal heart rate variation and identifying its episodic changes. Recently, using a development of the system for analysis on-line at the bedside, fetuses were identified as having the lowest 5th centile of variation[17]. Two points can be made. First there are some growth-retarded fetuses in which episodic variation is still present, but at a lower amplitude than normal[18]. Secondly there is a small group of otherwise normal fetuses (3%) with normal outcome at term of a normal infant, in which heart rate variation is low at 32 weeks and which stays low until after delivery.

We should contrast these two groups with those described by Visser *et al.*[15] as preterminal, in which the heart rate trace is flat other than for decelerations (often shallow) associated with uterine contractions. The point I want to make is that some of these fetuses may have lost their episodic behavioural pattern.

In adult medicine loss of such variation is normally described as coma. Episodic patterns of breathing and heart rate persist in fetal sheep whose brain stems have been sectioned at the inferior colliculus; they are absent if the pons and medulla are removed. We do not yet know the precise pathophysiology of these preterminal fetuses, nor how best to treat them other than by rapid caesarean delivery.

THE SITES OF DRUG ACTION

Finally, before leaving the subject of intrauterine behavioural patterns and sleep states, let me add a word or two about the action of drugs. Mild sedative barbiturates (such as pentobarbitone) and ethanol (ethyl alcohol) both arrest fetal breathing, in sheep and man; but it is fascinating to find that in sheep they do so by different mechanisms. Ethanol has a direct action on the medulla and/ or spinal cord, since its effect persists after cutting the brain stem in the upper pons. Pentobarbitone acts indirectly above the pons, since its effect is abolished by brain stem section. Similarly we used to think that hypoxia arrested fetal breathing movements by depression of the respiratory centre; in fact its primary effect is above the pons. So far as I know there are no clinical repercussions of these observations, yet. They, and other observations in perinatal physiology, have convinced us that we are dealing with a far more complex system in late fetal life than was supposed. The fetus is not a scaled-down miniature adult. It may be helpless at birth by adult standards, but the systems which regulate its homeostasis and behaviour have proved most complex.

LUNG GROWTH

The growth of the lung illustrates this complexity. When fetal breathing was rediscovered, and obstetricians could see by real-time ultrasound from 1976 onwards that it was a normal feature of fetal life, the question was then asked as to whether it had a purpose, perhaps in lung development. The answer appears to be that it does, since natural or experimental interference with the mechanisms which control it, in man or sheep, is associated with pulmonary hypoplasia[19]. As one might have expected, the growth of the lung also depends on factors other than the available space. The practical question then arises whether, if a condition normally associated with pulmonary hypoplasia (e.g. congenital diaphragmatic hernia) is detected prenatally, prenatal repair of that anomaly will lead to recovery of lung development. This question was debated and some evidence was offered and discussed at the Society for Fetal Medicine and Surgery at their meeting in Washington DC in June 1984. The result of that preliminary discussion was inconclusive. I mention it because the issue has a practical and intellectual appeal, whether or not a case can be made for such antenatal surgery which is ethically and medically sound.

CHEMORECEPTOR ADAPTATION

The ability of newborn infants to withstand gross deviations from normality is remarkable. It supports the view that the control mechanisms which support life are highly sophisticated. They are indeed. Within the past 2 years we have learnt to our surprise that the systemic arterial chemoreceptors, which determine the response of the cardiovascular system and ventilation to hypoxia and asphyxia in the adult, are unlikely to contribute to either response in the immediate newborn period. In the fetal lamb the aortic and carotid bodies are active over the fetal range of PaO_2 (about 23 mmHg) and $PaCO_2$ (about 45 mmHg); after birth the PaO_2 normally rises and the $PaCO_2$ falls. It takes 3 days in this species for the arterial chemoreceptors to reset and begin to function within the neonatal range of blood gas values[20]. Clinical practice will not, I expect, be altered one whit by this conclusion; but it may remove one obstacle to the better understanding of neonatal apnoea, and may explain why some newborn infants appear normal yet have a $PaO_2 < 60$ mmHg.

CONCLUSION

I became interested in perinatal physiology in 1950. It had the attraction that observations on animals and on the human infant before and after birth were both needed to provide a sound basis for clinical practice. Within the past 8 years real-time ultrasound and its applications (including the measurement of pulse velocity waveforms) have made possible remarkable developments in prenatal diagnosis, and there are clear signs that molecular biology will have an equally profound effect. The obstetrician and the pediatrician find that new sophisticated opportunities are now available for research and for the gradual translation of new ideas into clinical practice. I hope that we shall get as good or better support for these opportunities as we have had in the past 10 years.

References

1. Dawes, G. S. (1972). Animal physiology and perinatal medicine. In *Perinatal Medicine*: Third European Congress of Perinatal Medicine, pp. 3–12. (Bern: H. Huber)
2. Comroe, J. H. (1977). *Retrospectoscope. Insights into Medical Discovery*. (Menlo Park, California: Von Gehr Press)
3. Dawes, G. S. (1968). *Foetal and Neonatal Physiology*. (Chicago: Year Book Medical Publishers)
4. Roebuck, M. M., Castle, B., Vojcek, L., Weingold, A., Hofmeyr, G. J., Dawes, G. S. and Turnbull, A. C. (1984) The effects on the fetal lamb of nifedipine administration to the ewe. *Proc. Soc. Study Fetal Physiol.* 11th Annual Conference, p. 12
5. Lotgering, F. H., Gilbert, R. D. and Longo, L. D. (1984). The interactions of exercise and pregnancy: a review. *Am. J. Obstet. Gynecol.*, **149**, 560–8
6. Patrick, J., Natale, R. and Richardson, B. (1978). Patterns of human fetal breathing activity at 34 to 35 weeks gestational age. *Am. J. Obstet. Gynecol.*, **132**, 507–13
7. Dawes, G. S. (1973). Fetal physiology and the onset of labour. *Mem. Soc. Endocrinol.*, **20**, 25–36
8. Boddy, K., Dawes, G. S. and Robinson, J. (1974). Intrauterine fetal breathing movements. In Gluck, L. (ed.) *Modern Perinatal Medicine*, pp. 381–90. (Chicago: Year Book Medical Publishers)
9. Castle, B. M. and Turnbull, A. C. (1983). The presence or absence of fetal breathing movements predicts the outcome of preterm labour. *Lancet*, **2**, 471–3
10. Turnbull, A. C., Castle, B. M. and Dawes, G. S. (1984). Fetal breathing move-

ments and pre-term labour. *Proc. Soc. Study Fetal Physiol.* 11th Annual Conference, p. 26

11. Vince, M. A., Armitage, S. E., Baldwin, B. A., Toner, J. and Moore, B. J. C. (1982). The sound environment of the foetal sheep. *Behaviour*, **81**, 296–315

12. Rigatto, H., Moore, M., Horvath, L. and Cates, D. (1983). Further observations of the fetus in the chronic sheep preparation using a double wall plexiglass window. *Proc. Soc. Study Fetal Physiol.* 10th Annual Conference, p. 27

13. Nijhuis, J. G., Prechtl, H. F. R., Martin, C. B. and Bots, J. E. (1982). Are there behavioural states in the human fetus? *Early Human Dev.*, **6**, 177–95

14. Dawes, G. S., Houghton, C. R. S., Redman, C. W. G. and Visser, G. H. A. (1982). Pattern of the normal human fetal heart rate. *Br. J. Obstet. Gynaecol.*, **89**, 276–84

15. Timor-Tritsch, I. E., Dierker, L. J., Zador, I., Hertz, R. H. and Rosen, M. G. (1978). Fetal movements associated with fetal heart-rate accelerations and decelerations. *Am. J. Obstet. Gynecol.*, **131**, 276–80

16. Visser, G. H. A., Redman, C. W. G., Huisjes, H. J. and Turnbull, A. C. (1980). Non-stressed antepartum heart rate monitoring: implications of decelerations after spontaneous contractions. *Am. J. Obstet. Gynecol.*, **138**, 429–35

17. Lawson, G. W., Dawes, G. S. and Redman, C. (1984). Analysis of fetal heart rate on-line at 32 weeks gestation. *Br. J. Obstet. Gynaecol.*, **91**, 542–50

18. Henson, G. G., Dawes, G. S. and Redman, C. W. G. (1984). Characterization of reduced heart rate variation in growth-retarded fetuses. *Br. J. Obstet. Gynaecol.*, **91**, 751–5

19. Liggins, G. C. (1984). Growth of the fetal lung. *J. Dev. Physiol.*, **6**, 237–48

20. Blanco, C. E., Dawes, G. S., Hanson, M. and McCooke, H. B. (1984). The response to hypoxia of arterial chemoreceptors in fetal sheep and newborn lambs. *J. Physiol.*, **351**, 25–37

3

The importance of the infant's condition at birth

R. H. Usher

The importance of condition at birth is easiest to illustrate in the borderline viable child. A birth weight below 1500 g is compatible with survival in three-quarters of infants who require little or no resuscitation at birth, and almost never in those requiring prolonged resuscitation.

Table 1 Survival in infants weighing 500–1499 g by duration of ventilation required at birth, 1978–79

Duration of ventilation (min)	Number of livebirths	Percentage survival
0	43	74
1–3	30	77
4–10	25	52
>10	18	6

The complexity of the problem, or at least of its solution, is demonstrated by analysis of survival following caesarean section versus vaginal delivery for the under 1500 g infant. Caesarean section, on first analysis, appears to be a simple way to improve conditions at birth. It sems to decrease mortality by two-thirds. Further analysis, however, shows this to be totally dependent on a skewed gestational age distribution, with only the more mature infants being delivered by caesarean.

The role of recent obstetrical advances – particularly the more liberal use of caesarean section – to avoid birth asphyxia and trauma can be assessed by comparing condition at birth in high-risk infants delivered before and subsequent to these developments. Except for the borderline viable infant, mortality is not sufficiently sensitive as a reflector of outcome. Morbidity must become the

Table 2 Mortality rate by gestational age and route of delivery in the infant of 500–1499 g, 1978–79

Gestational age (weeks)	Caesarean birth		Vaginal birth	
	No. of livebirths	Percentage mortality	No. of livebirths	Percentage mortality
<26	2	100	23	87
26 and 27	5	20	20	60
28 and 29	7	0	7	14
30 and 31	11	33	9	11
32+	14	7	3	33
Total	39	18	62	56

major end-point to be examined.

Our studies at the Royal Victoria Hospital, a McGill University teaching unit in Montreal, have employed as a sensitive measure of depression at birth the duration of positive pressure ventilation required to produce sustained spontaneous independent respiratory activity by the newborn. Depression requiring more than 3 minutes of positive pressure ventilation is considered severe. Need for prolonged positive pressure ventilation at birth occurs much less often than low Apgar scores. One-minute Apgar scores of less than 4 are found in 67% of infants requiring more than 3 minutes' ventilation. This low Apgar score is, however, found overall in three times the number of infants than those who need prolonged ventilation.

We have identified certain high-risk groups of patients as follows:

1. full-size babies delivering as a breech,
2. macrosomic infants,
3. twins.

We have asked to what degree condition at birth and mortality have improved with modern obstetrics compared with 10–20 years earlier. What problems remain today? Unexpectedly we have also found some adverse effects of modern obstetrical approaches when comparing results in recent years with those predating these changes. Finally we have tried to answer the question: to what degree have overall rates of depression and trauma at birth improved, and what are current rates to be expected with various obstetrical complications?

These studies have been done on a consecutively delivered obstetrical population over 20 years, all of the outcome assignments having been made at the time of discharge by the speaker. Maternal, obstetrical, and neonatal data have been computerized throughout the period. Co-workers included Frances McLean, Robert Funnell, Paul Smith, Mark Boyd, Dawn Johansson, Ronald Cyr, Jeffrey Green and Douglas Bell. Much of the material to be presented has recently been published[1-4].

One of the issues we addressed was whether we could justify by improved condition at birth the increase in caesarean sections at our institution from 5%

Table 3 Indications for caesarean section, 1978–80

Indication	Percentage
Previous caesarean	7
Failure to progress	5
Malpresentation	4
Fetal distress	1
Other	2
Total	19

in 1961 to 19% today. Most of this increase occurred between 1974 and 1977, so that our studies compared patients delivered before and after this transition period. At the present time our 19% caesarean section rate has as the primary indication the conditions shown in Table 3.

The analysis of incidence of depression at birth (need for positive pressure ventilation) showed a worrisome increase in incidence with caesarean birth (Table 4).

Table 4 Incidence of depression at birth among full-size (2500 g+) infants by type of delivery, 1978–80

Delivery	No. of livebirths	Percentage depressed
Vertex, vaginal		
Spontaneous/low forceps	6459	2
Mid forceps	1173	5
Caesarean section		
Vertex: Repeat	673	6
Primary	719	10
Malpresentation	315	13

The increased frequency of depression after elective repeat caesarean birth was demonstrated to be due to general anaesthesia (10% depression), not present in cases delivered under epidural (2% depression). Of particular concern is the high incidence of depression in caesareans for breech presentation.

THE FULL-TERM BREECH

Over the past 6 years it has become the routine in our hospital to deliver by caesarean infants presenting as breech. We have analysed depression and trauma at birth following full-term breech delivery in 1963–73 when only 22% were delivered by caesarean, and in 1978–79 when 94% were so delivered. Excluding low birth weight and malformed infants, preterm and multiple births, and cases of maternal or fetal disease, there were 595 full-term breech

Table 5 Full-term breech delivery and depression at birth in two periods (percentages)

	1963–73	1978–79	Probability
Moderate depression (1–3 min)	14.5	15.4	NS
Severe depression (4 min+)	1.5	1.1	NS

deliveries in the early period with the low caesarean rate, and 175 in recent years with the high rate.

There was no improvement with a liberal caesarean policy. Of the three perinatal deaths in the early period, two during labour could have been avoided with better monitoring than was then available. There was only one delivery-related death among 595 cases which could have been avoided by caesarean birth. Seven cases of transient brachial palsy or clavicular fracture among the 595 might also have been similarly prevented.

The conclusion was that depression at birth associated with breech delivery is not reduced by caesarean section. Delivery of a breech presentation from above, as from below, is fraught with danger. Delivery-related perinatal deaths are extremely rare in the group delivered vaginally. Though no fractures and paralyses occurred in the 175 delivered during the liberal caesarean period, this does not represent a statistically significant change from the 1.2% incidence of the earlier period. It is difficult to justify as liberal a caesarean policy as exists here for the full-term breech.

MACROSOMIA

Several questions were asked regarding birth depression and trauma in the macrosomic infant, defined as weighing 4000 g or more. What is the incidence or mortality and morbidity, and specifically what is the type of morbidity associated with abnormal labour or difficult delivery in the large infant? What type of deliveries tend to produce depressed or injured macrosomic babies? To what degree has an increased caesarean rate improved the outcome?

In each period from 1963–65, and 1978–80, almost 1000 infants (10% of all births) were macrosomic. Caesarean section had increased in frequency 2.5 times between the periods, but at the same time the mid forceps rate had also increased (Table 6).

Table 6 Method of delivery of macrosomic infants

	1963–65	1978–80
No. macrosomic infants	955	942
Caesarean section – total	8%	21%
Primiparas for failure to progress	9%	19%
Multiparas for failure to progress	2%	2%
Mid forceps		
Primiparas	19%	29%
Multiparas	7%	11%

There was significant reduction in the frequency of depression at birth, and the frequency of birth trauma had in fact increased (Table 7). Though the perinatal mortality rate had decreased from 9.4 to 5.3 per 1000, none of the deaths in either period were related to birth asphyxia or trauma.

Table 7 Delivery-related complications in macrosomic infants compared to normal infants

	1963–65	1978–80	Probability
Depression at birth (ventilated)	64/1000	45	NS
Postasphyxic encephalopathy	8	4	NS
Meconium aspiration	5	14	NS
Brachial palsy	6	10	NS
Facial palsy	2	6	NS
Clavicular fracture	4	17	<0.01
Any of the above	22	34	NS

Table 8 Delivery-related complications in macrosomic compared to normal infants

	Birthweight (g) per 1000			
	2500–3999	4000–4499	4500+	Probability
No. infants	8452	811	131	
Depression at birth	36	45	46	NS
Post-asphyxic encephalopathy	2	5	0	NS
Meconium aspiration	2	12	23	<.001
Brachial palsy	1	9	15	<.001
Facial palsy	3	6	8	NS
Clavicular fracture	5	14	38	<.001
Total infants severely affected*	15	30	61	<.001

* Excludes moderate depression and clavicular fracture

Table 9 Delivery-related complications in macrosomic infants by type of delivery

Type of delivery	No. of livebirths	Incidence of severely affected infants* per 1000	Probability
Spontaneous vertex	919	14	NS
Low forceps	424	17	NS
Mid forceps	268	82	<0.01
Caesarean section	277	40	<0.01
Shoulder dystocia	70	143	<0.01

* Severe depression, encephalopathy, meconium aspiration, brachial or facial palsy

The types of complications which are more frequent among macrosomic infants delivered today are meconium aspiration syndrome, brachial paralysis, and clavicular fracture. These increased progressively with the degree of macrosomia. It is interesting to note no evidence of increased birth asphyxia in the macrosomic infant (Table 8).

The type of deliveries responsible for the increased risk to the macrosomic are mid forceps delivery (increases both asphyxia and trauma), caesarean section delivery, usually for failure to progress or fetal distress (increased birth asphyxia and meconium aspiration syndrome), and deliveries complicated by shoulder dystocia (increases brachial palsy).

An unexpected finding was that macrosomic babies delivered from multiparous women, for whom caesarean was seldom employed, had a much higher incidence of brachial palsy, and 60% as much overall morbidity as similar weight infants delivered to nulliparous women.

It was certainly clear from this analysis that freer use of caesarean section did not reduce the delivery risk to the macrosomic baby, which risk took the form of meconium aspiration syndrome, fractures and palsies. Prediction of excessive fetal size for age prior to term would be of potential benefit. It could lead to induction of labour before the infant became excessively large. Foreknowledge of macrosomia during labour would lead to more appropriate use of caesarean section for failure to progress, less ready recourse to mid forceps delivery, easier acceptance of failed forceps with resort to caesarean rather than use of dangerous degree of traction, and prediction of an increased risk of shoulder dystocia.

With regard to prediction, it was found that maternal diabetes was not a factor in 98% of macrosomics, but that three common risk factors played large roles. These were: (1) prepregnant weight above 70 kg (10% of mothers), (2) weight gain in pregnancy of more than 20 kg (11% of mothers), and (3) postdate pregnancy of 7 days or more (18%).

Table 10   Risk factors for macrosomia

	Incidence of macrosomia (%)
No risk factors	5
One risk factor	15
Two or three risk factors	32

Since macrosomia is present in only 2% of infants at 37 weeks, 12% at term, and 21% by 42 weeks, the role of judicious induction of labour for infants who on late pregnancy ultrasonography are found to be large for date is evident.

FULL-TERM TWIN DELIVERY

Next our attention was turned to the delivery of twins where a 4% caesarean rate in 1963–72 rose to a 46% caesarean rate in recent years (1978–83). Had this increase benefited the infants' condition at birth? This increase was predominantly for malpresentations (Table 11).

Mortality decreased among livebirths of 29 weeks or greater from 32 to 3 per

Table 11 Incidence of caesarean delivery in twin pregnancy, 1978–83

Presentation	No. of pregnancies	Incidence of caesarean (%)
Vertex/vertex	100	16
Vertex/malpresentation	64	69
Malpresentation/vertex	23	91
Malpresentation/malpresentation	34	91

1000, but this decrease was primarily due to the almost complete disappearance of RDS as a cause of death in the recent period. Birth asphyxia was not a factor in the death of any twin infant of 29 weeks or greater, either among the 530 infants delivered in 1963–72, nor in 342 delivered in 1978–83. The prevention of RDS death was accomplished by reducing the incidence with steroid prophylaxis, and improved therapy for the condition.

The incidence of depression at birth (need for positive pressure ventilation) in full-term twins did not decrease significantly with the increased caesarean rate in recent years (Table 12).

Table 12 Incidence of depression at birth in full-term twin infants

	1963–72		1978–83		
	No. of livebirths	Need for ventilation (%)	No. of livebirths	Need for ventilation (%)	Probability
First twin	152	3.9	101	2.9	NS
Second twin	153	11.1	102	9.1	NS

In part, the failure of caesarean section to produce its desired effect was due to the contribution of general anaesthesia for the operation to depression at birth (Table 13).

Severe depression did not occur more frequently in the earlier period when few caesareans were done. There was need for more than 3 minutes of positive pressure ventilation in 2.3% of twins delivered in 1963–72, and in 2.3% of those delivered in 1978–83, among infants of 28 weeks gestation or greater. There was only one instance in the two periods of severe depression occurring

Table 13 Depression at birth in full-term twins delivered by caesarean for malpresentation or elective repeat, by type of anaesthesia

Epidural		General		
No. of livebirths	Need for ventilation	No. of livebirths	Need for ventilation	Probability
70	3%	25	20%	0.005

among 163 twin infants presenting as a breech or other malpresentation who were delivered vaginally.

It must be concluded that among twins at term depression at birth is not reduced by caesarean section, that caesarean when employed should whenever possible be done under epidural anaesthesia, and that severe depression is rarely associated with breech delivery by the vaginal route. Birth asphyxia does not pose a major threat to twins delivered vaginally at term.

CHANGING PATTERNS OVER 20 YEARS

The births of 1960–62 in our institution were analysed by John O'Brien and George Maughan for the frequency of various forms of birth asphyxia and trauma, the primary cause of each case, and the obstetrical factors associated with them[5]. In order to understand to what degree the obstetrical advances of the past generation have affected this picture, Ronald Cyr and Frances McLean subjected the births of 1978–80 to the same methods of analysis. Once again the criterion for severe birth asphyxia was the need for more than 3 minutes of positive pressure ventilation after birth.

Table 14 Obstetrical management

	1960–62	1978–80
No. livebirths	10 995	9901
Caesarean		
Primary	3%	12%
Repeat	2%	7%
Low forceps	22%*	28%
Mid forceps	5%*	15%*
Electronic fetal monitoring	0%	75%
Opiate analgesia	48%	3%
Epidural analgesia/anaesthesia	22%	65%

* Percentage of vaginal deliveries

The perinatal mortality (500 g to discharge) was 22 per 1000 in the early period and 11 in the later. Among infants of 1000 g or more, birth asphyxia/trauma was responsible for 2.7 intrapartum fetal deaths per 1000 in the early period and 0.3 recently; for neonatal deaths 2.9 per 1000 in the 1960s and 0.3 now. Perinatal mortality due to birth asphyxia/trauma was therefore all but eliminated, decreasing from 5.6 to 0.6 per 1000. The relative contribution of increased use of caesarean delivery, fetal monitoring, epidural instead of opiate analgesia, and other obstetrical advances in this dramatic improvement is indeterminable.

Turning to neonatal morbidity, the improvement is less evident. There was no decrease in incidence of severe depression at birth, though post-asphyxic encephalopathy with or without seizures was reduced by 60% (Table 15).

The incidence of severe depression (ventilation required for more than 3

Table 15 Incidence of severe depression at birth and of post-asphyxic encephalopathy in two periods (rates per 1000)

	1960–62	1978–80	Probability
Birth weight 2500 g+			
Severe depression	5.2	4.8	NS
Abnormal cerebral signs	5.4	2.0	<0.05
Convulsions	1.8	0.7	<0.05
1000–2499 g			
Severe depression	56	47	NS
500–999 g			
Severe depression	500	595	NS

minutes) was intimately related to birth weight, with 10-fold increases between weight categories. The incidence approximated 1 in 200 births of 2500 g or more, 1 in 20 of 1000–2499 g, and 1 in 2 of 500–999 g. These rates were not affected by the 20 years of obstetrical advances. It was reassuring to find, however, that post-asphyxic encephalopathy, which carries with it a risk of permanent cerebral damage, was reduced by more than half.

Birth trauma showed no improvement, but an unexpected increase in frequency over the interval (Table 16).

Table 16 Incidence of birth trauma in two periods (rates per 1000)

	1960–62	1978–80	Probability
Skull fracture	0.2	0.9	0.05
Clavicular fracture	1.0	5.8	0.05
Brachial palsy	1.5	3.0	0.05
Facial palsy	2.4	4.1	NS
Infants traumatized	4.8	13.0	0.05
	(1 in 208)	(1 in 77)	

Many of the infants suffering trauma were also severely depressed at birth, developed encephalopathy, or had meconium aspiration.

Post-asphyxic encephalopathy rarely developed in infants requiring little or no ventilation after birth, but became increasingly frequent as ventilation required exceeded 3 minutes (Table 17).

The six infants requiring more than 10 minutes of ventilation at birth produced four of the seven infants in this population of some 10 000 who convulsed.

The primary obstetrical cause of severe depression or encephalopathy in infants of 2500 g or more delivered recently was most often mid forceps delivery, fetal distress of unknown cause, cord loops, prolapsed cord, shoulder dystocia, or general anaesthesia with elective caesarean section. In one-eighth of the cases, fetal pathology was the cause. These differ from primary cause assignment in 1960–62 when many were due to prolonged labour (CPD), and

Table 17 Duration of positive pressure ventilation at birth and post-asphyxic encephalopathy in the neonatal period

Duration of ventilation (min)	No. of livebirths	Incidence of encephalopathy (%)
0	9032	0.04
1–3	294	2
4–5	28	11
6–10	11	27
11+	6	100

some to opiates, though the contribution of mid forceps delivery was similar then to now.

Among infants of low birth weight, the primary cause of severe depression in recent years was often hypertensive disease of pregnancy, antepartum haemorrhage, intrauterine infection, or fetal malnutrition. Comparatively there was a more frequent contribution of malpresentation or opiate analgesia in the 1960s.

The role of mid forceps delivery in all types of morbidity except meconium aspiration was very apparent (Table 18).

Table 18 Neonatal morbidity with type of vaginal vertex delivery, 2500 g or more, 1978–80 (rates per thousand)

Type of delivery	No. of livebirths	Severe depression/ encephalopathy	Meconium aspiration	Fractures		Palsies		Total of infants affected
				Skull	Clavicle	Brachial	Facial	
Spontaneous	4355	1.8	3.4	0	3.3	0.7	1.8	10.3
Low forceps	2094	2.9	2.4	0	10.0*	2.9*	2.4	17.2*
Mid forceps	1171	11.1*	4.3	6.0*	16.2*	15.4*	20.4*	62.3*

* Different from spontaneous delivery, p <0.05

It was considered likely that the increased damage resulting from mid forceps delivery in recent years might be due to inexperience of recent obstetrical trainees. This generation had never needed to cope with the limited caesarean rate requiring great skill with forceps when descent or rotation was slow. Analysis of results in recent years by experience of the accoucheur showed this explanation to be erroneous. There was even a reverse tendency with increasing morbidity found in association with greater number of years in practice (Table 19).

Another possible explanation for the increased use of mid forceps and the increased trauma rate in recent years is the use of epidural analgesia/ anaesthesia in most vaginal deliveries. If the second stage of labour is slowed thereby, mid forceps may be used to expedite delivery even in the absence of fetal distress. The duration of second stage was therefore examined in 72 deliveries where mid forceps-related severe asphyxia/trauma occurred in the absence of fetal distress. The mean duration was 73 minutes in nullipara and

Table 19 Experience of the accoucheur and mid forceps related severe birth asphyxia/trauma for infants of 2500 g+, 1978–80

Years of experience	No. of deliveries	Primary caesarean rate (%)	Mid forceps rate (percentage vaginal)	Incidence of severe asphyxia/trauma (percentage mid forceps delivery)
14+	2737	12.7	15.3	8.5
6–13	3035	10.7	15.7	7.0
0–5	2532	13.2	18.7	5.3

35 minutes in multipara. In only 9 of the 72 did the obstetrician wait 'upper limit' of 2 hours in nullipara or 1 hour in multipara.

With regard to the contribution of forceps delivery to neonatal asphyxia/trauma, the following conclusions were drawn:

On the other hand the vast majority of forceps deliveries (98% of low forceps and 94% of mid forceps) produced healthy uninjured babies. Asphyxia and trauma caused by forceps use are presumably the result of excessive force and do not occur when low forceps or mid forceps delivery can be performed gently. To reduce birth asphyxia and trauma in the full-size baby, forceps deliveries must be used less often and more carefully. Improved training for childbirth and greater psychological support during labor could reduce the 65% incidence of patients requesting pain relief. The temptation to expedite delivery by use of mid forceps when second stage is slowed should be resisted unless a precarious fetal state demands it. When forceps delivery is attempted but is difficult to perform, Cesarean for failed forceps should not be considered as a professional defeat but as a more acceptable alternative than forceful rotation and extraction [Cyr's conclusions].

For the other factors possibly affecting the incidence of birth asphyxia and trauma, the following was found. A large fetus contributed to clavicular fracture, brachial palsy, facial palsy, and meconium aspiration. Fetal size was *not* a factor in producing severe depression or encephalopathy, or in skull fracture.

Nulliparous mothers' infants had more frequent fractures and palsies, but the same incidence of depression, encephalopathy, and meconium aspiration as those born to multipara.

Maternal age was not a factor.

Males had increased risk due solely to their higher birth weight.

Post-term infants were at higher risk, again solely because of their larger size.

Follow-up of infants with post-asphyxic encephalopathy, by Diana Willis and Gordon Watters, showed that those with abnormal cerebral signs were seldom damaged while those who convulsed in the newborn period were usually retarded or neurologically abnormal in infancy and childhood (Table 20).

Table 20   Follow-up at 2 years of infants with post-asphyxic encephalopathy as newborns

Neonatal signs	No. followed	No. abnormal
Abnormal cerebral signs alone	15	1
Convulsions ± abnormal signs	6	4
Totals	21	5

The toll taken by birth asphyxia/trauma in recent years can then be summarized as: six perinatal deaths and five brain-damaged infants in 9901 consecutive deliveries.

CONCLUSION

From all of these studies, what conclusions can be drawn with reference to the efficacy of modern obstetrical practice?

1. The severest forms of birth asphyxia resulting in death or permanent brain damage have been reduced to about 1 per 1000 births combined. Closer fetal monitoring may have played the major role in this improvement.
2. Caesarean sections have contributed little to reduction of asphyxia or trauma during delivery, and at the present time are employed much more often than can be justified.
3. Caesareans should not be performed under general anaesthesia if epidural is possible.
4. Forceps deliveries have a cost and should not be employed indiscriminately. Mid forceps deliveries especially should be performed only when there is evidence of fetal or maternal distress, and if criteria for safe forceps application have been met.
5. Caesarean delivery for failed forceps is highly preferable to forceful forceps extraction when difficulties are encountered with forceps delivery.
6. Epidural analgesia/anaethesia may be responsible for slowing the progress of second-stage labour. If so, it may also be responsible for forceps-related injuries if impatience leads to unnecessarily frequent use of midcavity forceps applications.
7. Modern obstetrics has created a much safer experience for the baby being born, but it has also brought with its technology some new hazards that need to be carefully monitored. Eternal vigilance is the price of safety.

References

1. Green, J., McLean, F., Smith, L. P. and Usher, R. H. (1982). Has an increased cesarean section rate for term breech delivery reduced the incidence of birth asphyxia, trauma and death? *Am. J. Obstet. Gynecol.*, **142,** 643
2. Boyd, M., McLean, F. and Usher, R. H. (1983). Macrosomia. *Obstet. Gynecol.*, **61,** 715

3. Cyr, R., McLean, R. and Usher, R. H. (1984). Changing patterns of birth asphyxia and trauma over 20 years. *Am. J. Obstet. Gynecol.*, **148,** 490
4. Bell, D., Johansson, D., McLean, F. and Usher, R. H. (1985). Birth asphyxia in twin deliveries (In preparation)
5. O'Brien, J. R., Usher, R. H. and Maughan, G. B. (1966). Causes of birth asphyxia and trauma. *Can. Med. Assoc. J.*, **94,** 1077

Section 2
Management of
Childbirth
in Normal Women

Chairman's introduction

P. M. Dunn

Welcome to this symposium on 'The Management of Childbirth in Normal Women'. A lay person might be forgiven for expressing surprise that so many obstetricians, midwives and paediatricians should have gathered to discuss such an apparently straightforward issue. We know that the great majority of women in developed countries are normal and healthy both in a general and in an obstetric sense. Presumably, therefore, childbirth might be expected to be uncomplicated and normal too.

But when we come to try to define normality and what is an intervention or a complication, then we immediately enter difficult and controversial ground. Everything from the upper limit of the normal-length labour, the posture adopted by the mother, how and when she should push, whether and when to cut the umbilical cord, and how the placenta is best delivered remains a battleground for opinion and practice. Even the way we monitor the progress of labour arouses strong conflict, some saying that you can only call labour normal in retrospect, while an opposing view suggests that even the most normal labour can be changed from physiology to pathology by overactive monitoring and the anxiety and other problems it may induce.

So when I was asked to chair and organize this symposium, I deliberately chose a team of experts, all well known, but with differing viewpoints and attitudes to this most important subject. The first speaker will be Professor O'Driscoll, who will speak of his philosophy on 'Active involvement in childbirth', evolved when he was the Master of the National Maternity Hospital here in Dublin. Then Professor Kubli, who heads the Obstetric Department of the University of Heidelberg, and is also Chairman of the FIGO Perinatal Committee and now Secretary General of IAMANEH, will speak on monitoring aspects of normal childbirth. Next comes Dr Odent from France, who has evolved his own style of management in Pithiviers which challenges a number of established medical and cultural attitudes. Then there will be my own paper on the third stage of labour and on how incorrect management may influence both fetal adaptation to extrauterine life and delivery of the placenta. Finally there will be Professor Kloosterman, until recently Head of Obstetrics and Gynaecology in the University of Amsterdam. He will, from his immense experience of midwifery and midwives, give us an overview from Holland.

4

Active involvement in Dublin

K. O'Driscoll and P. Crowley

The concept of active management of labour was evolved at the National Maternity Hospital, Dublin in the late 1960s. It represented a fundamental shift of emphasis in obstetric practice. Formerly, medical involvement in labour was essentially passive until full dilatation had been achieved, when almost any medical procedure aimed at vaginal delivery was acceptable. With the evolution of active management of labour, the involvement of senior obstetric staff began at the time of admission to hospital in an attempt to prevent emergencies arising in women who were normal at the start of labour. This increased medical involvement in the conduct of normal labour brought with it a heightened awareness of the woman's subjective experience of childbirth and its lasting effect on the psyche.

This fundamental reappraisal of medical involvement in normal labour necessitated a precise definition of terms of reference. A vocabulary was evolved which permits clarity and consistency in discussion of the management of labour. It should be made clear at the outset that the term active management of labour refers only to primigravidae in spontaneous labour at term with a singleton fetus in a vertex presentation. Induction of labour must not be confused with acceleration. Primigravidae and multigravidae are fundamentally different. The duration of labour is measured from the time of admission to the labour ward.

Active involvement in Dublin also led to a definition of norms. Criteria were laid down for the diagnosis of labour. The duration of labour was defined as less than 12 hours. Constant medical audit led to the definition of norms for obstetric interventions such as the use of oxytocin, forceps delivery and caesarean section.

The crucial limitation of the duration of labour is achieved by a number of processes. Accuracy in the diagnosis of labour is essential. Dystocia can result from inadvertent induction of labour following a 'false-positive' diagnosis of labour or from hesitancy in accelerating labour when a 'false-negative' diagnosis is made. Once labour has been diagnosed the commitment to delivery within 12 hours is emphasized by the use of a 12-hour partogram. The membranes are ruptured within an hour of admission. Cervical dilatation is the only criterion of progress considered. If there is no advance in cervical dilatation 1 hour after rupture of the membranes, a standard infusion of oxytocin is commended. Any mothers undelivered within 8 hours of admission are personally assessed by the senior resident on duty.

Communication with the mother is vital to the active management of labour. Ideally, this begins antenatally with a course of classes in preparation for childbirth. The commitment to delivery within 12 hours of admission is emphasized during the antenatal classes and again on admission to the delivery ward. The result of each assessment of cervical dilatation is communicated to the mother. Throughout labour she is cared for by a personal nurse.

The results of this active involvement in labour have been far-reaching. Cephalopelvic disproportion, once considered a significant problem in the Dublin population, has been virtually eliminated. Traumatic instrumental vaginal delivery with its attendant risks for both the mother and the baby has become unnecessary. Only 5% of mothers face a second pregnancy bearing the handicap of a caesarean section scar. The improvement in mothers' morale achieved by the limited duration of labour and the support of a personal nurse has dramatically reduced the requirement for analgesia. Productivity is increased as defined by the number of babies delivered per nurse. Job satisfaction for senior nurses is greatly enhanced by the ability to take responsible decisions in managing labour with the full support of senior medical staff. Student midwives enjoy the rewarding experience of one-to-one care of a woman in labour. Obstetricians are indelibly influenced for the better by constant observation of women in normal labour.

Bibliography

O'Driscoll, K. and Meagher, D. (1980). *Active Management of Labour*. (London: W. B. Saunders)

O'Driscoll, K., Jackson, R. J. and Gallagher, J. T. (1969). Prevention of prolonged labour. *Br. Med. J.*, **2**, 477–80

O'Driscoll, K., Jackson, R. J. and Gallagher, J. T. (1970). Active management of labour and cephalopelvic disproportion. *J. Obstet. Gynaecol. Br. Commonw.*, **77**, 385–9

O'Driscoll, K., Stronge, J. M. and Minogue, M. (1973). Active management of labour. *Br. Med. J.*, **3**, 135–40

O'Driscoll, K., Coughlan, M., Fenton, V. and Skelly, M. (1975). Active management of labour: care of the fetus. *Br. Med. J.*, **2**, 1451–3

5

Aspects of monitoring in normal labour

F. Kubli

GENERAL CONSIDERATIONS

Even after apparently normal pregnancy, labour and delivery still carry a certain risk. This is supported by:

1. Data from animal experiments such as those by Comline and Silver[1] on chronically instrumented fetal calves. These show stable fetal oxygenation and acid–base balance throughout the last weeks and days of pregnancy, but a fall in fetal pH and PO_2 during labour and delivery, which is very slight during the first stage and more pronounced during the second stage until delivery.

2. Epidemiological studies showing that non-risk pregnancy turns into risk-labour in 10–20% of cases; unpredicted problems during labour were observed in 17% in the Bavarian Perinatal Study[2] (1980).

3. Data published by Eskes[3] showing significantly lower cord pH values for home deliveries compared to monitored hospital deliveries.

4. The recent Dublin Study presented in detail by MacDonald in chapter 1, according to which convulsions in the neonatal period were significantly more frequent when apparent low-risk labours were not monitored compared to the randomized controls that were subject to electronic monitoring during labour.

This points to the fact that whereas modern clinical and para-clinical evaluation during pregnancy are useful risk predictors for labour, the diagnosis 'normal labour' nevertheless remains a *retrospective* and not a *prospective* diagnosis. On the other hand the remaining risk in term labour after normal pregnancy is quantitatively small. Interventions for monitoring should account for this fact and should be compatible with physical and psychological needs of the labouring women. In practical terms, that means monitoring in normal labour ideally should be compatible with:

1. ambulation and/or any change of position during labour, and
2. late rupture of membranes.

INSTRUMENTS

Continuous electronic monitoring of fetal heart rate during labour is still the only method of surveillance, which in practical terms provides virtually perfect safety with regard to the timely detection of intrapartum hypoxia. (It has to be noted that this is not synonymous with perfect diagnostic accuracy, since false-positive results do occur which need further diagnostic work-up.) However even with today's advanced technology, there is no single method of continuous FHR monitoring which would fulfil the above-mentioned criteria of 'non-intervention'. Thus, compromises have to be made and the available instruments should be used accordingly. If wirebound invasive continuous electronic monitoring is not accepted by the labouring woman, or not applicable for other reasons, the following procedures may be useful:

1. discontinuous recording by manually operated doppler instruments,
2. autocorrelation techniques for processing of abdominal wall signals,
3. telemetry.

Manually operated doppler instrument

Whenever discontinuous monitoring is preferred, this should be done by a doppler instrument and not by the traditional stethoscope because of its higher reliability and the lack of observer-dependence.

Autocorrelation techniques

These constitute a major step forward in signal-processing, allowing reliable continuous abdominal wall monitoring during most of the first stage. However, it has been shown by Rüttgers and Aver[4], as well as others, that the method is not reliable during an active second stage, and moreover in this situation carries a potential risk of misleading information and artefacts. Its use is therefore not recommended during the active second stage.

Telemetry

Telemetric transmission of fetal heart rate at present is without major technical problems and is practised in many hospitals as a routine procedure. It makes ambulation during labour very safe. Its disadvantages consist in that, for practical purposes, telemetry is still bound to invasive monitoring after rupture of membranes and that most transmitters are still relatively bulky. It is established as the method of choice for monitoring, when ambulation is desired after rupture of membranes. In a prospective randomized study[5] we could not find a significant effect on fetal outcome, nor on duration of labour, nor on the incidence of operative deliveries, when ambulation with telemetry was compared with wirebound monitoring; however the subjective evaluation by the patients was very much in favour of ambulation and telemetry.

STRATEGIES AND RECOMMENDATIONS

Policies and recommendations for monitoring normal labour should take into account the following observations:

1. with predicted 'normal labour' the remaining risk is real, but quantitatively small;
2. risk increases with advancing labour and is maximal during the active second stage. This has been shown in the animal experiment (see above) and in humans[6];
3. unrecognized pre-existing chronic fetal hypoxia may be accompanied by minimal fetal heart rate changes not detectable by discontinuous monitoring;
4. peracute intrapartum asphyxia not detectable by discontinuous monitoring may occur with a frequency of 1 : 1000 or less[7].

For practical purposes, the author's recommendations are as follows:

1. Continuous abdominal wall monitoring for at least 30 minutes is indispensable at entrance into the delivery floor ('entrance cardiotocogram').
2. Invasive monitoring is indicated during the active second stage, also in normal labour.
3. During the first stage, several options seem acceptable:
   (a) continuous abdominal wall monitoring (autocorrelation techniques) with intact membranes and non-ambulant mother,
   (b) telemetric continuous monitoring with ambulant patient after early spontaneous or artificial rupture of membranes in active labour (cervical dilatation ≥3–4 cm),
   (c) discontinuous abdominal wall monitoring seems to be an acceptable alternative. It can be done either for short periods (e.g. 15 minutes) of typical abdominal wall recording or by simple acoustic registration by means of a manually operated doppler machine. Intervals will have to depend on the situation, but should be relatively short with simple acoustic surveillance of FHR.
4. Invasive monitoring is mandatory during active labour, whenever predicted 'normal labour' turns into abnormal labour.

RESULTS

In the author's department continuous FHR monitoring by any of the described methods is usual also with non-risk labour. Between 1980 and 1983, 1461 (out of 5350) pregnant women went into labour without any detectable risk according to the history and course of pregnancy, and having had at least one antenatal visit at the department. The outcome was as follows:

Perinatal mortality: 1/1456 (0.7/1000);
1 minute Apgar score less than 5: 6/1450 (4/1000);
5 minute Apgar score less than 5: 0;
umbilical artery pH< 7.10: 6/1473 (4/1000);
marked true asphyxia, i.e. 1 minute Apgar score below 5 and pH umbilical artery < 7.10: 0/1000.

It is felt that individual monitoring policies should be continuously evaluated on the basis of these or similar outcome parameters.

References

1. Comline, R. S. and Silver, M. (1975). Placental transfer of blood gases. *Br. Med. Bull.*, **31**, 25
2. Selbmann, H. K. (1980). Münchner Perinatal-Studie 1975–77. *Deutscher Ärzteverlag*, Köln
3. Eskes, T. K. A. B. (1983) Das Risiko der Hausgeburt. *Arch. Gynecol.*, **235**, 624
4. Rüttgers, H. and Aver, L. (1983). Ergebnisse und Erfahrungen mit einem auto-korrelierenden Ultraschall-Kardiotokographen. *Z. Geburtsh. Perinat.*, **187**, 69
5. Wernicke, K., Kubli, F., Grothe, W. and Faul, B. (1982). Stellenwert der Telemetrie. In: Dudenhausen, J. W. and Saling, E. (eds.) *Perinatale Medizin*, Band IX. (Stuttgart: Thieme)
6. Kubli, F., Rüttgers, H. and Henner, H. (1972). Clinical aspects of fetal acid–base balance during labor. In Longo, L. D. and Bartels, H. (eds.) *Respiratory Gas Exchange and Blood Flow in the Placenta*. DHEW Publication (NIH) 73–361
7. Kubli, F. (1971). Zur Problematik der fetalen Intensivüberwachung. *Med. Mitt.*, **45**, 129

6

Management in Pithiviers

M. Odent

In any place where the priority is to facilitate the physiology of the birth process and to protect the mother–newborn relationship, the same points would be emphasized:

1. A labouring woman needs to feel that she belongs to a human group, to a community. This need is rarely satisfied in the context of modern hospitals, and also at a time when the family is commonly reduced to the nuclear family and when the young couples have often to go from one home to another, or from one job to another. That is why we encourage groups of parents, such as our singing groups, which may be considered as substitutes for the extended family.

2. A labouring woman needs privacy. An experienced and motherly midwife is commonly the best person to protect the right atmosphere of privacy.

3. A labouring woman can more easily release her inhibitions in a silent, warm, homely room, with a low soft light. More generally speaking the reduction of sensory stimuli is beneficial.

4. As early as during the first stage, a labouring woman must feel free to adopt any kind of posture. When a woman feels free about her movement, some positions are quite common. For example many women like to remain on all fours for a rather long time. This seems efficient for reducing pain, especially backache, and also works mechanically. When there is a posterior presentation this posture facilitates rotation inside the pelvis. The fetus tends to turn toward the front of the uterus as the heaviest part of it is its back. Moreover the woman on all fours 'focuses inwardly', and can thus more readily ignore what is going on around her. The resemblance of this position to a praying posture may help for achieving the appropriate state of consciousness; that is to say the right hormonal balance.

5. At the time of the second stage there is every indication that the reduction of the neocortical control facilitates the finding of physiologically and mechanically more favourable positions than the conventional lying or semi-sitting postures.

6. A supported squatting position is very common at the time of the very last contractions.

7. The mother–child relationship in the perinatal period and the expulsion of the placenta are closely connected with delivery conditions.

Our statistics show that such an attitude, which is radically different from the conventional obstetrical attitude, is a way to reconcile a low perinatal mortality rate and a low rate of caesareans and interventions in general (Table 1).

Table 1 1977 to 1983, 7054 births

Perinatal deaths	64 $(9.07^0/_{00})$
Caesareans	488 (6.90%)
Vacuum	322 (4.56%)
Manual removal of placenta	62 (0.87%)
Transfer pediatrics	119 (1.68%)

If we consider a shorter period, the percentages are approximately the same (Table 2).

Table 2 1982 to 1983, 1815 births

Perinatal deaths	14 $(7.70^0/_{00})$
Caesareans	125 (6.88%)
Vacuum	89 (4.90%)
Episiotomies	106 (5.84%)
Manual removal of placenta	16 (0.88%)
Transfer pediatrics	27 (1.48%)
Women with previous caesarean	66
Vaginal route after previous caesarean	36

Some data need a longer period to be better evaluated (Table 3).

Table 3 1968 to 1983, 11 462 births

Forceps	0
Maternal deaths	0
Ratio between primipara and multipara:	
Primipara	46%
Secundipara	35%
Para 3 (or more)	19%

Table 4 gives figures suggesting the importance of the personality of the midwives.

Table 4 M.C. and M.H. (two midwives), 1982 to 1983, 609 births

Caesareans	26 (4.26%)
Episiotomies	17 (2.79%)
Vacuum	23 (3.77%)
Manual removal of placenta	7 (1.15%)
Intrapartum deaths	0 –

We consider these last figures as the most important. They help us to remember a fundamental human need: a parturient needs first to be assisted by an experienced and motherly female.

7
The third stage and fetal adaptation

P. M. Dunn

The modern western management of the third stage consists of a series of interlocking interventions which are applied so routinely that many obstetricians now regard them as 'normal'. This management had its roots only 300 years ago when the dorsal position for delivery and cord traction were first introduced in France[1]. Now, once the baby has been delivered, the cord is divided with scissors between double clamps. Often triple clamps are used in order to ensure the availability of umbilical arterial and venous blood samples for acid–base and blood gas analysis. This division of the cord frees the infant for transfer to the resuscitation area, where all too often he or she is placed in the disadvantageous head-down position[2,3]. Meanwhile, in most developed countries, the third stage is usually managed actively[4]. An oxytocic agent, usually syntometrine, is given as the anterior shoulder delivers and, once the uterus is contracting, steady traction is exerted on the umbilical cord, while the free hand holds the uterus out of the pelvis. The aim of all these interventions is to reduce the risk of postpartum haemorrhage and retained placenta. Yet the fact remains that significant postpartum haemorrhage (> 500 ml) is commonly reported in 2–8% of hospital deliveries[5] and manual removal of the placenta in at least 1–2% of all cases.

To learn about the *normal* third stage without interventions, it is necessary to either to study the history *or* the anthropology of childbirth[6,7], or to work in the rural areas of developing countries that have not yet been penetrated by western obstetrics. Almost invariably the story is the same. The woman remains in the upright position; she may strain, but traction is never exerted on the cord. As the uterus contracts and retracts, the placenta is partly pushed and partly falls with the aid of gravity down alongside the baby, usually within 5 minutes. Meanwhile the cord remains unclamped and intact until well after the delivery of the placenta and until all pulsation in it has ceased, usually a period of 10–20 minutes. Only then is it divided with a blunt rather than a sharp instrument (presumably to encourage homeostasis).Neither end of the cord is ligated. Medical travellers have always been surprised to find that umbilical haemorrhage is not a problem. Nor are there apparently major problems with the delivery of the placenta.

In 1968 Botha described his experience working with the Bantu in rural South Africa over a 10-year period[8]. Attending some 26 000 deliveries he stated that a retained placenta was seldom seen and blood transfusion for a postpartum haemorrhage was never necessary. Botha went on to study the influence of clamping or not clamping the *placental* end of the cord. He showed that when it was not clamped, the mean duration of the third stage was reduced from 10.5 to 3.5 minutes ($p < 0.001$), and the blood loss was less than half as great ($p < 0.001$) as when this end of the cord was clamped.

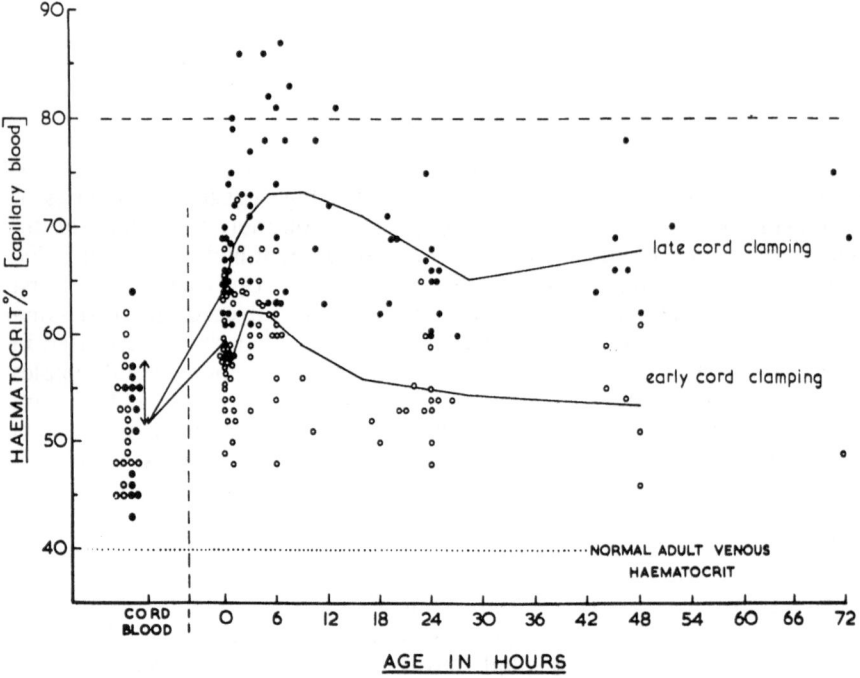

Figure 1   The umbilical cord and heel capillary blood haematocrit values of 32 infants, delivered normally at term, according to whether the umbilical cord was clamped at the instant of birth (< 1 s) or after a delay of at least 3 min. ○ = early clamping; ● = late clamping

Some years earlier, in the period 1961–1965, I had become interested in the same subject. At first my main interest was in the influence that cord clamping had on the infant and on adaptation to extrauterine life. Many clinical, haematological and biochemical parameters were measured and in every one of them the impact of cord clamping could be shown to be dramatic and significant. In Figure 1 may be seen the effect of immediate cord clamping (< 1 second) versus clamping delayed for at least 3 minutes on the term infant's haematocrit during the first 48 hours after birth[9]. Such changes should not surprise us, for in these studies the mean volume of blood transferred or not transferred from placenta to baby during this 3-minute period was 136 ml, which is equivalent to 49% of the normal blood volume of a term infant[10].

My studies revealed that the normal distribution of blood between fetus and placenta was altered during the second stage of labour with a net transfer of approximately 66 ml from baby to placenta at this time, presumably due to selective compression of the soft-walled umbilical vein[11]. If the cord was then clamped immediately at delivery, this blood (on average a total of 166 ml) is trapped within the placenta. The baby, not surprisingly, shows all the signs of hypovolaemia with a low blood pressure and intense peripheral vasoconstriction, while the placenta, on the other hand, is bulky, stiff, and engorged, as may be clearly seen on gross and microscopic examination[12]. A number of studies of the blood pressure within this vasculature were made at this time, and demonstrated that the mean residual pressure after delivery of the placenta and following immediate cord clamping was no less than 28 mmHg[13]. Thus the placenta was not only bulky, its volume being increased by perhaps 33% (compared with the blood evacuated status), but was also tense in the way any erectile vascular structure may be made rigid by blood under pressure.

My next step in 1964 was to try to study in more detail the mechanical problems presented by the passage of such a placenta through the retracting cervix after delivery of the baby. This was done by measuring the smallest hoop (I used pessary rings of known diameter) through which the placenta might be passed, first engorged with blood following early clamping, and, secondly, after draining out all the blood. At this point I noticed another factor which does not appear to have been described previously. This is the observation that, if traction is exerted on a cord inserted centrally into the placenta, the latter inverts like an inside-out umbrella and presents a much thicker diameter for passage through the ring (or cervix). The same does not apply if the cord is inserted into the margin of the placenta or if, in practice, traction is exerted directly, by say an inserted finger, on the lower edge of the placenta. This simple mechanical fact should have been obvious but, like the importance of gravity in childbirth, it seems to have escaped attention. One example will be given of these 1964 studies. Following early cord clamping, the placenta in this case weighed 725 g and would just pass through a ring with a diameter of 79 mm. After draining out 85 ml of blood the placenta passed through the ring with a diameter of 62 mm using central cord traction. When, however, traction was exerted to the edge of the placenta, it would pass through a ring with a diameter of 48 mm. This represents a 40% reduction from the original figure of 79 mm. Expressed in another way, the surface area enclosed within the largest ring was 1.7 times greater than that of the middle-sized ring and no less than 2.8 times greater than that of the smallest ring. We do not have to look further for justification for the practice of our forebears in neither clamping the umbilical cord nor exerting traction on it.

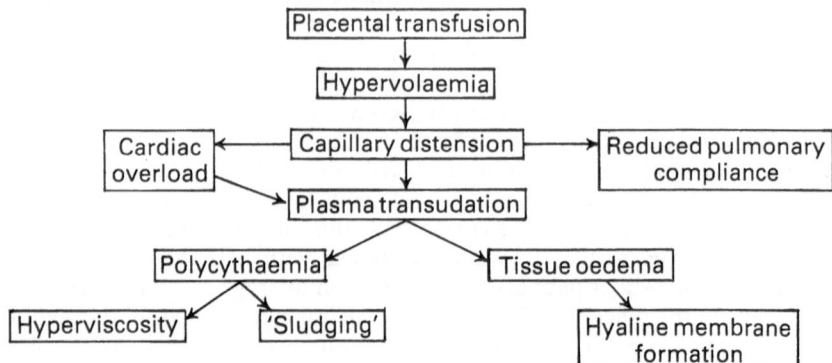

Figure 2 Diagram to indicate the cascade of events that may occur soon after birth when an infant becomes hypervolaemic due to a large placental transfusion

If we return to our delivery sequence, and do *not* clamp the cord immediately, the great bulk of the placental blood volume is transferred to the infant, impelled by gravity and uterine contraction[14,15]. If the cord is clamped at this point then the maternal surface of the placenta appears pink rather than purple, histological examination shows the capillaries to be empty of blood, and the vessels on the fetal surface are collapsed, the whole organ being limp, slippery and flexible. On the other hand, the infant, following late cord clamping, typically has the characteristic features of hypervolaemia and polycythaemia. Figure 2 shows diagrammatically the cascade of events that may result from a large placental transfusion and hypervolaemia. These include cardiac overload, capillary distension with reduced pulmonary compliance and plasma transudation with polycythaemia, hyperviscosity and sludging on the one hand, and tissue oedema, and possibly hyaline membrane formation in the preterm infant, on the other.

There is, however, an alternative to clamping the cord: that of not clamping it at all, as favoured by non-western practice, and then allowing the placenta to deliver and lie alongside the infant. This not only avoids the haemodynamic disturbance that may result from a marked rise in systemic blood pressure when pulsating umbilical arteries are clamped, cutting off the low-resistance placental circulation, but it also permits the placenta to provide a safety valve for any raised central venous pressure; for blood may flow backwards down the umbilical vein (there are no valves), hence providing the infant with the best opportunity for achieving a normal blood volume and haematocrit, and avoiding many of the problems of maladaptation to extrauterine life.

Those of you who were at the 3rd Congress in Lausanne in 1972 may just remember a paper I gave there on caesarean section and the prevention of respiratory distress syndrome of the preterm infant[16]. I showed that, in our experience, by delivering the infant with placental circulation intact at preterm caesarean section, and by then instituting appropriate resuscitative measures, we had been able to reduce the mortality of these high-risk infants by no less than 90%. My, in part, speculative hypothesis as to why this should be so has been reported elsewhere and is summarized in Figures 3 and 4. In brief, adaptation to extrauterine life depends on the achievement of adequate alveolar ventilation, accompanied by a fall in pulmonary vascular resistance, a greatly increased pulmonary blood flow and other secondary changes in the circulation. The key to successful adaptation appears to be the replacement of the lung fluid that fills the alveolus, prior to delivery, with air. Evacuation of this fluid is partially achieved during vaginal delivery by thoracic compression during the second stage of labour and, after birth, by pulmonary lymphatic drainage aided by the 'milking' action of respiratory movements and a low central venous pressure.

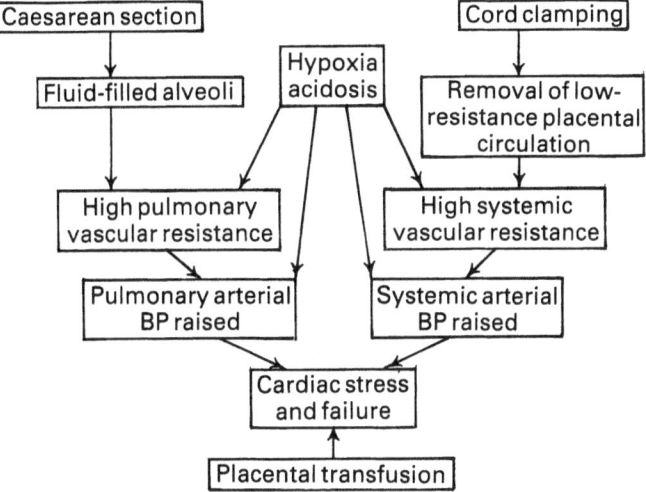

Figure 3 Diagram to indicate possible mechanisms at and soon after delivery that may lead to transitory cardiac overload and failure

Clearance of lung fluid is often inadequate when the preterm infant is delivered by caesarean section, particularly when the latter is elective. The baby has been deprived of the vaginal squeeze to the thorax and respiratory movements may be weak or absent because of such factors as maternal anaesthesia, a compliant rib cage, and increased airway resistance, as well as lack of surfactant. In addition, cord clamping at delivery of vigorously pulsating umbilical vessels will cut off the low-resistance placental circulation and might be expected to cause a sharp rise in systemic blood pressure. In the presence of a continuing high pulmonary vascular resistance, the heart may exhibit transitory 'failure' with raised pulmonary and central venous pressures.

Raised pulmonary venous pressure might then be expected to lead to pulmonary oedema with the extravasation of plasma proteins causing inactivation or displacement of surfactant and hyaline membrane formation. Meanwhile, a raised central venous pressure would impede pulmonary lymphatic drainage, a situation which would be exacerbated if the infant were then resuscitated in the head-down position[17].

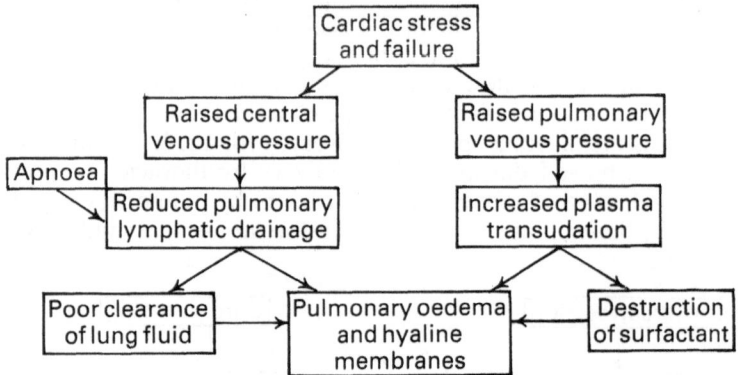

Figure 4 Diagram to indicate possible mechanisms whereby transitory cardiac strain and failure immediately after delivery may lead to respiratory distress syndrome of the newborn

Since introducing this technique of delivering the baby with its placental circulation intact, first in Birmingham and Warwick in 1961–63 and subsequently in Bristol, a number of observations have appeared in the literature that lend support to the hypothesis[18-26]. It must be added that Landau and his colleagues[27] also recommended a similar practice in 1950. He believed that the problem in the baby was due to lack of blood transfusion and recommended raising the placenta above the baby, as have others since[28,29]. Two earlier papers are relevant too[30,31].

Before leaving the third stage there is one other matter that needs mentioning. The release of oxytocin which takes place following suckling was demonstrated by Chassor Moir in studies made many years ago[32], thus providing physiological justification for the practice widely found among non-western cultures of putting the infant to the breast while waiting for the placenta to deliver.

This has been the briefest of reviews of a large and complex subject. Many aspects, especially concerning the effect that cord clamping may have on the infant, have had to be omitted. Let me just end with a quotation made by a British obstetrician 200 years ago when discussing this very subject[33]. He wrote:

There is yet in all things a perfectly right as well as a wrong method; and though the advantage or disadvantage of either may be overlooked, the propriety and advantage of the right method must be evidently proved by individual cases, and of course by the general result of practice. In this, as well as in many other points, we have been too fond of interfering with art, and have consigned too little to nature, as if the human race had been destined to wretchedness and disaster, from the moment of birth, beyond the allotment of other creatures.

References

1. Mauriceau, F. (1752). *Diseases of Woman with Child and in Childbed*, 8th edn. Transl. by H. Chamberlen. (London)
2. Dunn, P. M. (1973). The newborn, now or never. *J. Irish Med. Assoc.*, **66**, 585–92
3. Emery, J. R. and Peabody, J. L. (1982). Head position is critical to intracranial pressure in asphyxiated infants (Ab.). *Paed. Res.*, **16**, 334
4. Hull, M. G. R., Turner, G. and Joyce, D. N. (1980). In Dixon, G. (ed.) *Undergraduate Obstetrics and Gynaecology*, p. 223 (Bristol: John Wright)
5. Stirrat, G. M. (1981). *Obstetrics*, p. 152. (London: Grant McIntyre)
6. Engelmann, G. L. (1882). *Labour among Primitive Peoples* (St. Louis: Chambers)
7. Ploss, H. H., Bartels, M. and Bartels, P. (1935). *Woman: An Historical Gynecological and Anthropological Compendium* (ed. Dingwall, E. G.), vols 1–3. (London: Heinnemann)
8. Botha, M. C. (1968). The management of the umbilical cord in labour. *S.A. J. Obstet. Gynaecol.*, **6**, 30–3
9. Dunn, P. M. (1970). Neonatal polycythaemia (Ab.) *Arch. Dis. Childh.*, **45**, 273
10. Dunn, P. M. (1984). Reservations about the methods of assessing at birth the predictive value of intrapartum fetal monitoring, including premature interruption of the feto-placental circulation. In Rolfe, P. (ed.) *Fetal and Neonatal Physiological Measurement*, Vol. 2. (Guildford: Butterworths). (In press)
11. Dunn, P. M. (1967). Alterations in the distribution of blood between the fetus and placenta during and after delivery. Manuscript of paper given at the Canadian Paediatric Society Centennial Commonwealth Meeting, Toronto, September 3–9
12. Dunn, P. M., Fraser, I. D. and Raper, A. B. (1966). Influence of early cord ligation on the transplacental passage of fetal cells. *J. Obstet. Gynaecol. Br. Commonw.*, **73**, 757–60
13. Dunn, P. M. (1966). The placental venous pressure during and after the third stage of labour following early cord ligation. *J. Obstet. Gynaecol. Br. Commonw.*, **73**, 747–56
14. Usher R., Shephard, M. and Lind, J. (1963). The blood volume of the newborn infant and placental transfusion. *Acta Paediatr. Scand.*, **52**, 497–512
15. Yao, A. C. and Lind, J. (1982). *Placental Transfusion*. (Springfield, Illinois: C. C. Thomas)
16. Dunn, P. M. (1973). Caesarean section and the prevention of respiratory distress syndrome of the newborn. In Bossart, H. *et al.* (eds) *Perinatal Medicine,* 3rd Europ. Congr. Perinatal Medicine, Lausanne, 1972, pp. 138–45. (Bern: Hans Huber)
17. Dunn, P. M. (1985). In the delivery room. In Fleming, P. J. *et al.* (eds) *Neonatal Vade Mecum.* (London: Lloyd Luke) (In press)
18. Brady, J. P. and James, L. S. (1962). Heart rate changes in the fetus and newborn infant during labor, delivery and the immediate neonatal period. *Am. J. Obstet. Gynecol.*, **84**, 1–12
19. Dawes, G. S., Jacobson, H. N., Mott, J. C., Shelley, H. J. and Stafford, A. (1963). The treatment of asphyxiated, mature foetal lambs and rhesus monkeys with intravenous glucose and sodium carbonate. *J. Physiol.*, **169**, 167–84
20. Oh, W., Lind, J. and Gessner, I. H. (1966). Circulatory and respiratory adaptation to early and late cord clamping in newborn infants. *Acta Paediatr. Scand.*, **55**, 17–25
21. Arcilla, R. A., Oh, W. and Lind, J. (1966). Portal and atrial pressures in the newborn: a comparative study in infants born with early and late clamping of the cord. *Acta Paediatr. Scand.*, **55**, 615–25
22. Oh, W., Wallgren, G., Hanson, J. S. and Lind, J. (1967). The effects of placental

transfusion on respiratory mechanics of normal term infants. *Pediatrics*, **40**, 6–12
23. Dawes, G. S. (1966). Pulmonary circulation in foetus and newborn infant. *Br. Med. Bull.*, **22**, 61–5
24. Lanweryns, J. M., St Classens, B. and Boussauer, L. (1968). The pulmonary lymphatics in neonatal hyaline membrane disease. *Pediatrics*, **41**, 917–30
25. Klein, M. (1972). Asphyxia neonatorum caused by foaming. *Lancet*, **1**, 1089–91
26. Adamson, T. M., Boyd, R. D. H., Hill, J. R., Normand, I. C. S., Reynolds, E. O. R. and Strang, L. B. (1970). Effect of asphyxia due to umbilical cord occlusion in the foetal lamb on leakage of liquid from the circulation and on permiability of lung capillaries to albumin. *J. Physiol.*, **207**, 493–505
27. Landau, D. R., Goodrich, H. B., Franka, W. F. and Burns, F. R. (1950). Death of Caesarean infants: A theory as to its cause and a method of prevention. *J. Pediatr.*, **36**, 421–6
28. Secher, O. and Karlberg, P. (1962). Placental and blood transfusion for newborns delivered by Caesarean section. *Lancet*, **1**, 1203–5
29. Vardi, P. (1965). Placental transfusion. An attempt at physiological delivery. *Lancet*, **2**, 12–13
30. Gunther, M. (1957). The transfer of blood between baby and placenta in the first minutes after birth. *Lancet*, **1**, 1277–80
31. Mahaffey, L. W. and Rossdale, P. D. (1959). A convulsive syndrome in newborn foals resembling pulmonary syndrome in the newborn infant. *Lancet*, **1**, 1223–5
32. Moir, C. J. (1964). The obstetrician bids, and the uterus contracts. *Br. Med. J.*, **2**, 1025–9
33. Denman, T. (1801). *An Introduction to the Practice of Midwifery*, 3rd edn, p. 254. (London)

8

The Netherlands as an obstetric experiment

G. J. Kloosterman

One of the most intriguing questions concealed in the title of this symposium is: what are normal women?

The answer to this question will depend on the persons asked. Poets, painters, judges or psychiatrists will hold different views and even if we consult obstetricians there will be a great variety of opinions, among other things influenced by the moment of pregnancy and/or labour when we ask the question.

If we accept that the woman must be able to bring a healthy child spontaneously into the outer world, then everybody will agree that we only can call a woman normal a few days after delivery; but it is also true that the great majority of pregnant women afterwards appears to belong to this group, especially so if we consider women who, after a well-controlled pregnancy, showed no signs of abnormality and in whom labour started spontaneously after the 37th and before the 43rd week of pregnancy (after 259 and before 295 days).

That the majority of all women has always been able to bring a healthy child into the world without any assistance is a fact, recognized from time immemorial.

In 1701 the famous Dutch obstetrician Hendrik van Deventer[1] defined a natural or easy birth as a birth accomplished by Nature alone, without any intervention or assistance; a birth not in need of any help of midwife or doctor. He compared one of his clients even with a waffle-iron, from whom the children rolled out as easily as the waffles from the waffle-iron.

In 1752 the founding father of British obstetrics, William Smellie[2], wrote in his famous *Treatise on the Theory and Practice of Midwifery*: 'I call that a natural labour in which the head presents and the woman is delivered by her pains and the assistance commonly given.

55

Smellie also gave statistical data. He estimated that 92% of all births could be called natural, 7% laborious or unnatural (the head comes with difficulty and must be assisted either with the hand or with instruments) and 1% praeternatural (the child is brought by breech or feet).

Statistical data were also given by the Dutch midwife Schrader[3], who lived from 1656 to 1746 and practised from 1693 to 1745. She assisted in 3060 deliveries and gave a short description in her diary of every confinement. From this unique document we can learn that natural childbirth occurred in 94%. Manual help, mostly version and extraction and/or manual removal of the placenta, occurred in 5.5% and instrumental assistance, mostly the crotchet, was necessary in 0.5%. These results are the more striking since her practice contained more pathology than could be expected in a random sample of the population (in her material multiple pregnancy was 2.4%, placenta praevia totalis 2%oo, etc).

If 250 years ago more than 90% of all women with a full-grown pregnancy were able to bring their child into the world spontaneously without any assistance other than sympathy and encouragement, it seems utterly improbable that this power nowadays should be lost in women, who without any doubt are in a better state of general health.

But when we look around us, we must conclude that, especially in our part of the world, also called the industrialized (or rich or first) world, the faith in the existence of healthy or normal women seems to be lost.

A delivery without any form of analgesia (from pethidine or gas and air to epidural or general anaesthesia), without an episiotomy, without outlet forceps or vacuum extraction, without injections of oxytocin – such a delivery has become exceptional. At the same time obstetricians seem to agree that all children should be born in hospitals, where doctors can cope with most sorts of emergencies, and in the past 20 years total hospitalization is achieved in almost all countries of this industrialized world on both sides of the Iron Curtain.

In the same period there has taken place an impressive and incomparable advance in obstetric results, measured by maternal and perinatal mortality, and many obstetricians attribute this progress to this new kind of management of natal care, including the disappearance of home confinements and the disappearance of the independent midwife.

But not everybody is convinced of this connection, and especially among the consumers there is no full acceptance of the new hospital routines. Many regard childbirth as an intense personal experience to be shared by other members of the family, and a strong protest is heard against the restricted, sterile conditions of the labour and delivery rooms, the immense 'gadgetry' and the ever-increasing caesarean section rate.

Some women go so far as to turn their back on the obstetric profession, stay at home, and accept the attendance of unqualified lay midwives to escape the strict rules of hospitals. In doing so they accept a risk for themselves and their child. The bad results of these non-institutionalized home confinements are (mis)used by the profession to justify their stark type of obstetric organization, whereas it would be much better to accept that many healthy and self-confident women wish to experience childbirth as a natural, creative art without unnecessary interference.

Mistrust and antagonistic views between public and profession are not new. Smellie[2] wrote (p. 241):

A general outcry hath been raised against gentlemen of the profession, as if they delighted in using instruments and violent methods in the course of their practice; and this clamour hath proceeded from the ignorance of such as do not know that instruments are sometimes absolutely necessary, or from the interested views of some low, obscure and illiterate practitioners, both male and female, who think they find their account in decrying the practice of their neighbours. It is not to be denied that mischief has been done by instruments in the hands of the unskilful and unweary, but I am persuaded that every judicious practitioner will do everything for the safety of his patients before he has recourse to any violent method, though cases will occur, in which gentle methods will absolutely fail.

It is therefore necessary to explain those reinforcements which must be used in dangerous labours though they ought by no means be called in, except when the life of the mother or child or both is evidently at stake. For my own part I have always avoided them as far as I thought consistent with the safety of my patients.

In my opinion Smellie hit the nail on the head by stating that every interference must be justified by some pathological condition, and asks for an explanation.

This is also true for the present-day type of obstetric organization. Whereas it is self-evident that nowhere can pathology of pregnancy and labour be handled better than in a large well-equipped hospital by a highly specialized staff, there is no proof that normal women have any advantage in such surroundings. There are even voices heard that perinatal death could be increased by delivery in hospital because of the surgical and pharmacological intervention practised there[4,5].

Quite rightly Murphy et. al.[6] point to the fact that it is extremely difficult to obtain unbiased estimates of the risk of perinatal problems directly attributable to alternative places of delivery (and the same holds true for the different persons – midwives, GPs or obstetricians – responsible for obstetric care).

In the industrialized world on both sides of the Iron Curtain only the Netherlands still stick to the idea that pregnant women have to be considered healthy and normal till the opposite is proven. As long as everything stays normal they can be controlled and assisted by midwives, and have a free choice to stay at home or go to hospital for delivery under the care of the same midwife who controlled the pregnancy.

Since 1958 the number of home confinements decreased from 70% to 35%, but since 1978 this percentage did not drop further, and in 1982 it was even slightly higher than in 1978. The number of confinements under the care of a registered midwife only (at home or in hospital) is 40%, and this percentage is the same as 20 years ago.

The data of 1982 are given in Tables 1–3 and show that a well-selected group of apparently normal women can deliver in simple surroundings without electronic monitoring and without sophisticated means with very good results. A perinatal mortality of 2 per thousand (including of course all transfers to hospital during labour), 7 times lower than the perinatal mortality in hospital and 5 times lower than the average for the whole country, is in striking contrast with

Table 1 Babies born in the Netherlands, 1982

Place of Delivery	Births	Percentages
At home	61 205	35.4
Hospitals	106 911	61.8
Maternity units	2188	1.3
Midwife schools	2156	1.2
Abroad	621	0.4
Totals	173 081	100.0

Data from Kloosterman, *Management of Childbirth in Normal Women*

Table 2 Babies born at home, 1982

	Births	Percentages
With maternity home help	56 785	92.5
With other kind of help	4420	7.2
Total	61 205	100.0

Data from Kloosterman, *Management of Childbirth in Normal Women*

Table 3 Maternity home help (MHH) (total births: 56 785, at home)

Stillbirths	47	
First week mortality		
At home	33	
Hospital	34	
Perinatal mortality, MHH	114	(2.0‰)
1982: Perinatal mortality, Netherlands:		10.0‰

Data from Kloosterman, *Management of Childbirth in Normal Women*

the results reached in countries where home confinements went down to less than 1 or 2% and where perinatal mortality of home confinements is sometimes 4 times higher than in hospital[7]. But showing that home confinements are much more acceptable than many obstetricians think is not enough. The same holds true for sharing obstetric care with midwives. Where are the advantages? The advantages are: a far greater amount of complete spontaneous births without any form of anaesthesia or instrumental or pharmacological interference. Whereas caesarean section rates in almost all countries with total hospitalization are above 10%, and in some countries even 16–18%, this proportion was 4.7% in 1980 in the Netherlands and forceps and vacuum extractions were 5.9% in 1982.

A very thorough study by Dr Van Alten in Wormerveer, a village 15 miles north of Amsterdam, covering a group of 4804 women during the period January 1970 till January 1977, confirmed the conclusion that selection during pregnancy makes it possible to define a low-risk group with a very good prognosis, a group with more than 94% complete spontaneous deliveries and a caesarean section rate of 1%. This study is still being continued, and in this book Dr M. Eskes and Dr M Knuist also give data of the pH of arterial umbilical cord blood and of the so-called Prechtl score, in women who delivered out of hospital, at home or in a simple maternity clinic.

It was not my intention to make propaganda for the Dutch system of obstetric organization. I am convinced that it will be very difficult, and perhaps even dangerous, to introduce such a system in a country where it never existed. I am also convinced that staying at home as a protest against a prevailing system of total hospitalization without adequate professional care is dangerous and rejectable.

I only give these data to show that nowadays more than 90% of all women can deliver spontaneously and are, as in the time of Smellie and Van Deventer, only in need of encouragement and sympathy.

If the healthy, normal parturient does not stay at home, then she must be in a hospital that is as homely as possible, in surroundings with a maximum of freedom to choose her company and posture, surroundings with a minimum of rules and prescriptions.

References

1. Deventer, H. van. (1701). *Nieuw Ligt voor Vroedmeesters en Vroedvrouwen*, p. 88. ('s-Gravenhage).
2. Smellie, (1752). *A Treatise on the Theory and Practice of Midwifery* pp. 193–6. (London)
3. Schrader, C. G. *Memory Boeck van de Vrouwens* (1745). Adapted and re-edited by Kloosterman, G. J. and Van Lieburg, M. (1984) (Amsterdam: Rodopi)
4. Tew, M. (1978). The case against hospital deliveries: the statistical evidence. In Kitzinger, S. and Davies, J. A. (eds). *The Place of Birth*, pp. 55–6. (Oxford: Oxford University Press).
5. Tew, M. (1980). Facts, not assertions of belief. *Soc. Serv. J.*, **90**, 1194–7
6. Murphy, J. F., Dannery, M., Gray, O. P. and Chalmers, I. (1984) Planned and unplanned deliveries at home: implications of a changing ratio (1984). *Br. Med. J.*, **288**, 1429–32
7. Kloosterman, G. J. (1983). The Dutch experience. In Zander and Chamberlain (eds.) *Pregnancy care for the 1980's*, pp. 115–26. (The Royal Society of Medicine and Macmillan Press)

Chairman's summary

P. M. Dunn

We have had a useful discussion. For all the arguments and different points of view, we would all agree that the common aim is that mother and baby be safely delivered in good health, and that the experience be as happy and as fulfilling as possible. Where we differ at times is how best to achieve this aim. At one end of the spectrum are those who believe that Nature always knows best, while at the other end are those who believe that pregnancy and childbirth should be regarded as a 9-month disease that must be fought with all the medical knowledge at our command. Most of us hold views somewhere in the middle. It is a matter of getting the balance right between watchful expectancy on the one hand, and maintaining the confidence and normal physiology of the mother on the other.

As a paediatrician I am inevitably a bystander to some extent in the drama of childbirth, but it has always seemed to me that one of the great dangers of interventions *when all is normal* is that complications or disordered physiology may be deemed as justification for the initial intervention and indeed for further interventions. Professor Kloosterman is always saying 'You just cannot improve on Nature when she is performing well – you can only make things worse.'

Nowhere are the devastating effects of over-intervention more obvious than when western-style obstetrics is introduced into Third World countries where they so often have inadequate resources and knowledge to deal with the problems that may result. This Bantu lady in a western-style obstetric unit was struggling to maintain an upright position during labour as she would in her own kraal, but was repeatedly told to lie down by the staff. The caesarean section rate in this hospital was 24%, or 8 times higher than that for women in the surrounding rural areas. A Bantu midwife who had been trained in the modern obstetrics told me:

The mothers always deliver on their backs because we make them – but in their kraals they kneel. I believe you, doctor, when you say the upright position is better, because when labour is slow, I get them to kneel and they deliver well. I didn't know I was doing right.

But progress is being made and steadily we professionals are learning to listen to mothers as well as to Nature, and gradually we are achieving a better balance.

May I now draw this session to a close by first thanking the members of our panel for their contributions and you for your questions, and then by reading a quotation by Euripedes which is a particular favourite of mine:

> Happy the man whose lot it is to know
> The secrets of the earth. He hastens not
> To work his fellow's hurt by unjust deeds,
> But with rapt admiration contemplates
> Immortal Nature's ageless harmony,
> And how and when her order came to be.

Section 3
Antenatal Fetal Assessment

9

Fetal and neonatal assessment

G. Rooth

FETAL

The following is a plea for better understanding of the value of intrauterine pressure (IUP) monitoring. When IUP should be done is another problem, which will not be dealt with here.

Usually whether intra- or extrauterine pressure is monitored during labour it is mainly used to diagnose late decelerations. In view of the value justly ascribed to IUP already in the first description of the technique by Caldeyro Barcia and Alvarez[1] it is surprising that this information has not been systematically better used. The continuous fetal transcutaneous measurements during labour have confirmed Caldeyro Barcia's initial observations.

Every single uterine contraction, if above a certain level (usually about 20 mmHg), leads to a fall in fetal Po_2[5]. This is due to obstruction of the placental circulation during the contractions. As fetal fall in Po_2 is due to its own oxygen consumption, and as the monitoring system – skin electrode – induces a delay, the fall in fetal Po_2 begins about 50 seconds after the onset of a contraction. Therefore, fetal Po_2 may be at a peak value during the beginning of the contractions (Figure 1).

The stronger the contractions the more marked will the fall be. Still, if the uterine activity is normal the fall in fetal Po_2 rarely exceeds 3 mmHg and gradually returns to the precontraction level during the interval. The relationship between the intensity of the contractions and the fall in fetal Po_2 is highly significant[3]. If the contractions are clustered there is no time for fetal Po_2 to recover and each contraction will further depress fetal Po_2. If the interval between contractions is too short the recovery after one contraction is not complete and fetal Po_2 will gradually fall to a lower level (Figure 2). These observations are not anecdotal but are consistent. Fetal heart rate also reacts to too strong or too frequent contractions. However, as expected, fetal Po_2 falls

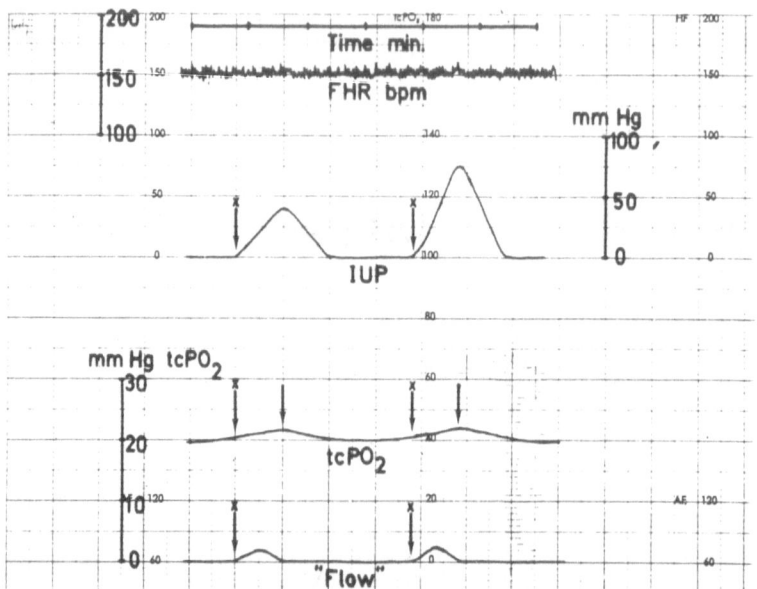

Figure 1 The arrows marked × indicate when the contraction starts. The unmarked arrow 50–60 seconds later is the beginning of the fall in fetal Po$_2$ (data from ref. 2)

before any changes are seen in fetal heart rate.

Thus, from comparisons between IUP changes and fetal tcPo$_2$ (transcutaneous technique) it is evident that the former strongly and systematically influence the former. If IUP is performed valuable information may be obtained from these observations.

NEONATAL

Using the oxygen cardiorespirogram we have monitored more than 3000 newborn infants non-invasively in the first week of life in order to define the range of normality of oxygen tension, heart rate, heart rate variability, respiratory excursions and respiratory rate[4]. Mainly quiet newborn infants with a birthweight 2500 g, Apgar score 7 and without signs of disease, were studied. Oxygen was monitored with the transcutaneous technique (tcPo$_2$). The highest tcPo$_2$ values were seen in the second half of the first hour of life, corresponding to the intense ventilation needed to eliminate the surplus of CO$_2$ and lactic acid accumulated during delivery. The level of tcPo$_2$ varies markedly and the mean difference between the highest and the lowest values during 1 hour of recording was 15 mmHg. During crying tcPo$_2$ falls in 98% of the cases. The median fall is about 15 mmHg, but it may be as large as 40–55 mmHg in the individual case. This fall during crying persists during the whole of the first week of life.

Heart rate was also highest in the first hour of life and then gradually fell

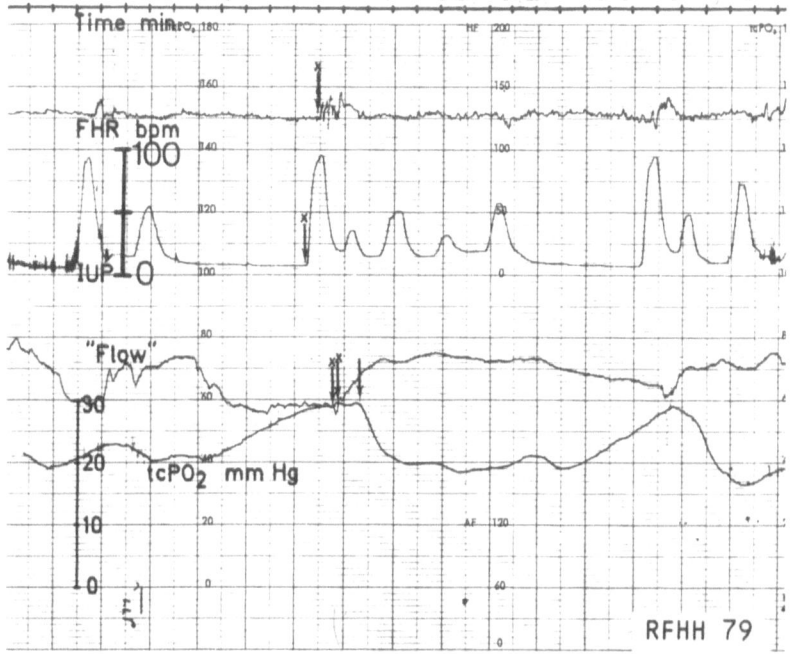

Figure 2 Same arrows as in Figure 1. When several contractions appear clustered without relaxation in between, fetal tcP_{O_2} falls markedly but recovers in the interval, provided this is long enough (data from ref. 2)

from a mean of 135 bpm to 111 bpm 3–4 hours after birth. At about 4 days after birth heart rate again increased. There was a gradual increase in both long-term and short-term variability during the first week of life. Respiratory rate showed such marked range that the mean value of 40 breaths per minute gives no useful information.

The most important observation studying all the parameters simultaneously was to see how they varied with the activity state of the infants. Thus, although detail of the influence of activity state is best observed under the rigid conditions of Prechtl and others, the influence of activity in the clinical situation itself is not only marked, it dominates the changes seen in the oxygen cardiorespirogram.

In order to obtain an oxygen cardiorespirogram only standard equipment, today available in every neonatal unit, is needed, i.e. a transcutaneous P_{O_2} equipment, beat-to-beat heart rate monitor and a transthoracic impedance monitor. Preferably all signals should be displayed on one single recorder using a standard chart speed of 1 cm/min and standard amplifications of the individual signals.

Several pathological conditions may readily be seen in the oxygen cardiorespirogram. Most important from a practical point of view is probably congenital heart abnormalities. In these patients, who may appear healthy,

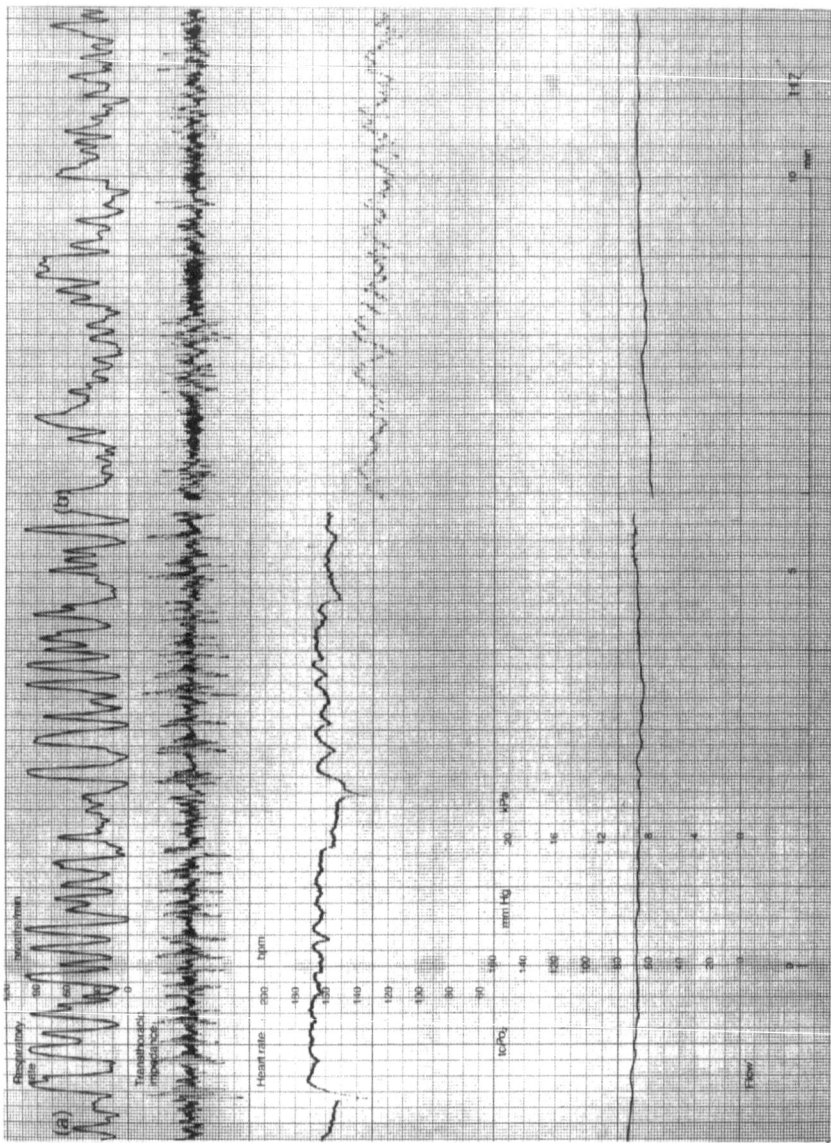

Figure 3 Oxygen cardiorespirogram at (a) 30 minutes and (b) 24 hours after birth. The curves are (from the top): respiratory rate, respiratory excursions, beat-to-beat heart rate, and tcPo$_2$. The infant was awake and unquiet both times. The periodic breathing in (a) had disappeared in (b). Note also the marked fall in heart rate and the, albeit small, reduction in tcPo$_2$ (from Huch, R. Huch, A. and Rooth, G. *An Atlas of Oxygen Cardiorespirograms in Newborn Infants* (Wolfe Medical Publications))

$tcPo_2$ is almost invariably low and only increases little during an oxygen test.

References

1. Caldeyro-Barcia, R. and Alvarez, H. (1952). Abnormal uterine action in labor. XIII British Congress of Obstetrics and Gynaecology. *Obstet. Gynecol.*, **59**, 646–56
2. Rooth, G., Fall, O., Huch, A. and Huch, R. (1979). Integrated interpretation of fetal heart rate, intrauterine pressure and fetal transcutaneous Po_2. *Gynecol. Obstet. Invest.*, **10**, 265–80
3. Huch, R., Huch, A. and Rooth, G. (1981). Monitoring fetal oxygen tension: In Barson, A. J. (ed.) *Laboratory Investigation of Fetal Disease*, pp. 17–50. (Bristol: John Wright & Sons)
4. Huch, R., Huch, A. and Rooth, G. (1983). *An Atlas of Oxygen Cardiorespirograms in Newborn Infants*. (London: Wolfe Medical Publications)

References

10

The value and interpretation of fetal heart rate patterns

H. P. van Geijn

INTRODUCTION

In the development of a new test for use in clinical practice, Grant[1] distinguishes the following phases: technical improvements, definition of abnormal test results (validity), choice of appropriate clinical applications (efficacy) and appropriate management policy (effectiveness). In this regard the current status of electronic fetal heart rate monitoring (EFM) can be summarized as:

1. availability of proper techniques resulting in accurate and repeatable heart beat frequencies;

2. cardiotocography can potentially prevent adverse outcome, certainly if combined with additional monitoring techniques such as fetal microblood sampling;

3. a good negative but poor positive predictive outcome, i.e. a normal test is a good indicator of fetal well-being but an abnormal test is a poor predictor of presence of fetal hypoxia/distress;

4. a low interobserver agreement in reading and interpretation of cardiotocographic tracings and

5. an effectiveness that improves with increasing risk factors.

VALUE OF ELECTRONIC FETAL HEART RATE MONITORING

In this section some aspects in the evaluation of fetal heart rate monitoring will be discussed in more detail.

Interobserver variability in reading of cardiotocograms

In a recent study[2], performed within the framework of the European Community Project 'Perinatal Monitoring', experts from nine EC countries were asked to describe two fetal heart rate tracings in a very simple way: (a) indicate a segment with a single feature, (b) indicate start and end of this feature and (c) define feature as baseline, acceleration, deceleration or other. The agreement among the experts on the classification and start and end of a segment was as low as 48 and 57% in the initial trial. This figure improved to 64 and 69% after the experts had been allowed to adapt themselves to the majority coding. The interobserver agreement in reading of fetal heart rate tracings has also been studied by Trimbos and Keirse[3], Di Renzo and Galli[4] and Lotgering and co-workers[5]. Whichever evaluation parameter was used, either a CTG-scoring system or visual assessment, interobserver agreement never exceeded 64%.

Validity of cardiotocography

The diagnosis of fetal distress by means of EFM and/or determination of fetal pH was recently studied in Oxford[6] and Nijmegen[7]. Both groups compared operative deliveries for fetal distress with the condition of the newborn infant at birth. Neonatal acidosis was defined as umbilical artery $pH < 7.12$ and $BE < -12$[6] respectively $pH\ 7.16$ and $BE < -11.3$[7]. In both the Oxford and the Nijmegen studies the correct identification of those having the abnormal condition, i.e. fetal distress, was disappointing (sensitivity 12 respectively 19%, positive predictive value 12 and 28%); while the identification of the labours without fetal distress gave far better results (sensitivity 92 respectively 96%, negative predictive value 91% and 93%). These figures depend on the cut-off values for pH and base excess to define neonatal acidity. Another bias is caused by obstetric interventions performed following the diagnosis of fetal distress.

Risk categories and effectiveness of cardiotocography

Neutra and co-workers[8] studied cardiotocography in comparison to intermittent auscultation for various risk categories. They calculated neonatal death rates for the lowest, low, medium, high and highest risk categories. A beneficial effect from electronic fetal monitoring was apparent in the highest and high risk categories – neonatal death rates 304 and 81 per thousand in the unmonitored groups, versus 195 and 40 in the monitored groups – but could not be demonstrated in the lowest risk category: 0.5 versus 1.1 neonatal deaths per thousand.

INTERPRETATION OF FETAL HEART RATE PATTERNS

One of the reasons why the current status of fetal heart rate monitoring does not fulfil the expectations imposed at its introduction, may be the fact that many factors influence the firing frequency of the sinoatrial node and so complicate the reading and interpretation of fetal heart rate patterns. Among the factors influencing fetal heart rate and variability[9] are maternal medication, fever, infection, hyperthyroidism, body position, convulsions and shock, and fetal age, circadian rhythms, behavioural states, congenital anomalies, cardiac innervation, brain damage and hypoxia. This chapter will focus on the relationship between fetal heart rate and maternal use of drugs, fetal age, behavioural states, congenital anomalies and hypoxia.

Table 1 Drugs affecting fetal heart rate variability

Decrease		Increase
Alphaprodrine	(Nisentil)	Ephedrine
Atropine		Magnesium sulphate
Diazepam	(Valium)	Physostigmine (Antilirium)
Hydroxyzine	(Atarax)	Phentolamine (Regitine)
Meperidine	(Demerol)	
Mephobarbital	(Mebaral)	
Morphine		
Phenobarbital	(Luminal)	
Promethazine	(Phenergan)	
Propiomazine		
Propanolol	(Inderal)	
Scopolamine		
Late response to paracervical blockade		Initial response to paracervical blockade

From: van Geijn, H. P. (1984). In Finster, M. and Eskes, T. K. A. B. (eds.). *Pregnancy and Drugs* (In press)

Maternal use of drugs

Drugs with a known influence on fetal heart rate variability are summarized in Table 1. Among these, the influence of maternal diazepam medication has been studied by us in more detail. Diazepam is a lipid-soluble drug with a small molecular weight that crosses the placenta rapidly. In the fetus, as in the mother, it is distributed with a preference for certain tissues, i.e. body fat, central nervous system and gastrointestinal tract. Particularly following long-lasting administration, the tissues act as a reservoir from which diazepam and its equally active metabolites are slowly released[9]. Within a few minutes following intravenous administration to the mother, both long-term and short-term (beat-to-beat) variability of fetal heart rate decrease[10]. After a single dose of 10 mg i.v. this effect lasts for about 60 minutes. After oral use of diazepam at the end of pregnancy (e.g. 3 times daily 5 mg) the effect on fetal heart rate variability during labour is even more profound and a decrease in beat-to-beat variability is observed in the newborn infant during the first 2–3 days following birth[10].

Fetal age

With increasing fetal age the following changes have been described in the

fetal heart rate[11-13]. Baseline heart rate decreases; the incidence of decelerations decreases; the incidence, duration and amplitude of accelerations
increase and there is an increase in beat-to-beat and long-term variability of
heart rate.

Fetal behavioural states

In the newborn infant, behavioural states are recognized on the basis of
observable criteria[14]: breathing movements, body movements, open/closed
eyes and vocalization. The newborn infant is 95% of the time asleep and states
1 (quiet, NREM sleep) and 2 (active, REM sleep) alternate in a cyclic fashion.
An episode of quiet sleep does not last more than 40 minutes in the healthy
newborn infant.

Table 2 Criteria for fetal behavioural states

	Eye movements	*Body movements*
1F (quiet sleep)	Absent	Occasional
2F (active sleep)	Present	Periodic
3F (quiet awake)	Present	Absent
4F (awake)	Present	Continuous

Nijhuis and co-workers[15] have demonstrated the presence of behavioural
states in the near-term fetus similar to those observed in the newborn infant.
In recent years we studied heart rate and body movements during these behavioural states in the near-term fetus[16-18]. Recordings were continuous for 2
hours. Fetal movements were identified by two observers each handling an
ultrasound transducer, one directed to the fetal head, the other to the fetal
trunk. Movements were recorded with coded event-markers, while visibility
of fetal orbit and trunk were indicated with a foot-pedal. Fetal behavioural
states were defined applying the criteria described in Table 2. The fetus, like
the newborn infant, spends 95% of the time either in state 1F (quiet sleep;
30%) or 2F (active sleep; 65%). Episodes of these sleep states alternate with a
duration for 1F of 21 ± 6 minutes and 2F of 49 ± 22 minutes. State 1F (quiet
sleep) is characterized by a relatively stable baseline, presence of beat-to-beat
variability and only occasionally short-lasting increases in heart rate during
quick fetal movements (startles) (see Figure 1). During state 2F (active sleep),
the fetus has a baseline heart rate slightly higher than during 1F, accelerations
occur periodically with fetal body movements and beat-to-beat variability between these accelerations is more pronounced than in 1F (see Figure 2).
Figure 3 shows a transition from a state 1F (quiet sleep) to a state 2F (active
sleep). These patterns in heart rate and heart rate variability concomitant with
alternating fetal behavioural states have also been observed during active
labour[17].

Fetal congenital anomalies

Navot and co-workers[19] studied the antenatal fetal heart rate in 20 fetuses with

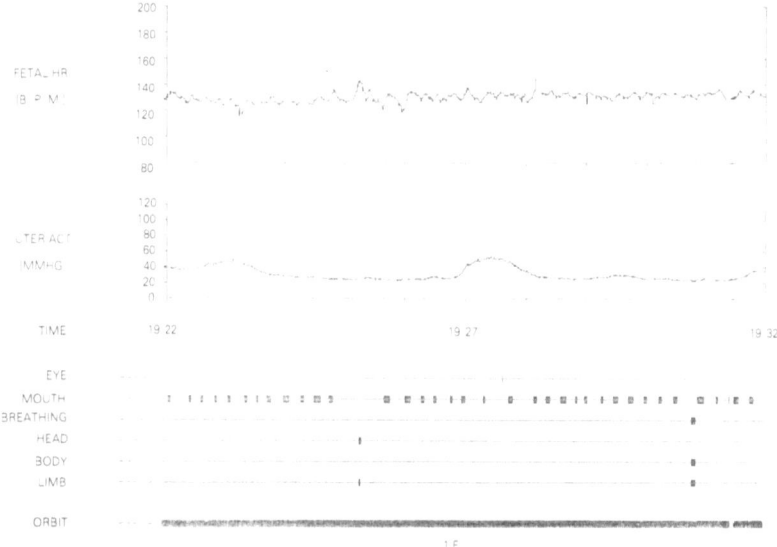

Figure 1 A recording during behavioural state 1F (quiet sleep). Horizontal axis: time axis in minutes. Vertical axis: fetal heart rate, maternal uterine activity; observed fetal eye, mouth, breathing, head, body and limb movements and visibility of a fetal orbit

major congenital malformations, while 40 normal fetuses served as matched controls. Loss of long-term variability appeared in 55% of the malformed fetuses versus 3% in the controls, decelerations in 65% (versus 5%), a non-reactive fetal heart rate pattern in 75% (versus 8%). Normal heart rate variability was present in only 20% of the malformed fetuses in comparison to 93% in the controls. Powell Phillips and Towell[20] found, in the presence of major congenital malformations, an abnormal heart rate recording in 51% and a further 24% had a suspicious recording. Before acting on such an abnormal heart rate, systematic real-time echoscopic examination of the fetal organs/tissues, amount of amniotic fluid, etc. is recommended when a pregnancy is suspect for fetal congenital anomalies, e.g. early intrauterine growth retardation, polyhydramnios[21].

Fetal hypoxia

The most ominous fetal heart rate pattern is characterized by absence of accelerations, decreased long-term and short-term variability and/or late decelerations, frequently no more than a few heart beats[22]. If this terminal heart rate pattern is correlated to fetal outcome (neonatal acidosis), a high positive predictive value will be found. Earlier signs of fetal compromise are a transient increase in fetal heart rate variability[23] and the pure and atypical variable decelerations[24]. Krebs and co-workers[24] found a significantly lower pH when variable decelerations had one or more of the following features: loss of initial

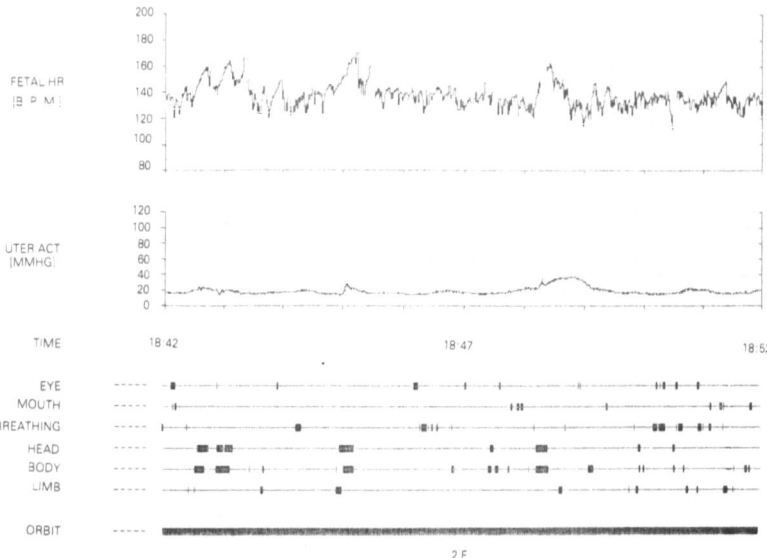

Figure 2 A recording during state 2F (active sleep). For explanation of horizontal and vertical axes, see Figure 1

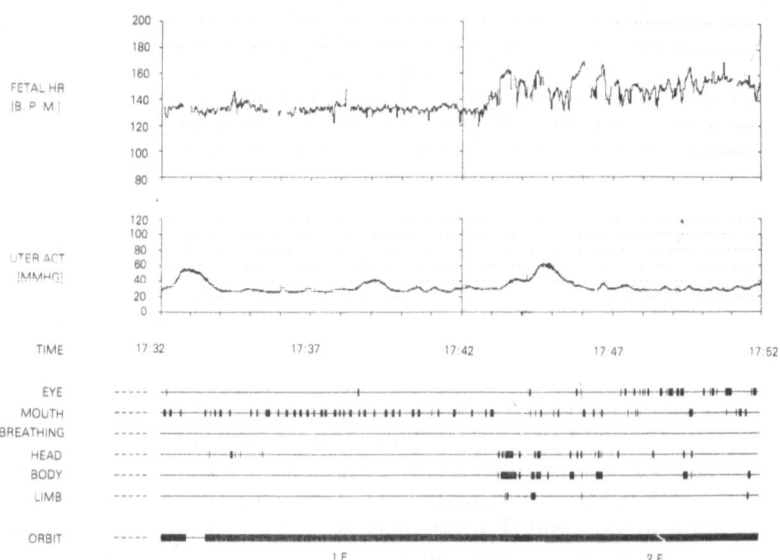

Figure 3 A transition from a state 1F (quiet sleep) to 2F (active sleep) at 17.43 hours. For explanation of horizontal and vertical axis, see Figure 1

acceleration, slow return to baseline fetal heart rate, loss of secondary acceleration, prolonged secondary acceleration, biphasic deceleration, loss of variability during deceleration and continuation of the baseline at a lower level.

COMMENTS

The current rather disappointing validity, efficacy and effectiveness of fetal heart rate monitoring can partially be attributed to problems in the interpretation of heart rate patterns caused by the many factors influencing fetal heart rate and variability. A normal heart rate pattern reliably predicts absence of fetal hypoxia, but cardiotocography is of limited value in the prediction of presence of fetal hypoxia. The result is a high false-positive rate of abnormal tracings. So, there is a need for a better (patho-)physiological background of fetal heart rate and variability and for additional, preferably non-invasive, monitoring techniques.

In the healthy near-term fetus the antepartum heart rate, and in many instances also the heart rate during the first stage of labour, reflects primarily the continuously changing fetal behavioural states, in particular the quiet and active sleep states. The use of such names as non-stress test, extended non-stress test, passive test, arousal test and fetal acceleration test, has the danger that understanding of the basic physiological phenomena remains hidden, while nothing is really being tested. Furthermore, CTG-scoring systems are useful to teach how to look at fetal heart rate tracings, but are of limited value for the recognition of fetal hypoxia, since they do not consider such factors as maternal use of drugs, fetal age, fetal behavioural states, presence of fetal anomalies, etc.

Continuous carbon dioxide monitoring, determination of fetal blood velocity wave forms and in a lesser degree nuclear magnetic resonance are among the techniques identified to be promising for future wide-scale application in perinatal medicine[25]. We must, however, do our best to avoid the problems which have arisen with electronic fetal heart rate monitoring. Prospective studies need to be carried out under well-defined conditions, so that a new technique can be properly assessed before general implementation.

References

1. Grant, A. (1984). Principles for clinical evaluation of new methods for perinatal monitoring. *J. Perinat. Med.*, **12**, 227–31
2. Jongsma, H. W., Rooyakkers, J. C. and Martin, C. B. (1983). Summary of the results of the first perinatal monitoring trial on the visual description system of the cardiotocogram. In van Geijn, H. P. (ed.) *Perinatal Monitoring, 2nd progress report*. Commission of the European Communities, Medical and Public Health Research
3. Trimbos, J. B. and Keirse, M. J. N. C. (1978). Observer variability in assessment of antepartum cardiotocograms *Br. J. Obstet. Gynaecol.*, **85**, 900–6
4. Di Renzo, G. C. and Galli, P. A. (1984). Score and test in perinatal monitoring. Presented at *Controversies in Perinatal Medicine*, 31 May–2 June, Assisi, Italy
5. Lotgering, F. K., Wallenburg, H. C. S. and Schouten, H. J. A. (1982). Interobserver and intraobserver variation in the assessment of antepartum cardiotocograms. *Am. J. Obstet. Gynecol.*, **144**, 701–5

6. Sykes, G. S., Molloy, P. M., Johnson, P., Stirrat, G. M. and Turnbull, A. C. (1983). Fetal distress and the condition of newborn infants. *Br. Med. J.*, **287**, 943–5

7. Eskes, T. K. A. B. (1984). Natural childbirth and operative obstetrics. Presented at *Controversies in Perinatal Medicine*, 31 May–2 June, Assisi, Italy

8. Neutra, R. R., Fienberg, S. E. and Greenland, S. (1978). Effect of fetal monitoring on neonatal death rates. *N. Engl. J. Med.*, **299**, 324–6

9. Van Geijn, H. P. (1980). Studies on fetal and neonatal baseline heart rate variability. *Thesis*, Nijmegen

10. Van Geijn, H. P., Jongsma, H. W., Doesburg, W. H., Lemmens, W. A. J. G., de Haan, J. and Eskes, T. K. A. B. (1980). The effect of diazepam administration during pregnancy or labour on the heart rate variability of the newborn infant. *Eur. J. Obstet. Gynecol.*, **10**, 187–201

11. Wheeler, T. and Murrills, A. (1978). Patterns of fetal heart rate during normal pregnancy. *Br. J. Obstet. Gynaecol.*, **85**, 18–27

12. Visser, G. H. A., Dawes, G. S. and Redman, C. W. G. (1981). Numerical analysis of the normal human antenatal fetal heart rate. *Br. J. Obstet. Gynaecol.*, **88**, 792–802

13. Natale, R., Nasello, C. and Turlink, R. (1984). The relationship between movements and accelerations in fetal heart rate at twenty-four to thirty-two weeks gestation. *Am. J. Obstet. Gynecol.*, **148**, 591–5

14. Prechtl, H. F. R. (1974). The behavioural states of the newborn infant (a review). *Brain Res.* **76**, 185–210

15. Nijhuis, J. G., Prechtl, H. F. R., Martin, C. B. and Bots, R. S. G. M. (1982). Are there behavioural states in the human fetus. *Early Human Dev.* **6**, 177–95

16. Van Geijn, H. P., Griffin, R. L. A., Caron, F. J. M., Sollie, J. E. and Arts, N. F. Th. (1983). Heart rate and behavioral states in the near term fetus. In *Abstracts Xth Conference on Fetal Breathing and Other Fetal Measurements*, Malmö, 6–8 June, p. 55

17. Griffin, R. L., Caron, F. J. M. and van Geijn, H. P. (1984). Behavioural states in the human fetus during labour. *Abstracts XIth Annual Conference of the Society for the Study of Fetal Physiology*, Oxford, 21–22 July, C 16. *Am. J. Obstet. Gynecol.*, (In press)

18. Van Woerden, E. E., van Geijn, H. P., Caron, F. J. M., Griffin, R. L. and Arts, N. F. Th. (1984). Distribution of movements within behavioral states of the human fetus. *Abstracts IXth European Congress of Perinatal Medicine*, Dublin, 2–5 September, p. 52

19. Navot, D., Mor-Yosef, S., Granat, M. and Sadovsky, E. (1984). Antepartum fetal heart rate patterns associated with major congenital anomalies. *Obstet. Gynecol.*, **63**, 414–17

20. Powell Phillips, W. D. and Towell, M. E. (1980). Abnormal fetal heart rate associated with congenital abnormalities. *Br. J. Obstet. Gynaecol.*, **87**, 270–74

21. Sollie, J. E., van Geijn, H. P., Exalto, N. and Arts, N. F. Th. (1984). Ultrasound scanning for fetal congenital abnormalities in obstetric practice. *Abstracts IXth European Congress of Perinatal Medicine*, Dublin, 2–5 September, p. 63

22. Tushuizen, P. B. Th., Stoot, J. E. G. M. and Ubachs, J. M. H. (1974). Fetal heart rate monitoring of the dying fetus. *Am. J. Obstet. Gynecol.*, **120**, 922–31

23. Martin, C. B. (1982). Physiology and clinical use of fetal heart rate variability. *Clin. Perinatol.*, **9**, 339–52

24. Krebs, H. B., Petres, R. E. and Dunn, L. J. (1983). Intrapartum fetal heart rate monitoring. Atypical variable decelerations. *Am. J. Obstet. Gynecol.*, **145**, 297–305

25. Project on Perinatal Monitoring (1984). Symposium on New Methods in Perinatology (Falck Larsen, J., ed.). *J. Perinat. Med.*, **12**, 221–84

11
Antenatal assessment of fetal health using dynamic real-time ultrasound

P. F. Chamberlain

INTRODUCTION

Methods used for the antenatal assessment of fetal health have undergone major changes in recent years. The monitoring of fetal biophysical variables, such as fetal heart rate (FHR) and fetal movements (FM) has to a large extent replaced assays of pregnancy hormones (urinary oestrogens) for this purpose. The introduction of dynamic real-time ultrasound into obstetrics offers a further potential tool for the antenatal assessment of fetal condition. The use of ultrasound to this end is greatly aided by recent improvements in ultrasound technology, especially picture resolution and instrument portability.

Before any method of antepartum fetal monitoring is applied, consideration of those factors associated with altered perinatal outcome is warranted. Based upon a review of the patterns of perinatal mortality as we see them in the Province of Manitoba, we have adopted a real-time ultrasound-based method of antenatal fetal health assessment as we feel it is best suited to detect some of those conditions likely to be associated with altered perinatal outcome.

It is the purpose of this paper to review the patterns of altered perinatal outcome as seen in the Province of Manitoba and to outline why we feel a real-time ultrasound-based system of fetal monitoring best addresses the antenatal detection of some of these. Following this, the method of antenatal fetal assessment using dynamic real-time ultrasound that we use will be described, and the results we have recorded when this method is applied to a large high-risk obstetric population will be reported.

BACKGROUND

In 1982 the total perinatal mortality in the Province of Manitoba was 12.4/1000. When divided into its component parts, the stillbirth and neonatal death rates were almost identical being 6.3/1000 and 6.1/1000 respectively[1]. When

79

the aetiology of these perinatal deaths was reviewed, three major sub-categories were noted to account for 74% of the total perinatal mortality. These were hypoxia (30%), congenital anomalies (24%) and respiratory complications (20%). The remaining 26% of the total perinatal mortality was attributed to a variety of causes, including unclassified (12%), placental (7%) and other causes (7%).

More detailed review of these three major subcategories of perinatal deaths showed the following:

1. In the hypoxia subcategory, 68% of these deaths occurred in fetuses with a birth weight of ≥ 1000 g and 52% in fetuses with a birth weight of ≥ 1500 g. The vast majority of these hypoxic perinatal deaths occurred in the form of antepartum stillbirths.

2. In the major congenital anomaly subcategory, structural congenital defects, either alone or in combination with other structural or chromosomal abnormalities, accounted for 82% of these deaths. Of these, multiple defects (38%), isolated cardiac (26%), CNS (15%) or renal (3%) defects were the most common. These deaths were evenly divided into antepartum stillbirths and neonatal deaths.

3. In the respiratory-related death subcategory, hyaline membrane disease accounted for 89% of the deaths. Meconium aspiration syndrome was responsible for the remaining 11%.

From these data it is evident that perinatal mortality is multifactorial, with frequently more than one process being operant, and that the ideal method of fetal assessment would accurately identify the hypoxic fetus, the fetus with a major structural congenital defect and the fetus destined to develop respiratory-related complications in the neonatal period.

With diagnostic real-time ultrasound it is possible to assess a variety of parameters of fetal condition. These include biophysical variables such as fetal breathing movements (FBM): FM; and fetal tone (FT); amniotic fluid volume (AFV) and fetal structure and growth.

These parameters may be divided into acute, subacute and chronic indices of fetal health based upon the rapidity with which alteration in their behaviour occurs in response to a fetal insult. For example, the presence of normal FBM, FM, and FT may be interpreted as indicative of normal fetal oxygenation and integrated fetal CNS function at the time of examination. Abrupt cessation of these parameters in response to fetal hypoxia has been demonstrated in the chronic animal preparation[3]. Similarly, the presence of normal fetal growth is indicative of normal antecedent fetal development on a more long-term scale. AFV would appear to have a time scale intermediary between the above two, being more susceptible to change than fetal growth but less so than the acute variables such as FBM, FM, and FT.

The concept of assessment of multiple variables to arrive at a decision on fetal condition is not new, but simply represents the application of principles of extrauterine physical diagnosis to the fetus *in utero*. This is a major advantage of real-time ultrasound and forms the basis of our hypothesis that simultaneous assessment of multiple parameters of fetal condition allows for a more accurate determination of fetal health or compromise than single variable assessment alone.

METHOD

When performing our examination we divide it into two parts:

1. Assessment of acute and subacute parameters of fetal condition by means of the biophysical profile score (BPS) in order to assess the risk of fetal hypoxia or asphyxia.
2. Assessment of fetal structure and the pattern of fetal growth as a more long-term index of preceding fetal development.

Criteria for a normal BPS, as originally described by Manning, Platt and Sipos, are shown in Table 1[4].

Table 1 Biophysical profile scoring: technique and interpretation[4]

Biophysical variable	Normal (score = 2)	Abnormal (score = 0)
1 Fetal breathing movements	At least one episode of FBM of at least 30 seconds duration in 30 minutes observation	Absent FBM or no episode of ≥30 seconds in 30 minutes
2 Gross body movement	At least three discrete body/limb movements in 30 minutes (episodes of active continuous movement considered as a single movement)	Two or fewer episodes of body/limb movements in 30 minutes
3 Fetal tone	At least one episode of active extension with return to flexion of fetal limb(s) or trunk; Opening and closing of hand considered normal tone	Either slow extension with return to partial flexion or movement of limb in full extension or absent fetal movement
4 Reactive FHR	At least two episodes of FHR acceleration of ≥15 BPM and of at least 15 seconds duration associated with fetal movement in 30 minutes	Less than two episodes of acceleration of FHR or acceleration of <15 bpm in 30 minutes
5 Qualitative AFV	At least one pocket of AF that measures at least 1 cm in two perpendicular planes	Either no AF pockets or a pocket <1 cm in two perpendicular planes

FBM, Fetal breathing movement; FHR, fetal heart rate; AFV, amniotic fluid volume; AF, amniotic fluid

In the 30-minute observation period at least one episode of FBM ≥ 30 seconds duration, three discrete body/limb movements, one episode of limb/trunk extension with return to flexion and one pocket of AFV ≥ 1 cm in two perpendicular planes are required.

These sonographic findings, combined with a reactive NST, constitute a normal BPS. Each parameter is arbitrarily assigned a score of 2 if normal and 0 if abnormal. A completely normal examination thus results in a score of 10, and if completely abnormal in a score of 0.

Management is based upon the BPS as shown in Table 2[5].

Table 2 Biophysical profile scoring: management protocol[5]

Score	Interpretation	Management
10	Normal infant, low risk for chronic asphyxia	Repeat testing at weekly intervals; repeat twice weekly in diabetics and patient ≥42 weeks gestation
8	Normal infant, low risk for chronic asphyxia	Repeat testing at weekly intervals; repeat testing twice weekly in diabetics and patients ≥42 weeks; oligohydramnios an indication for delivery
6	Suspect chronic asphyxia	Repeat testing in 4–6 hours; deliver if oligohydramnios present
4	Suspect chronic asphyxia	If ≥36 weeks and favourable then deliver; if <36 weeks and L/S <2.0 repeat test in 24 hours; if repeat score ≤4 deliver
0–2	Strong suspicion of chronic asphyxia	Extend testing time to 120 minutes; if persistent score ≤4, deliver, regardless of gestational age

L/S, amniotic fluid lecithin : sphingomyelin

The association between the BPS and perinatal mortality has been reported by us and other investigators[4,6].

Assessment of fetal growth is performed using standard curves for head circumference (HC), abdominal circumference (AC), HC:AC ratio and fetal weight for gestational age[7-9]. Failure of growth in these parameters or in estimated fetal weight as derived from AC documented on successive examinations 2–3 weeks apart is considered an indication for delivery regardless of the BPS score.

Screening for structural congenital defects is performed by a detailed ultrasound examination of the fetus.

RESULTS

Biophysical profile score-based fetal assessment has been the primary method of fetal health assessment employed in the University of Manitoba since the Fall of 1979. As of January 1984, 12 620 high-risk obstetric patients referred by both obstetricians and family physicians for the purposes of antenatal fetal health assessment have been seen[10].

The mean gestational age of this study population was 34.3 weeks (range: 26–42+ weeks). The most frequent referral indications were suspect growth retardation (20.8%), hypertension (17.5%) and suspect post-dates pregnancy (11.6%), accounting for 49.9% of the total study population.

The total perinatal mortality (PNM) was 7.37/1000 and when corrected for major congenital anomalies and severe Rh disease was 1.90/1000.

The corrected stillbirth rate and corrected neonatal death rate was 1.18/1000 and 0.72/1000 respectively. Congenital anomaly (66.6%) and severe Rh disease (7.7%) accounted for 74.3% of the total perinatal mortality. The low corrected neonatal death rate (0.72/1000) is most probably a function of the gestational age of the study population (mean: 34.3 weeks).

The relationship between a falling BPS and a rising PNM was again noted. Corrected PNM with a normal BPS was 0.652/1000 as compared to 187/1000 with a BPS of 0. In total, 26 257 tests were performed on the 12 620 patients (mean: 2.1). When the test score distribution was examined 25 606 (97.5%) were normal while only 651 (2.5%) were either equivocal or abnormal. This test score distribution differs significantly from that seen with either the NST (89% normal) or the CST (84.6% normal)[11].

This high incidence of normal examinations with its low PNM and the strong relationship between a falling BPS and rising PNM makes us feel that this method of fetal assessment accurately differentiates the healthy from sick fetus. Repeat examinations, frequently required with antepartum FHR monitoring, are seldom needed. More importantly, the false-negative test rate is low (0.634/1000), comparable to that reported with the CST (0.4/1000) and considerably lower than that of the NST (3.2/1000)[12].

Ninety per cent of the major structural congenital anomalies that occurred in this study population were identified in the antepartum period.

CONCLUSIONS

A method of antepartum fetal well-being assessment using real-time ultrasound directed towards the antenatal detection of the hypoxic fetus and the fetus with a major structural congenital defect has been described. Hypoxia and congenital anomalies are major contributors to total perinatal mortality and their antenatal detection is important if perinatal mortality is to be reduced.

References

1. Perinatal and Maternal Welfare Committee; The College of Physicians and Surgeons of Manitoba, 1982
2. Perinatal and Maternal Welfare Committee, The College of Physicians and Surgeons of Manitoba, 1981
3. Dawes, G. S., Fox, H. E., Leduc, B. M., Liggins, G. C. and Richards, R. T. (1970). Respiratory movements and paradoxical sleep in the fetal lamb. *J. Physiol.*, **210**, 47P
4. Manning, F. A., Platt, L. D. and Sipos, L. (1980). Antenatal fetal evaluation: development of a fetal biophysical profile score. *Am. J. Obstet. Gynecol.*, **136**, 787
5. Manning, F. A., Morrison, I., Lange, I. R., Harman, C. and Chamberlain, P. F. (1984). Fetal biophysical profile scoring. The concept, method and results. *Contemp. Obstet. Gynecol.* **64**, 326
6. Vintzileos, A. M., Campbell, W. A., Ingardia, C. J. and Nochimson, D. J. (1983). Score and its predictive value. *Obstet. Gynecol*, **62**, 271

7. Campbell, S. and Thomas, A. (1977). Ultrasound measurement of the fetal head to abdomen circumference ratio in the assessment of growth retardation. *Br. J. Obstet Gynaecol.*, **84**, 165

8. Campbell, S. and Wilkin, D. (1975). Ultrasonic measurement of the fetal abdominal circumference in the estimation of fetal weight. *Br. J. Obstet. Gynaecol.*, **82**, 689

9. Usher, R. and McLean, F. (1969). Intrauterine growth for live-born Caucasian infants at sea-level: standards obtained from measurements in seven dimensions of infants born between 25 and 44 weeks of gestation. *J. Paediatr.*, **74**(6), 901

10. Manning, F. A., Morrisson, I., Lange, I. R., Harman, C. and Chamberlain, P. F. (1985). Fetal assessment based upon fetal biophysical profile scoring: experience with 12,620 referred high-risk pregnancies. I. Perinatal mortality by incidence. *Am. J. Obstet. Gynecol.*, **151**, 343

11. Schifrin, B. S., Foye, G. Amato, J. *et al.* (1979). Routine fetal heart rate monitoring in the antepartum period. *Obstet. Gynecol.*, **54**, 21

12. Freeman, R. E., Anderson, G. and Dorchester, W. (1982). A prospective multi-institutional trial of antepartum fetal heart rate monitoring. 1. Review of perinatal mortality and morbidity according to AFHR test results. *Am. J. Obstet. Gynecol.*, **143**, 771

12

Assessment of adaptation to extrauterine life in clinics without integrated neonatology

G. Duc

This chapter presents a clinical protocol which has been used to assess neonatal adaptation to extrauterine life in the following perinatal situation: delivery of a baby presenting with subtle signs of adaptation difficulty, in a hospital without a neonatal intensive care unit.

The question is: can the baby stay with the mother, or does he have to be transferred to a neonatal intensive care unit? This type of question is asked in every country in the world independently of the organization of perinatal care. The answer is particularly important in countries without a centralized perinatal care system, where most of the deliveries occur in hospitals without a neonatal care unit.

Switzerland, my country, is such an example, with 73 000 births a year, 99% of which are delivered in hospital. These deliveries are widely distributed. Twelve hospitals deliver less than 50 babies a year. This represents 0.5% of the total. One hundred and thirty five hospitals have less than 500 babies a year and represent almost half the total deliveries in the country. We have 10 obstetric clinics with a full-time neonatal service covering 20% of the total deliveries.

Moreover, the organization of perinatal care is not homogeneous. Switzerland is made up of 26 cantons, each one with its own perinatal care system. The highest number of deliveries per canton occurs in Zürich with about 12 000/ year; the lowest in Appenzell with 200/year. Transferring high-risk pregnancies to obstetric clinics with an integrated neonatal department is complicated by differences in hospitalization costs between cantons and by reimbursement difficulties through health insurances.

Optimal screening methods to detect babies who should be transferred are particularly important in Switzerland's geographical situation (high mountains) where expensive helicopter transport is sometimes required.

Our programme is aimed at clinics without a neonatal unit or neonatologist on duty. Such clinics are usually in close contact with a neonatal intensive care unit where a neonatologist can be reached for consultation at any time by telephone. As such clinics lack medical personnel trained in the use of neonatal monitoring devices, it is evident that the protocol should not require specialized training or sophisticated technology. Moreover, in order to avoid causing anxiety to the mother, the observations should be possible at her bedside.

Consider the following example: baby Fritzli is born in a regional hospital at 35 weeks gestation, with birth weight of 2040 g and an Apgar score of 6 at 1 min and 8 at 5 and 10 min. At 15 min he is tachypnoeic with a respiratory rate of 90/min, discrete grunting and retractions. Apart from these symptoms, Fritzli is pink, does not require oxygen supplementation, is alert and does not show any other pathological findings. The mother's history does not reveal any increased risk of infection. The hospital is located 112 km (= 70 miles) from the neonatal intensive care unit and is separated from it by steep mountains. Fritzlis' delivery in this hospital was fully justified. The obstetrical team (one chief and three residents on training) deliver about 700 babies a year. Ultrasound, cardiotocography and scalp pH sampling are available. Evidently at 15 min of life baby Fritzli cannot be considered as having adapted perfectly to extrauterine life. On the other hand, emergency transportation, possibly requiring the use of a helicopter, is not justified at this point. A period of systematic observation is necessary before a decision can be made.

Fritzli is placed in an incubator at the mother's bedside. The doctor, or the nurse or the midwife who has been involved in the delivery, may be more motivated to take care of the observations and may also help prevent unnecessary anxiety to the mother.

The duration of this observation period should not exceed 2–3 h. If symptoms persist the decision to transfer the infant should be discussed with the ICU neonatologist.

The following data are recorded by the observer. First, general information regarding complications of pregnancy and delivery together with gestational age, birth weight, Apgar score and resuscitation procedures. This basic information should be communicated to the neonatologist. Vital parameters are assessed every 15–20 min and registered in a protocol included in every newborn chart. For example: to evaluate respiratory adaptation the following parameters are observed and registered: respiratory rate, grunting, retractions, nasal flaring, skin colour. An analogous scheme is used to evaluate the circulatory system: heart rate, heart murmur, capillary filling, temperature and colour of the extremities.

A simple test to judge capillary filling has been shown to be particularly sensitive in detecting peripheral circulatory disturbances associated with the early onset of bacterial infection. With gentle thumb pressure a region of the baby's leg is blanched. The duration of capillary filling is then evaluated and should not be longer than 4–6 s. At a time when some obstetricians turn off the light in the delivery room, it is important to remember that the detection of cyanosis and peripheral circulatory disturbances necessitate optimal and constant illumination of the room where the observation has to be made.

Regarding neurological status, we limit our observations to detecting changes in muscle tone and absence, or abnormality of grasping and Moro reflexes. Rectal and incubator temperatures are registered at regular intervals.

We advise our obstetric colleagues to limit their laboratory investigations to capillary pH, if possible, together with pCO_2 and BE, as well as capillary haematocrit and glucose determinations. A pH below 7.25, a haematocrit below 40% or above 70% and glucose levels below 2 mmol/l are indications for consultation with the ICU.

The data are systematically collected in a protocol (as represented in Table 1), which is part of the baby's chart. Decision to transfer the baby is taken by the ICU neonatologist together with the obstetrician at the referring clinic. It is easier for the mother to understand this decision when she herself has taken part in observing the child.

In our experience this simple tool has proved useful in avoiding unnecessary transfer and has improved communication between obstetricians, midwives and nurses of referring clinics and the neonatal ICU team. Exchanging infor-

Table 1 Evaluation of neonatal adaptation in delivery room

Postnatal age					
Respiration					
Respiratory rate					
Grunting					
Retractions					
Nasal flaring					
Cyanosis					
Circulation					
Heart rate					
Heart murmur					
Capillary filling					
Cold extremities					
Pale extremities					
Neurological status					
Muscle tone					
Moro reflex					
Grasping					
Thermoregulation					
Rectal temperature					
Laboratory investigations					
Acid–base status					
Haematocrit					
Reflotest					
Incubator temperature					
FiO_2					
Breast feeding					
Bottle feeding					

The clinical parameters are checked every 15–20 min; duration of observation: maximal 3 h

mation, experiences and ideas over the telephone resulted in an integration of different levels of care, where neonatal consultation extended to discussion on prenatal problems and led to increasing early transfer of very high-risk mothers to the perinatal centre.

Bibliography

Ackermann-Liebrich, U., Duc, G., Paccaud, F. and Romanens, M. (1984). Die neonatale Mortalität in der Schweiz. *Schweiz. Aerztezeitung*, **65**, 443–7

Duc. G. and Mieth D. (1978). Versorgung des Neugeborenen im Gebärsaal. In Bachmann, K. D. *et al.* (eds.) *Pädiatrie in Praxis und Klinik*. Bd 1, pp. 163–70. (Stuttgart/New York: Gustav Fischer Verlag; Stuttgart: Georg Thieme Verlag)

Section 4
Asphyxial Brain Damage

Chairman's introduction

G. Duc

The scientific committee of the present meeting has decided to devote this Symposium to brain damage associated with perinatal asphyxia in the term infant.

In past meetings of this society we have concentrated on the cerebral pathology associated with prematurity and have, in a way, neglected the brain of the term infant. New aspects of this pathology are worthwhile discussing.

First, the neonatologist is now armed with new technology such as ultrasound which allows the detection and follow-up of the anatomical alterations of the brain secondary to asphyxial events at the bedside. As these alterations are not homogeneously distributed, it is important that the clinician is well aware of their characteristic localizations. This is going to be Dr J. S. Wigglesworth's subject. Dr Wigglesworth is a perinatal pathologist and particularly an expert in this field. He will summarize for us the anatomopathological findings in the acute phase of asphyxia, as well as the chronic evolution of the brain lesions.

The importance of intrauterine asphyxia as a cause of cerebral disturbances is still difficult to assess qualitatively because we still don't know which biochemical or clinical parameters are to be considered as specific markers of intrauterine events.

As cord blood pH is one of the most widely used parameters to assess intrapartum asphyxia, studies on the association between cord blood pH and neurological outcome are of great interest, particularly for obstetricians. Dr Touwen, developmental neurologist, will present original data on the subject and discuss the methodological aspects of neurological assessment.

As regards treatment of post-asphyxial conditions, control of intracranial pressure and cerebral blood flow represent the most promising new developments. Dr M. Levene, neonatologist, will sum up the state of the art of monitoring these parameters and discuss the available therapeutic interventions.

The last word on perinatologic problems belongs to the follow-up team. Dr Claudine Amiel-Tison, developmental neurologist and neonatologist, is one of the pioneers in this field. Dr Amiel-Tison will discuss the changing patterns of postnatal asphyxial neurological anomalies and stress the importance of the methodology used when results from different sources are compared.

13

Pathophysiological aspects of asphyxial brain damage

J. S. Wigglesworth

A major problem in understanding perinatal brain asphyxial damage is presented by the wide spectrum both of clinical presentation and of pathological findings. In order to consider the pathophysiology of asphyxial brain damage it is necessary to define the range of lesions to be included. The major lesions in this group are set out in Table 1. Massive destructive lesions often occur *in utero* and are otherwise merely extreme examples of the others, so they will not be discussed here. The two major types of damage are those involved under the term 'selective neuronal necrosis' and 'periventricular leukomalacia' and these will form the subject of the present discussion.

SELECTIVE NEURONAL NECROSIS

A wide variety of sites can be affected by selective neuronal necrosis[1]. These include the cerebral cortex (especially hippocampus), diencephalon, basal

Table 1 Major lesions associated with asphyxial brain damage

Massive destructive lesions of prenatal and perinatal period	Hydranencephaly
	Porencephaly
	Multicystic encephalomalacia
Patterns of selective neuronal necrosis	Cortex – white matter – thalamus
	Thalamus – brainstem
Periventricular leukomalacia	
Status marmoratus: associated with selective necrosis	
Parasagittal cerebral injury: mainly in older infants	

ganglia, midbrain, pons, medulla and cerebellum. A problem is presented by
the fact that in any one infant severe damage can occur at some of the sites
while others remain unaffected. A number of different patterns of damage
have been described by neuropathologists but only two major ones will be
mentioned here.

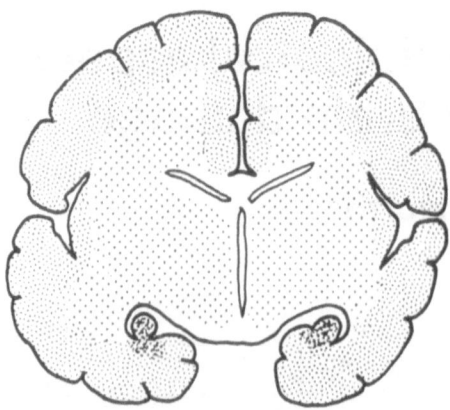

Figure 1   Distribution of asphyxial brain damage affecting cortex, white matter and
thalamus. Density of shading indicates severity of damage

The classic type of asphyxial brain damage occurring in the relatively
mature infant is that which affects the cerebral cortex in association wth cerebral oedema and seizures. The pattern of damage is indicated in Figure 1. The
most severely affected region is the hippocampus and visual cortex, but the
whole cortex may be involved and hypoxic damage usually involves also the
future white matter region. There may be generalized cerebral softening as
well as swelling, and focal infarction is relatively frequent. The latter event is
apparently due to occlusion of individual cerebral arteries following brain
swelling (e.g. occlusion of the posterior cerebral artery by pressure against the
tentorium with resultant occipital infarction). On histological examination the
ischaemic neurones have shrunken acidophilic cytoplasm and pyknotic nuclei.
Involvement of the developing white matter area is indicated by astrocytic
hypertrophy. Extension of neuronal necrosis to the thalamus is a frequent
finding. The other distinct pattern of selective neuronal necrosis is that involving the brainstem and thalamus (Figure 2). Severe damage may occur involving spinal cord, grey matter, olivary nuclei and nuclei in pons, midbrain
(especially inferior colliculi) and up to the thalamus with no significant cortical
involvement. If this form of injury occurs *in utero* there may be severe gliosis
of the areas involved by the time of delivery.

Until recently the cortical–thalamic pattern of selective neuronal necrosis
was the only one known in human infants. Yet early experiments achieved
necrosis in midbrain grey matter in fetal monkeys subjected to asphyxia by delivery within an intact sac[2]. Studies by Myers and associates have succeeded in
causing cerebral oedema and extensive cortical necrosis in experimental

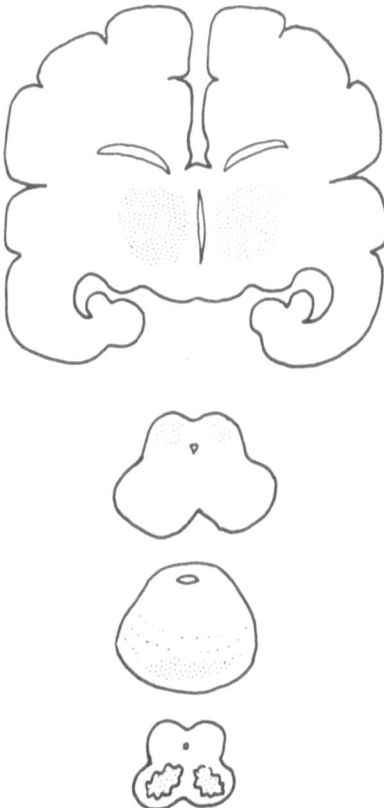

Figure 2 Distribution of asphyxial brain damage affecting brainstem, midbrain and thalamus

fetuses by prolonged severe hypoxia rather than acute total anoxic stress[3]. The importance of local lactic acid build-up in determining neuronal damage in cerebral hypoxia is stressed by Myers[4]. The thalamic and brainstem form of damage is visualized as resulting from an acute anoxic stress such as results from umbilical cord occlusion. The neurones in the affected sites normally receive a good blood supply and have a high metabolic rate, which renders them unduly vulnerable to circulatory arrest. The developing cerebral hypoxia has a number of differing effects on the brain as shown in Figure 3. An immediate effect is to cause a rise of blood pressure and redistribution of organ flows. The hypoxia and hypercarbia interfere with cerebral autoregulation and may result in increase or decrease of regional flow according to the level of the blood pressure. Myers' belief that hypoxia directly causes cerebral oedema by a cytotoxic effect is not universally accepted. Prolonged hypoxia will eventually interfere with myocardial function and cause a fall in BP and fall in cerebral blood flow. Cerebral blood flow studies in monkeys have shown that flow to cortex and white matter falls more than that to the basal ganglia. Increasing local lactic acid will contribute to the development of neuronal necrosis. Cerebral oedema will occur as a result of neuronal necrosis and lead into a vicious cycle of increased brain-swelling, decreased blood flow and increasing tissue necrosis. In practice the two patterns of selective neuronal necrosis are not totally separate as failure of cardiac function may occur at any stage and lead to circulatory arrest and necrosis of grey nuclei.

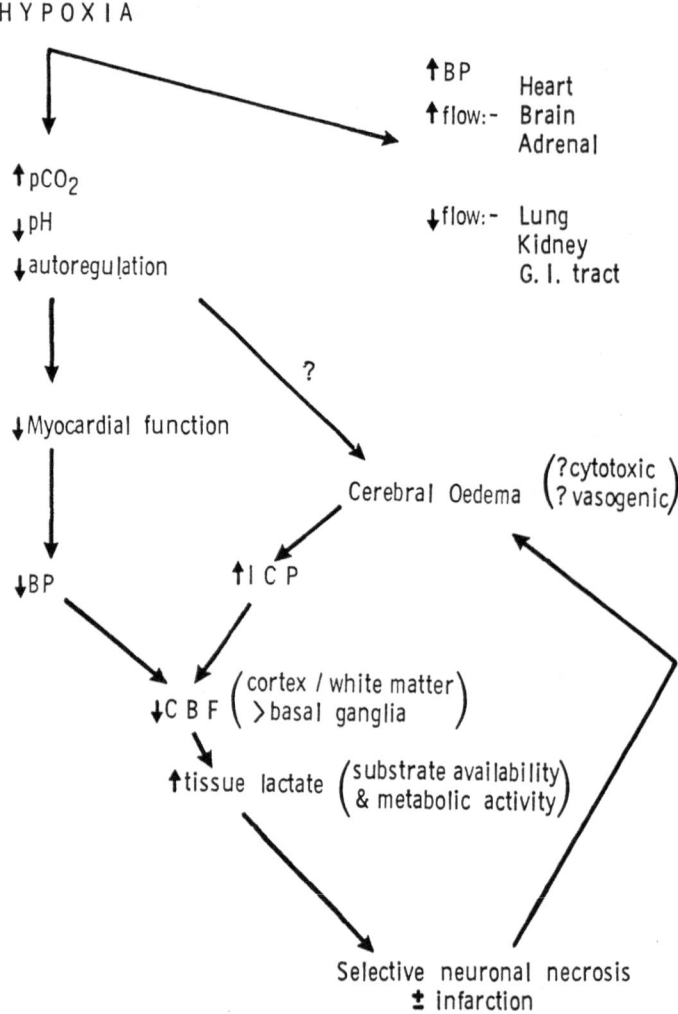

Figure 3 A scheme to illustrate sequence of events in perinatal asphyxia and the development of asphyxial brain damage

PERIVENTRICULAR LEUKOMALACIA

Periventricular leukomalacia (PVL) is the other common pattern of asphyxial brain damage to the perinatal period. Areas involved include the frontoparietal and parieto-occipital white matter (Figure 4). The condition develops most frequently in newborn preterm infants although it sometimes develops *in utero* and is sometimes recognized in the term infant. The early stage involves swelling and disintegration of axis cylinders or larger areas of coagulation necrosis. As the lesion evolves the damaged tissue may become infiltrated with lipid-filled macrophages and larger areas of necrosis may break down to form cystic spaces. The sites where the lesions occur are at the boundary between the anterior and middle, and the middle and posterior, cerebral arteries, and also at the boundary between arterial branches penetrating from the cortex and those supplying the basal ganglia, thalamus and ependyma[5,6]. Thus the lesions can be regarded as occurring at a sort of double boundary zone.

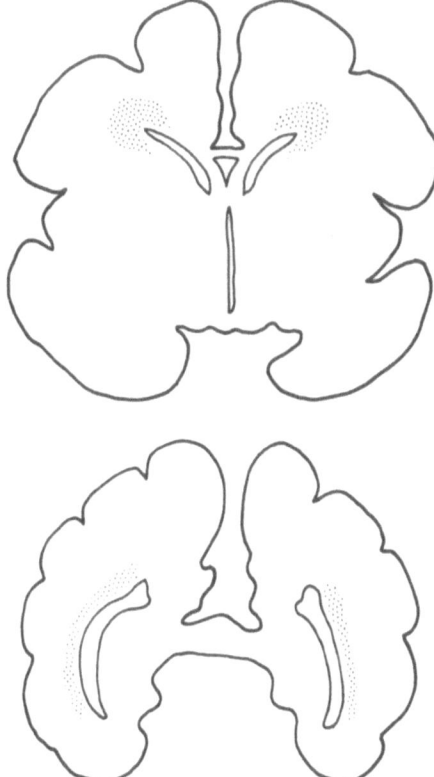

Figure 4   Distribution of damage in periventricular leukomalacia

It has been widely accepted since the studies of De Reuck and colleagues that periventricular leukomalacia is caused by hypotension. There is, however, no clear evidence for this in the human infant, although blood flow studies on newborn puppies provide some support for the concept[7].

If we consider the fetus *in utero* it is apparent that there are several sites at which factors may operate to impair fetal cerebral circulation and oxygenation. Maternal cardiac or respiratory disorders, diabetes, drugs or obstetric complications may influence the efficiency of uteroplacental circulation or placental transfer. Direct interruption of placental function may stem from abruptio placentae, placental infarction or umbilical occlusion. Within the fetus, as in the neonate, the status of cardiac function may be critical in determining whether the brain is damaged by the variety of influences operating at maternal or placental level. A high proportion of infants who die with anoxic–ischaemic brain damage of any type show areas of ischaemic damage within the myocardium irrespective of whether the asphyxia has developed before or after birth.

References

1. Volpe, J. J. (1981). *Neurology of the Newborn*, p. 185. (Philadelphia: W. B. Saunders)
2. Ranck, J. B. and Windle, W. F. (1959). Brain damage in the monkey, *Macaca mulatta*, by asphyxia neonatorum. *Exp. Neurol.*, **1**, 130
3. Myers, R. E. (1977). Experimental models of perinatal brain damage: relevance to human pathology. In Gluck, L. (ed.) *Intrauterine Asphyxia and the Developing Fetal Brain*, pp. 37–97. (Chicago: Year Book Medical Publishers, Inc.)
4. Myers, R. E. (1979). Lactic acid accumulation as cause of brain edema and cerebral necrosis resulting from oxygen deprivation. In Korobkin, R. and Guilleminault, C. (eds.) *Advances in Perinatal Neurology*, pp. 84–114. (New York: Spectrum Publishers)
5. De Reuck, J., Chatta, A. S. and Richardson, E. P. Jr. (1972). Pathogenesis and evolution of periventricular leukomalacia in infancy. *Arch. Neurol.*, **27**, 229–36
6. Shuman, R. M. and Selednick, L. J. (1980). Periventricular leukomalacia. *Arch. Neurol.*, **37**, 231–5
7. Young, R. S. K., Hernandez M. J. and Yagel, S. K. (1982). Selective reduction of blood flow to white matter during hypotension in newborn dogs: a possible mechanism of periventricular leukomalacia. *Ann. Neurol.*, **12**, 445–8

14

Acidaemia and its neurological effects

B. C. L. Touwen and H. J. Huisjes

Acidaemia means a decreased pH in the infant's blood. Clinically we speak of acidaemia when the pH of the blood in the umbilical vein is less than 7.20. A common cause of acidaemia at birth is asphyxia, leading to hypoxaemia or/and ischaemia. In both instances glucose uptake increases and anaerobic glycolysis occurs, followed by accumulation of lactate. If perfusion at that moment is insufficient – especially in ischaemia – a circulus vitiosus may occur and intracellular acidaemia may destroy cells, especially in the brain which is so strongly dependent on adequate perfusion by well-oxygenated blood.

Acidaemia may arise suddenly, during delivery, or may already have existed for a longer period of time, as in intrauterine asphyxia. In general, acidaemia can be considered as the end-result of a complex set of negative factors which were present during pregnancy and delivery. It is rarely an isolated or an aetiologically simple condition. Is it, therefore, reasonable to expect unequivocal effects? In this paper I will show that the effect of a low pH in the umbilical blood is not so distinct as we should like it to be. Acidaemia – and asphyxia – are significant only when considered in the context of the complex obstetric condition – pregnancy and delivery – taken as a whole.

The data which I present are derived from the Groningen Perinatal Project, a Project which was started in 1975 in the Obstetric Department of the Groningen University Hospital, with the aim of searching for relations between obstetric difficulties and neonatal and later neurological outcome. From June 1975 onwards during 3 years all the newborns were neurologically examined – in the case of prematurity at term age – using the technique described by Prechtl[1]. Data on obstetric history, present obstetrics, sociogenetic background, and the baby's condition immediately after birth were collected and stored on computerfile[2-4].

The total group consisted of 3162 live-born single infants (2991 FT; 171 PT), from these a reliable PH was known in 2771 cases, 2623 full-terms and 148 pre-

99

term infants. What were the neurological findings in these infants?

Table 1 presents the neurological findings, categorized as normal or abnormal, for the full-term infants, subdivided into intrauterine growth retardation, acidaemia, the combination of these two, and the absence of these. The presence of acidaemia or growth retardation increases the risk of neurological abnormalities, but there are two things which are noteworthy: In the first place, this risk – taken in absolute terms – is not very high: the majority of infants turned out to be normal, even in the presence of acidaemia or/and growth retardation. Secondly the increased risk appeared to be largest in the combination group: acidaemia together with growth retardation caused a risk that appeared to be three times higher, whereas acidaemia by itself increased the risk but slightly.

The subdivision of the prematurely born infants resulted in very small groups. Obviously the results are less propitious than in the group of full-terms, but the numbers are too small to warrant definite conclusions. It is clear, however, that the presence of acidaemia increases the risk of neurological abnormality (Table 2).

It can be concluded that acidaemia in the newborn infant is related with some increase of neurological morbidity. The question remains whether this is

Table 1 Neurological abnormality in relation to acidaemia and intra-uterine growth retardation in full-term infants

	Normal	Abnormal	
	(n)	n	Percentage
Growth-retarded	251	24	8.7
Acidaemic	258	15	5.5
Growth-retarded and acidaemic	51	7	12.1
Neither growth-retarded nor acidaemic	1962	68	3.3
pH umb. v. unknown	347	21	5.7
Total	2869	135	4.5

Table 2 Neurological abnormality in relation to acidaemia and intra-uterine growth retardation in preterm infants

	Normal	Abnormal	
	(n)	n	Percentage
Growth-retarded	18	5	21.7
Acidaemic	10	4	28.5
Growth-retarded and acidaemic	12	3	20.0
Neither growth-retarded nor acidaemic	85	11	11.4
pH umb. v. unknown	20	3	13.0
Total	145	26	15.2

a specific relationship. In order to analyse the specific significance of acidaemia we made use of Prechtl's (1968) optimality concept.[5]

For a set of 74 variables which described pregnancy and delivery representa-
tively, an optimal range was defined, and the number of variables lying within
this optimal range was called the obstetrical optimality score. Thus a quantifi-
cation of the obstetrical condition was reached. A classification was made into
four classes, comprising the upper and lower deciles (respectively 74–66 and
≤54 optimal variables) and the remaining 80% divided into two equal classes
(respectively 65–61 and 60–55 optimal variables).

The neurological findings were also quantified according to the optimality
concept, with the use of 60 representative items, for which an optimal range
was defined. The neurological optimality score consisted of the number of
items lying within this predefined optimal range. Again a classification was
made into four classes: the most optimal class consisted of the infants with
optimality scores 60 and 59, the second class 58–56, the third class 55–50 and
the fourth and least optimal class consisted of the infants with scores less than
50. This last class can be considered comparable to a neurological diagnosis
abnormal.[6]

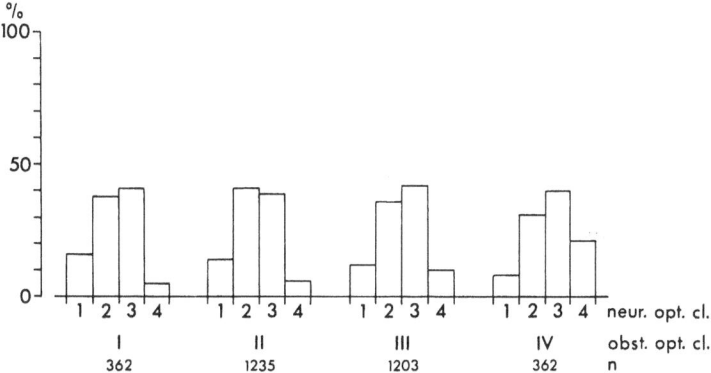

Figure 1 The distribution of four neurological optimality classes (1–4) within each of
four obstetrical optimality classes (I–IV). Neurological optimality: 1: 60–59; 2: 58–56;
3: 55–50; 4: ≤ 49 neurological variables within the optimal range.
Obstetrical optimality: I: 74–66; II: 65–61; III: 60–55; IV: ≤ 54 obstetrical variables
within the optimal range.
The proportion of neurological least optimal infants (class 4) increases in the least
optimal obstetrical class (IV)

In Figure 1 the distribution of the neurological classes within the obstetrical
classes is shown, and it is evident that there is an increase of neurological morbidity parallel to a decreasing obstetrical optimality. This relationship is statistically significant (χ^2 94.90, d.f. 9, p 0.001). The distribution of the
neurological findings within the obstetrical optimality classes for infants with
or without acidaemia (Figure 2), shows two unexpected things: In the first
place, only 15 from 360 infants with acidaemia belong to the highest obstetrical
optimality class and within this subgroup the neurological morbidity seems
even smaller than in the comparable obstetrical class of non-acidaemic infants.

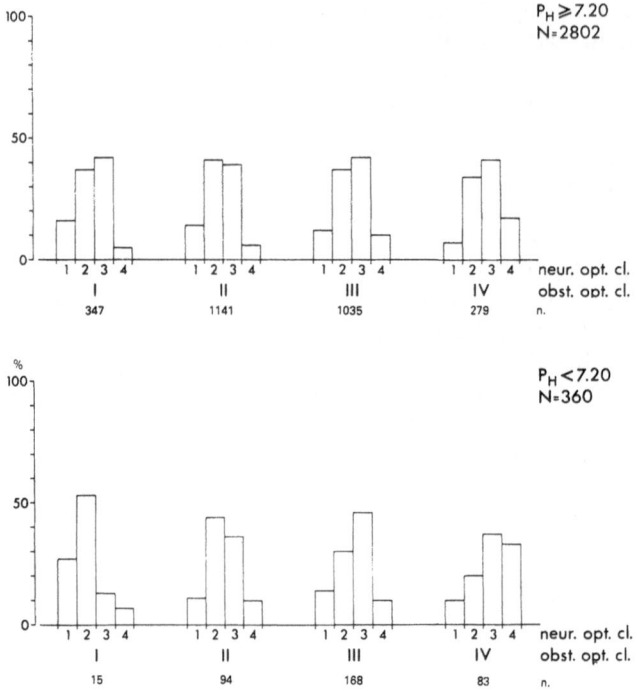

Figure 2   The distribution of the four neurological optimality classes within each of the four obstetric optimality classes in a group of infants with pH of the umbilical vein above 7.20, and a group with pH below 7.20. In both groups neurological non optimality (class 4) is more frequent in the least optimal obstetric class IV

In the second place, only in the lowest obstetrical class is the neurological morbidity of the acidaemic subgroup clearly increased. As, however, in the class with the lowest obstetrical optimality many other obstetrical variables beside pH are non-optimal, it is very difficult to appreciate the specific role of acidaemia. Only if the obstetric condition, regardless of acidaemia, deviates widely from optimal, does the effect of acidaemia on the risk for neurological morbidity increase.

The neurologically abnormal infants ($n=160$) were re-examined at 4–6 years, together with a control group of 160 neonatally normal infants. Six of the originally abnormal children had died, against two of the control group – there was no relation with the presence or absence of acidaemia at birth. Another seven could not be re-examined due to emigration and, in some cases, refusal of the parents to cooperate. So an originally abnormal group of 150 remained, with a control group of 155. Fifteen (10%) of the originally neurologically abnormal children were found to be severely abnormal at 4–6 years (e.g. CP, mental retardation) against none of the control group. Mild non-handicapping neurological abnormalities were found in 28 children of the originally abnormal group (±17%) against 11 in the control group (±7%). So there was an evident relationship between the neonatal neurological condition and the later outcome, although the majority of infants recovered. There was no relationship with the presence of acidaemia at birth, however, nor with growth retardation or preterm birth[6].

Our conclusion is that acidaemia in the newborn increases the risk of neonatal morbidity, but only in concurrence with other obstetrical problems. There is a distinct relationship between neonatal and later neurological morbidity, but a specific effect of acidaemia on the neurological condition at 4–6 years cannot be demonstrated. For the neonatal neurological condition the complexity of obstetrics has to be taken into account. The relationship between obstetrics and later neurological outcome is an indirect one, however, in which the neonatal neurological condition plays a preponderant role.

Acknowledgement

The Perinatal Project Groningen (heads: Professor Dr H. J. Huisjes and Professor Dr B. C. L. Touwen) was supported by the Praeventiefonds (grant no. 28–266), the Netherlands and partly by the Prinses Beatrixfonds, the Netherlands.

References

1. Prechtl, H. F. R. (1977). *The neurological examination of the fullterm newborn infant*. Second revised and enlarged edition. Clinics in Developmental Medicine, no. 63. (London: Heinemann)
2. Jurgens-Van Der Zee, A. D., Bierman-Van Eendenburg, M. E. C., Fidler, V. J., Olinga, A. A., Visch, J. H., Touwen, B. C. L. and Huisjes, H. J. (1979). Preterm birth, growth retardation and acidemia in relation to neurological abnormality of the newborn. *Early Hum. Devel.*, **3**, 141–54
3. Huisjes, H. J., Touwen, B. C. L., Hoekstra, J., Van Woerden-Blanksma, J. T., Bierman-Van Eendenburg, M. E. C., Jurgens-Van Der Zee, A. D., Fidler, V. J. and Olinga, A. A. (1980). Obstetrical–neonatal neurological relationship. A replication study. *Eur. J. Obstet. Gynecol. Reprod. Biol.*, **10**, 247–56
4. Touwen, B. C. L., Huisjes, H. J., Jurgens-Van Der Zee, A. D., Bierman-Van Eendenburg, M. E. C., Smrkovsky, M. and Olinga, A. A. (1980). Obstetrical condition and neonatal neurological morbidity. An analysis with the help of the optimality concept. *Early Hum. Devel.*, **4**, 207–28
5. Prechtl, H. F. R. (1968). Neurological findings in newborn infants after pre- and paranatal complications. In Jonxis, J. H. P., Visser, H. K. A. and Troelstra, J. A. (eds.). *Aspects of Praematurity and Dysmaturity*. Nutricia Symposium, pp. 303–21. (Leiden: Stenfert Kroese)
6. Touwen, B. C. L., Lok-Meijer, T. Y., Huisjes, H. J. and Olinga, A. A. (1982). The recovery rate of neurologically deviant newborns. *Early Hum. Devel.*, **7**, 131–48

15

The role of technology in detection and management – techniques of investigation

M. I. Levene

In the management of the asphyxiated newborn, careful clinical assessment is essential. As an aid to this assessment a variety of investigative methods have recently become available. Advances in technology and imaging now give the clinician a wide range of methods by which to look at the asphyxiated newborn in order to better manage these infants. These methods are employed either to make a more definitive diagnosis of pathology or to detect complications early in order to institute appropriate treatment. Imaging and monitoring methods will be discussed separately.

IMAGING

There are four methods of imaging the brains of severely asphyxiated newborns; computerized X-ray tomography (CT), ultrasound, nuclear magnetic resonance imaging (NMRI) and radioisotope scanning (RIS). CT is the method most widely used and is most reliable in the diagnosis of cerebral oedema. In full-term infants CT reveals areas of parenchymal hypodensity corresponding to oedema[1]; this, however, is unreliable in premature infants. Real-time ultrasound does on occasions show diffuse cerebral echodensity associated with cerebral oedema but is much less reliable than CT[2]. More recently NMRI has been reported to detect intracerebral water associated with hypoxic–ischaemic encephalopathy[3, 4]. This is important because NMRI appears to be safe and the infants can be repeatedly scanned to follow evolution of the lesion. Radioactive technetium has been used to assess the severity of cerebral insults following birth asphyxia[5]. Technetium is retained in areas where the blood–brain barrier has been damaged and abnormalities may correlate with outcome.

As well as cerebral oedema the asphyxiated newborn infant may develop a number of intracranial complications that are also detectable by imaging techniques. These include subdural and subarachnoid haemorrhages, intraventricular and primary intraparenchymal haemorrhage, and arterial infarction. Real-time ultrasound is a useful screening investigation to exclude these conditions but if they are suspected on ultrasound examination then further investigation by CT, NMRI or RIS may be necessary.

SEIZURE ACTIVITY

Only one-quarter of infants with electroconvulsive activity on EEG show signs of clinical seizures[6]. Undiagnosed epileptic activity probably renders the brain more likely to further damage. Two techniques exist for continuous EEG monitoring; the cerebral function monitor and the Oxford instruments continuous two-channel EEG system[6]. The latter is more satisfactory as it is far less movement-sensitive because the pre-amplifiers are miniaturized and adherent to the infant's head. Early recognition of epileptogenic activity and rapid treatment may reduce further cerebral impairment in these infants.

BLOOD PRESSURE MONITORING

Hypotension occurs commonly in severely asphyxiated infants and intermittent blood pressure measurements are not sufficient to recognize the need for treatment. Continuous measurement of arterial blood pressure from the radial artery or the aorta is a relatively simple technique. Continuous readout or ideally a computer-based trend analysis of blood pressure will alert the clinician to early hypotension, and treatment can be directed towards prompt and efficient maintenance of arterial perfusion.

INTRACRANIAL PRESSURE MEASUREMENT

Traditionally the management of birth asphyxia has been largely directed towards the avoidance of raised intracranial pressure (ICP), but no reliable methods have been available for accurate measurement of ICP. Recently Levene and Evans[7] have reported a simple method for continuous monitoring of ICP by means of a fine cannula in the subarachnoid space. This method appears to be remarkably free from complications. A micro-computer then calculates the cerebral perfusion pressure (CPP) from the mean blood pressure (MAP) and the ICP: $CPP = MAP - ICP$. The ICP and CPP can be continuously displayed and treatment initiated to maintain the CPP or reduce the ICP.

The application of these new methods allows the clinician to maintain the asphyxiated newborn infant in optimal condition and to detect complications early in order to initiate effective treatment. Although our aim must be to avoid perinatal asphyxia its management, once it has occurred, should be undertaken in well-equipped centres with staff experienced in neurologically orientated intensive care.

References

1. Flodmark, O., Fitz, C. R. and Harwood-Nash, D. C. (1980). CT diagnosis and short-term prognosis of intracranial hemorrhage and hypoxic/ischaemic brain damage in neonates. *J. Comput. Ass. Tomogr.*, **4**, 775–87
2. Levene, M. I., Williams, J. L. and Fawer, C.-L. (1985). *Ultrasound of the Infant's Brain*. (London: Spastics International Medical Publications)
3. Levene, M. I., Whitelaw, A., Dubowitz, V. *et al.* (1982). Nuclear magnetic resonance imaging of the brain in children. *Br. Med. J.,* **285,** 774–6
4. Johnson, M. A., Pennock, J. M., Bydder, G. M. *et al.* (1983). Clinical NMR imaging of the brain in children. Normal and neurologic disease. *Am. J. Neurorad.*, **4**, 1013–26
5. O'Brien, M. J., Ash, J. M., and Gilday, D. L. (1979). Radionuclide brain-scanning in perinatal hypoxia/ischaemia. *Devel. Med. Child Neurol.*, **21**, 161–73
6. Eyre, J. A., Oozeer, R. L. and Wilkinson, A. R. (1983). Diagnosis of neonatal seizure by continuous recording and rapid analysis of the electro-encephalogram. *Arch. Dis. Child.*, **58**, 785–900
7. Levene, M. I., and Evans, D. H. (1983). Continuous measurement of subarachnoid pressure in the severely asphyxiated newborn. *Arch. Dis. Child.*, **58**, 1013–15

16

Outcome and long term follow-up

C. Amiel-Tison

There has been a great deal written on asphyxial brain damage in the full-term newborn; both animal experiments and clinical observation have shown that all degrees of damage, from mild to severe, can be the consequence of perinatal asphyxia. However the selection of cases included in studies of perinatal asphyxia and prediction of outcome has not been satisfactory because of the poor delineation of causative circumstances and the non-specific definition of the resulting hypoxic–ischaemic encephalopathy. Certainly asphyxia is bad for the full-term brain, the question is how bad?

THE OUTCOME IN RECENT SERIES: DIFFICULTIES IN COMPARING RESULTS

Data from six studies published in the past 15 years are summarized in Table 1; these are the most frequently cited publications and involve only full-term newborns[1-6]. *Universal standards for presenting this sort of data do not exist.* Therefore, for example it is sometimes impossible to determine the actual mortality rate due to variability in the time of inclusion into the study, variability in the time of death and the fact that ethical considerations and their effects on the number of deaths are not taken into account.

The criteria for inclusion into a study are never the same

Neurological signs and symptoms are always a factor, but the nature and severity of symptoms are variable from one study to another, and often insufficiently defined. Asphyxia (represented by documented intrapartum fetal distress or immediate neonatal distress with low Apgar score, or the need of

Table 1 Data from six studies published in the past 15 years

Publications	Criteria for selection of cases	Initial cohort	Neonatal or later death	Follow-up available	Sequelae (severe & moderate)	Normal outcome or mild sequelae	Duration of follow-up
Amiel-Tison, 1969[1]	Neurological signs only	41	4 (10%)	25	10 (40%)	15 (60%)	2 to 5 years
Brown et al., 1974[2]	Neurological signs and asphyxia	94	20 (22%)	73	39 (53%)	34 (47%)	Mean 21 months
Sarnat and Sarnat, 1976[4]	Neurological signs and EEG	21	4 (19%)	17	5 (30%)	12 (70%)	6 to 12 months
De Souza and Richards, 1978[3]	Neurological signs and asphyxia	59	6 (10%)	53	11 (21%)	42 (79%)	2 to 5 years
Finer et al., 1981[5]	Neurological signs and asphyxia	89	6 (7%)	83	25 (30%)	58 (70%)	Mean 19 months
Fitzhardinge et al., 1981[6]	Neurological signs and asphyxia	65	0 —	62	34 (55%)	28 (45%)	2 years

immediate resuscitation) is a criterion for selection in all the series except my own[1], in which documented asphyxia was clearly present in only 19 cases out of 41.

The techniques for follow-up studies used and the duration of the studies are very variable

Some of them do not last more than 12 months; in most of the series the results are presented at various ages; the definitions of sequelae are strictly subjective in each publication, some have only considered abnormal versus normal, some have two, three or four categories of abnormalities from severe to probably insignificant. None has reached school age. It is clearly impossible to make valid comparisons between results of these studies.

PROPOSALS FOR COLLECTING COMPARABLE NEONATAL DATA

The first major difficulty in the neonatal period and later is that there is *no specific sign to define hypoxic–ischaemic encephalopathy*. There are many signs and symptoms of various levels of brain dysfunction. There is a particular evolution in signs with the clinical course moving in a fairly stereotypical way[1,7], a delay between birth and the onset of seizures, with progressive stupor and coma and subsequent improvement in vital functions, consciousness and activity. This pattern is in contrast to the more static course observed in fetopathies or malformations.

Therefore a careful daily observation throughout the first week of life is necessary; the data may be easily collected on a grid[8], and a gradation[9] is established on these clinical data, at the end of the first week; the three grades are summarized on Table 2.

Table 2 Gradation of neurological signs and symptoms observed throughout the first week of life in the full-term newborn (from Amiel-Tison et al.[9])

Grade 1: mild signs	Hyperexcitability and abnormal tone (seizures excluded)
Grade 2: moderate	CNS depression (seizures included)
Grade 3: severe	Repeated seizures and coma

Although the use of ultrasound has now become routine in the neonatal ICU, we have not modified our clinical gradation to include these data, as for the full-term newborn, this three-level gradation of symptoms is sufficient for correlation with outcome. Another attempt at clinical classification was proposed by Sarnat and Sarnat[3]: these two attempts to classify neurological signs in the neonatal period have many common points: the presence or absence of signs of CNS depression, the presence or absence of seizures. Besides EEG and CT scan, new functional investigations (PET scan, CBF measurements, NMR spectroscopy) will help in the future to better define ischaemia.

As the clinical approach is becoming more satisfactory than before, and as many cases of hypoxic–ischaemic encephalopathy are from prenatal origin, then it becomes improper to include asphyxia in criteria for selection of cases: including asphyxia means on the one hand taking into account many cases carrying a low risk of brain damage, and on the other hand excluding ischaemic lesions of prenatal origin with no asphyxic episode at birth.

In conclusion, being more confident than before in the clinical observation, it becomes less satisfactory to use documented birth asphyxia as a criterion for identification of hypoxic–ischaemic encephalopathy in the neonatal period: if birth asphyxia is present, it helps; absent, it does not eliminate the diagnosis.

Using a clinical gradation of neurological signs in the neonatal period, I have been able to demonstrate the *level of safety of full-term birth* achieved in two obstetrical tertiary care centres in Paris.

The incidence of *grade 3 type* (severe anoxic lesions) was very low 20 years ago[1], approximately 2 per 1000, and has been gradually decreasing to 0.7 per 1000 in the 1980s[10]. At the same time there has been a shift to prenatal injuries of unknown mechanism[10]. Intrapartum death, which was around 1 per 1000, is now approaching zero.

A decreasing incidence of *grade 2 type* (moderate lesions) was observed as well[11]. This was demonstrated in Port-Royal between 1975 and 1978, with an incidence going from 6 per 1000 to 2 per 1000. This is associated with the intrapartum monitoring of fetal heart becoming a routine procedure and the increasing incidence of caesarean section. In 1981–82 at Baudelocque the incidence of grade 2 was 2 per 1000, the caesarean section rate[10] was 20%.

The incidence of the *grade 1 type* (mild lesion or dysfunction) has also been decreasing[11] towards an 'acceptable' rate of 4 to 6 per 1000; complete eradication of these borderline cases would result in a further increase of caesarean section; as the risk of mild sequelae is very low in most of these cases, it appears reasonable to tolerate such a rate of mild dysfunction.

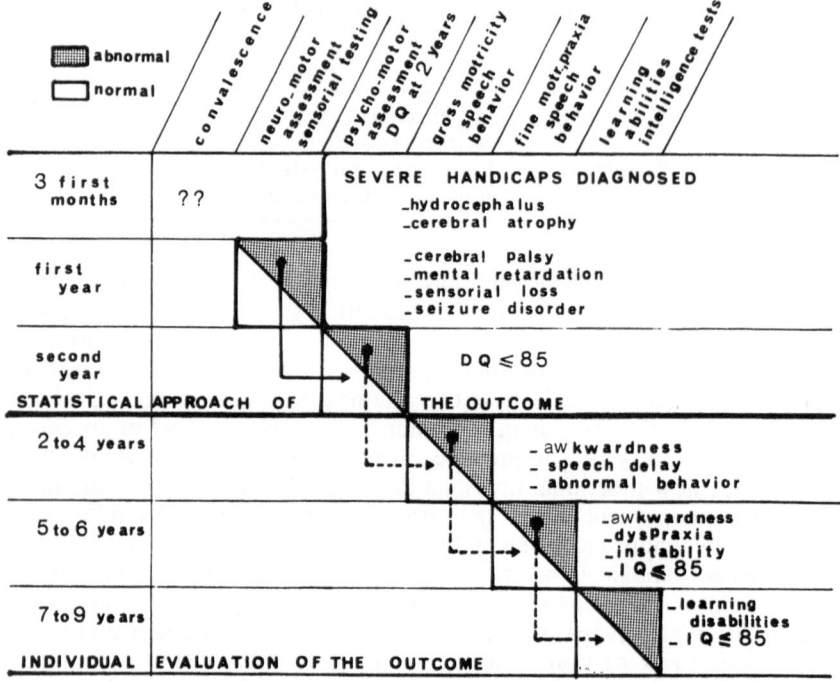

Figure 1   Summary of a stepwise evaluation of outcome from birth to 9 years. A statistical approach of the outcome is achieved at 2 years; however individual prediction is unwise at this age except when a severe handicap is present. Arrows indicate 'normalization'; dotted lines indicate that more data are needed

PROPOSAL FOR COLLECTING COMPARABLE FOLLOW-UP DATA

The second major difficulty is in the *methodology of the follow-up*. The brain develops very rapidly during infancy and childhood; the neurologist and the psychologist have to follow this development step by step and cannot evaluate any specific function before the time of its normal appearance. Therefore when one produces data on outcome, every child in the cohort should be evaluated at specific ages. The definition of severe or moderate sequelae, like definition of normalcy itself, will be clearly different at 2, 5 or 9 years of age. As there is not a specific clinical picture of hypoxic–ischaemic encephalopathy in the newborn, nor is there a specific handicap later on, evaluations on outcome have to explore *every cerebral function* to detect possible sequelae. Figure 1 describes what kind of testing[12-15], can be done according to age, and what kind of sequelae can be gathered as the child is getting older. Unfortunately, at this time, there are not enough long-term data based on neonatal gradation of neurological signs. In my series[1], the outcome grade 3 was very poor, 63% of severe encephalopathy; the same results as for Fitzhardinge[6], 55% of severe sequelae. The outcome for grade 2 is much better, 20–30% with mild or moderate handicaps[1,16]; grade 1 carries a low risk of about 10% of mild handicaps[16].

CONCLUDING REMARKS

As a conclusion, what kind of information can a high-risk perinatal centre expect from the follow-up clinic?

1. The majority of severe handicaps are diagnosed during the first year of life[12,17].
2. Reasonably good statistical risk of 'minimal brain damage' can be based on neuromotor abnormalities within the first year and/or low DQ at 2 years[12,17].
3. Individual outcome cannot be firmly defined before 8–9 years of age, when learning disabilities can be detected[15,16].
4. The longitudinal observation is necessary to establish the relationship between perinatal risk factors and school performances or behavioural problems as there is no specificity in these difficulties[16,18].
5. As a consequence, the results of any preventive effort in perinatal care can be measured by short-term follow-up studies (2 years); however an individual prediction of late outcome is not possible at this stage. The follow-up clinic can furnish feedback to the perinatal centre with yearly data concerning the cohort born 2 years previously, organized in 3 groups:
   severe sequelae;
   at risk for moderate or mild sequelae at school age; and
   normal.

When abnormalities have been observed in the 2 first years, the follow-up will go on and will allow therapeutic and educational programmes to be applied. These data will help to demonstrate the ongoing link between birth asphyxia and later difficulties encountered by some of these children, a link which cannot be established in a retrospective way.

References

1. Amiel-Tison, C. (1969). Cerebral damage in full-term newborn. Etiological factors, neonatal status and long term follow-up. *Biol. Neonate*, **14**, 234–50
2. Brown, J. K., Purvis, R. J., Forfar, J. O. and Cockburn, F. (1974). Neurological aspects of perinatal asphyxia. *Dev. Med. Child Neurol.*, **16**, 567–80
3. Sarnat, H. B. and Sarnat, M. S. (1976). Neonatal encephalopathy following fetal distress: a clinical and electroencephalographic study. *Arch. Neurol.*, **33**, 696–705
4. De Souza, S. W. and Richards, B. (1978). Neurological sequelae in newborn babies after perinatal asphyxia. *Arch. Dis. Child.*, **53**, 564–9
5. Finer, N. N., Robertson, C. M., Richards, R. T., Pinnell, L. E. and Peters, K. L. (1981). Hypoxic–ischemic encephalopathy in term neonates: perinatal factors and outcome. *J. Pediatr.*, **98**, 112–17

6. Fitzhardinge, P. M., Flodmark, O., Fitz, C. R. and Ashby, S. (1981). The prognostic value of computed tomography as an adjunct to assessment of the term infant with post asphyxial encephalopathy. *J. Pediatr.* **99**, 777–81
7. Volpe, J. (1973). Neonatal seizures. *N. Engl. J. Med.*, **2**, 413–16
8. Amiel-Tison, C. (1979). Birth injury as a cause of brain dysfunction in full-term newborns. In Korobkin, R. and Guilleminault, C. (eds.) *Advances in Perinatal Neurology*, Vol. I, pp. 57–83. (New York: Spectrum)
9. Amiel-Tison, C., Henrion, R., Esque-Vaucouloux, M. T., Firtion, G., Tchobroutsky, C. and Varangot, J. (1977). La souffrance cérébrale du nouveau-né à terme. Résultats d'une enquête prospective. *J. Gynécol. Obstet. Biol. Reprod.*, **6**, 971–89
10. Lebrun, F., Amiel-Tison, C. and Sureau, C. (1985). Sécurité de la naissance à terme et taux de césariennes. *Arch. Fr. Pédiatr.* **42**, 391–6
11. Amiel-Tison, C., Dalisson, C. and Henrion, R. (1980). Evolution de la pathologie cérébrale du nouveau-né à terme. *Arch. Fr. Pédiatri.*, **37**, 87–92
12. Amiel-Tison, C. and Grenier, A. (1983). *Neurological Evaluation of the Newborn and the Infant.* (New York: Masson)
13. Rapin, I. (1982). *Children with Brain Dysfunction*, pp. 138–40. (Raven Press: New York)
14. Ellison, P. H., Prasse, D. P., Siewart, J. and Browning, C. A. (1983). Correlations of neurologic assessment in infancy with fine motor, gross motor and intellectual assessment at four years in a neonatal intensive care population. In Sterr, L., Bard, H. and Friis-Hansen, B. (eds.) *Intensive Care in the Newborn.* Vol. IV, pp. 241–6. (New York: Masson)
15. Hunt, J. V. (1979). Longitudinal research: a method for studying the intellectual development of high risk preterm infants. In Field, T. M., Sostek, A. M., Goldberg, S. and Shuman, H. H. (eds.) *Infants Born at Risk: Behavior and Development*, pp. 443–60. (London: Spectrum)
16. Amiel-Tison, C., Dubé, R., Garel, M. and Jequier, J. C. (1983). Outcome at age 5 years of full-term infants with transient neurologic abnormalities in the first year of life. In Stern, L., Bard, H. and Friis-Hansen, B. (eds.) *Intensive Care in the Newborn*, Vol. IV, pp. 247–58. (New York: Masson)
17. Fitzhardinge, P. M. (1980) Current outcome of NICU Population. In Brann, A. W. and Volpe, J. J. (eds.), *Neonatal Neurological Assessment and Outcome*, pp. 1–5. Ross conference on pediatric research. (Columbus: Ross Laboratories)
18. Rutter, M. (1982). Syndromes attributed to 'minimal brain dysfunction' in childhood. *Am. J. Psychiatry*, **139**, 21–33

Section 5
Hypertension in Pregnancy

Chairman's introduction

J. Bonnar

INTRODUCTION

Despite the advances in the care of pregnant women, pregnancy hypertension remains one of the major causes of maternal death and morbidity. In developing countries eclampsia remains a serious problem with a high mortality rate. The reported maternal and fetal morbidity and mortality rates for pregnancy hypertension vary throughout the world due to the lack of uniformity in diagnosis and incomplete international statistics. Even in the developed countries the maternal and fetal death rates due to hypertensive disorders of pregnancy are usually under-reported.

The eastern countries have the highest maternal mortality rates for eclampsia. The rates for western countries vary between 3 and 5 per 100 000 births in the British Isles and slightly higher in North America.

Pregnancy hypertension is also responsible for a major proportion of the overall fetal mortality rate but the specific contribution of pregnancy hypertension is difficult to define because of the confusion in diagnosis in most hospital reports.

On the other side of the picture there have been in some countries policies of active intervention, particularly with respect to the early induction of labour. Mild hypertension on its own at term has been a common indication to induce labour. In many obstetric services this has contributed to an increase in the caesarean rate. Mild hypertension at term without any proteinuria is usually a benign condition which is not associated with any increase in the perinatal mortality rate. Indeed some studies have shown that the perinatal mortality rate in this group is lower than that found in normal pregnancy.

The occurrence of proteinuria in association with significant increases of blood pressure in late pregnancy is associated with an increased fetal and neonatal mortality rate. The most serious problem occurs when severe hyper-

117

tension and proteinuria occur before or early in the third trimester. In this situation the obstetrician has to provide a precise and continuing control of the maternal blood pressure and so avoid the dangers of uncontrolled hypertension on the maternal vasculature. If this can be achieved the pregnancy can be continued with all the benefits of increasing maturity for the fetus.

There remains no cure for severe pre-eclampsia except delivery of the patient. In those cases, therefore, where the blood pressure cannot be controlled despite potent hypotensive drug therapy, further delay is unwise and delivery is advisable irrespective of the gestation.

In the workshop we have experts from several countries who have a wealth of experience in the management of hypertension in pregnancy. In the following papers the most important aspects of the diagnosis and management of pregnancy hypertension are discussed, and those areas where further knowledge is required to elucidate this complex disease process.

17

The follow-up of patients with severe pre-eclampsia

B. U. Ihle, J. N. Oats and P. A. Long

INTRODUCTION

The syndrome of pre-eclampsia may be due to that condition peculiar to pregnancy but it may be superimposed on an underlying and often unsuspected medical disorder[1]. Detection of such an underlying cause may not be possible for weeks or even months after the termination of the pregnancy as time may be needed both for the superimposed pre-eclampsia to abate and/or the normal physiological changes of pregnancy to assume the non-pregnant state.

Chronic renal disease has long been recognized as an important associated disease but its accurate identification and diagnosis usually requires an invasive and potentially harmful renal biopsy. Fairley and Birch[2] have shown that detection of microscopic glomerular haematuria using phase contrast technique is a highly sensitive and specific indicator of glomerulonephritis. This test can be used to screen an at-risk population and identify those patients in whom a renal biopsy is likely to be beneficial.

Follow-up of patients who had severe pre-eclampsia is therefore necessary to identify patients with underlying medical disorders so that after identification and categorization of those with a serious, or potentially serious, condition appropriate therapy or surveillance can be instigated. Without such an assessment it is not possible to define accurately the spectrum of the syndrome in one's community. For these reasons a follow-up clinic was instituted at the Mercy Maternity Hospital, Melbourne and this paper is a preliminary report of the findings in the first 131 patients referred to the clinic.

PATIENTS AND METHODS

Patients with either early-onset pre-eclampsia (signs appearing before 37 weeks' gestation) or severe or recurrent pre-eclampsia in late pregnancy, were referred to the follow-up clinic during, or at the end of, the puerperium. Documentation was made of their past medical and obstetrical history with particular emphasis being placed on personal and family history of hypertensive and renal disorders. A clinical evaluation was performed.

At least two 24-hour creatinine clearance and total urinary protein estimations were made, together with analysis of plasma sodium, potassium, chloride and urea concentrations. Phase contrast microscopy was performed to detect microscopic glomerular haematuria on at least three separately collected specimens of urine from each patient. An intravenous pyelogram was carried out in all patients with abnormal findings on urine microscopy.

A renal biopsy was performed if the glomerular red cell count was greater than 20 000/ml (normal < 8000/ml) 6 weeks or more postpartum. The biopsy was taken at least 6 months after delivery because of the difficulty in interpreting renal histology earlier in the postpartum period when there may be superimposed pre-eclamptic changes. Renal biopsy was not performed in patients with late-onset disease; a presumptive diagnosis of renal disease being made if significant glomerular haematuria persisted for at least 6 weeks postpartum.

Essential hypertension was diagnosed when no abnormality was found on phase contrast urine microscopy *together* with a recorded elevation of blood pressure before 20 weeks' gestation *or* known hypertension antedating the index pregnancy *or* if the patient required antihypertensive medication for more than 3 months postpartum.

True or idiopathic pre-eclampsia was diagnosed only after exclusion of renal disease and essential hypertension.

Perinatal mortality was defined as infants delivered after the 20th week of pregnancy and whose birthweight was greater than 400 g, who were stillborn or who died within 28 days of birth[3]. Patients with multiple pregnancies have been excluded from this analysis.

RESULTS

In the first 15 months of the clinic, 59 patients with early-onset and 72 patients with late-onset pre-eclampsia were referred for follow-up assessment. The incidence of pre-eclampsia at the Mercy Maternity Hospital is 9.9%, and 23.5% exhibit the signs of the syndrome before 37 weeks' gestation[4], so approximately 40% of those with early-onset and 15% of those with late-onset pre-eclampsia were seen.

The clinical details of the patients attending the clinic are summarized in Table 1. As expected the disease was more severe and the perinatal mortality was much higher in the early-onset in comparison with the late-onset group. The overall hospital perinatal mortality for that period was 2%.

Early-onset pre-eclampsia

The final diagnoses in the 59 patients with early-onset pre-eclampsia are listed in Table 2. Significant glomerular haematuria was detected in 31 of the 59 (53%) and renal biopsy confirmed an abnormal finding in *all* patients.

Table 1   Clinical details of patients

	Onset of pre-eclampsia	
	Before 37 weeks	After 37 weeks
Mean gestation at delivery	33 ± 3.2 weeks	39.3 ± 1.3 weeks
Primiparas	56%	76%
Diastolic BP >100 mmHg	58%	16%
Proteinuria >0.3 g/day	40%	15%
Eclampsia	3.4%	0%
Perinatal mortality	16.6%	0.1%

Table 2   Final diagnosis in patients with early-onset pre-eclampsia

	Primiparas	Multiparas
Renal disease		
IgA GN	9	8 (5)*
Non-IgA GN	4	4 (2)
SLE	2	1 (0)
Diabetic	1	2 (2)
Reflux	3	2 (2)
Polycystic kidneys	2	0
Essential hypertension	8	7 (5)
Idiopathic pre-eclampsia	4	2 (0)
Total	33	26 (16)

GN, Glomerulonephritis; SLE, systemic lupus erythematosus
* Numbers in parentheses indicated no. of patients with recurrent pre-eclampsia

The most common finding was IgA nephropathy (55%, 17 of 31). All these patients had normal creatinine clearances, two did not have significant proteinuria postpartum and only two required antihypertensive medication after delivery.

Non-IgA nephropathy was found in eight patients (26% of those biopsied). All these women were normotensive and none had significant proteinuria postpartum. Three patients had systemic lupus erythematosus based on clinical, serological and renal histological features.

Histological changes consistent with diabetic nephropathy were found in the remaining three women biopsied. Although these three had gestational diabetes during the index pregnancy, none had required insulin therapy and in all three the postpartum glucose tolerance test had returned to normal values.

Intravenous pyelography demonstrated reflux nephropathy in five and polycystic kidneys in two patients.

Essential hypertension was diagnosed in 15 patients. Five of the seven multiparous patients had a past history of pre-eclampsia and three of the primiparous patients had been found to be hypertensive whilst taking oral contraceptive therapy. All 15 patients required antihypertensive medication following delivery.

No underlying disease was found in six women, four primiparas and two multiparas, thus giving a presumptive diagnosis of idiopathic or 'true' pre-eclampsia in 12% of the primiparas and 8% of the multiparas.

Sixteen of the 26 multiparous patients had pre-eclampsia in one or more previous pregnancies. All 16 had an underlying disorder, 11 (69%) had chronic renal disease and five (31%) had essential hypertension.

Late-onset pre-eclampsia

Chronic glomerular nephropathy, as indicated by persistently elevated glomerular red cell counts, was present in eight (15%) of the primiparas and four (24%) of the multiparas. Essential hypertension was diagnosed in four (7%) of the primiparas and 10 (59%) of the multiparas. By exclusion 43 (78%) of the primiparas and three (18%) of the multiparous patients had idiopathic pre-eclampsia.

DISCUSSION

The detection of glomerular haematuria by phase contrast urine microscopy has made it possible to select those patients who have glomerulonephritis for definitive diagnosis by renal biopsy without subjecting others to the procedure. Consequently the true incidence of chronic renal disease in a high-risk population can be determined accurately. If only biochemical indices of renal function are used to detect renal impairment the incidence of chronic renal disease will be grossly underestimated.

From the patients' viewpoint, definitive diagnosis enables a more informed prognosis to be given for future pregnancies. It also indicates both to the woman and her medical attendants when there is a need for surveillance of renal function in the long term so that therapy can be instigated if and when indicated. What impact such surveillance will have on the natural history of the various nephropathies identified remains conjectural. Similarly for the patient who has been diagnosed as having essential hypertension, regular assessment of her blood pressure should prove to be beneficial.

For the research worker trying to unravel the aetiology and pathophysiology of pre-eclampsia it is obviously important to identify those patients with an underlying medical disorder, which may be asserting a major effect on the pathogenesis of the syndrome.

There have been a number of follow-up studies of patients with pre-eclampsia and these have been elegantly reviewed by Chesley[1]. Direct comparison of their findings is difficult because of differing definitions employed, and particularly when trying to assess the incidence of chronic renal disease, the types of investigations used.

McCartney[5] reported that in 62 renal biopsies taken from primaparas with 'acute hypertension in pregnancy'[7] (the gestation was not stated) 26% had chronic renal disease and 70% had glomerular endotheliosis said to be pathognomonic of pre-eclampsia. In contrast only 3% of the 152 multiparas had glomerular endotheliosis, 43% had chronic renal disease. Comparison of McCartney's findings with those from this report can only be approximate but similar trends are apparent.

We were surprised at the biopsy findings of diabetic nephropathy in the three patients who had gestational diabetes since they had not required insulin and their postpartum glucose tolerance tests were normal. Gonzalez-Gonzalez et al.[6] reported similar findings in eight women with mild diabetes in pregnancy, four of whom developed pre-eclampsia. All eight had biopsy evidence of diabetic nephropathy.

Other surveys[1] have reported that only a small proportion of multiparous patients have true or idiopathic pre-eclampsia which is in accord with the 12% so identified in this study. However the finding that 88% of primiparous patients with early-onset disease had an identifiable underlying cause is at variance with these surveys with the exception of one report by Bellar and Dame[7] from West Germany. This may represent a real difference in the aetiology of the syndrome in Australia, or may only be reflecting a difference in investigative methodology.

This study has shown that a presumptive diagnosis of true or idiopathic pre-eclampsia is likely to be correct only in primigravid patients who develop the signs late in pregnancy. In all others a careful search for an underlying medical disorder has a high probability of being rewarded with a positive finding.

References

1. Chesley, L. C. (1978). *Hypertensive Disorders in Pregnancy*. (New York: Appleton-Century-Crofts)
2. Fairley, K. F. and Birch, D. F. (1982). Haematuria: a simple method for identifying glomerular bleeding. *Kidney Int.*, **21**, 105–8
3. The Consultative Council on Maternal and Perinatal Mortality. Survey of Perinatal Deaths in Victoria. 21st Annual Report for the Year 1982. Health Commission of Victoria, 1983
4. Beischer, N. A. and Abell, D. A. (1983). Third Clinical Report, Mercy Maternity Hospital Melbourne for the Years 1978–1980 (Melbourne: Ramsay Ware)
5. McCartney, C. P. (1964). Pathological anatomy of acute hypertension of pregnancy. *Circulation*, **29–30**(II), 37–42
6. Gonzalez-Gonzales, L., Lopez-Llera, M., Gonzalez-Angulo, A., Linares, G. R. and Sneider, G. B. (1971). Diabetes mellitus and toxaemia of pregnancy, electron microscopic study of renal biopsies. *J. Reprod. Med.* **7**, 133–8
7. Bellar, F. and Dame, W. (1976). Morphological alterations in the kidneys during pre-eclampsia: a preliminary communication. In Lindheimer, M. D., Katz, A. I. and Zuspan, F. P. (eds) *Hypertension in Pregnancy*, pp. 155–6. (New York: John Wiley and Sons)

18

Hypertension-related perinatal mortality in Alberta

J. J. Boyd

This presentation is an attempt to discover if there is a different rate of occurrence of high blood pressure in pregnancy in Canada (using the figures from the province of Alberta) compared with Britain and the USA. I point out at the outset that the Canadian figures have been obtained retrospectively and are crude at best, but useful for a rough comparison. It has been my own clinical impression from 14 years in Canada that the incidence of hypertension in pregnancy is much less than my previous clinical experience in Scotland.

In 27 years (1955–81) in Alberta there were 939 706 pregnancies and 381 maternal deaths. The commonest single reasons for maternal death were infection, haemorrhage and embolism. Cerebrovascular accident was the fifth-commonest while death involving eclampsia was the eighth (18 deaths).

The two main hospitals in Edmonton, the University and the Royal Alexandra, deliver about 7000 women per year; they serve as referral hospitals for high-risk obstetrics. At the University Hospital over 7 years (1977–83) there were 14 518 deliveries. Pre-eclamptic toxaemia was recorded in 440 first pregnancies (7.9%), and other forms of hypertension in 202 of the remainder (1.4%). The Royal Alexandra Hospital delivered 6053 women in 1983, of whom 360 had problems with hypertension (6%). This was divided into 306 mild PET, five with severe PET and two with eclamptic seizures. There were three perinatal deaths in these patients.

For a wide general view (see Table) three groups have been compared, admittedly from different years and with the US and British studies being prospective. The Alberta study uses the Physicians Activities Study (PAS) computer data collected by medical records librarians for women having babies in our province in 1983. This is extracted from medical summaries and I suspect underestimates the number with milder hypertensive conditions. The International Disease Classification (IDC) codes covering all types of hypertension in pregnancy have been used.

Table

	'The women . . .'[a] Niswander, 1959–65	'British births'[b] 1970	Alberta (PAS)* 1983
Pregnancies	37 667	16 815	30 490
All HBP	9 119 (24.2%)	4 383 (26%)	987 (3.2%)
Mild PET	7 376		588
PET	723	2 659	98
Eclampsia	26	181	16

* Retrospective computer using IDC codes 642.0–642.9
[a] *The Women and their Pregnancies*, Niswander and Gordon. (W. B. Saunders, 1972)
[b] *British Births 1970* (Heinemann, 1978)

Study of this table confirms the clinical suspicion that the incidence of all forms of high blood pressure, and in particular the more severe forms of PET and eclampsia, occur with less frequency in the Canadian and American groups. Canada would seem to have the lowest incidence. It must be emphasized again that these groups are separated by 20 and 10 years.

19

The effect of hypertension on the uteroplacental vasculature

B. L. Sheppard and J. Bonnar

INTRODUCTION

In pregnancy, fetal well-being is dependent on an adequate flow of maternal blood to the intervillous space of the placenta. The blood supply to the endometrium of the non-pregnant uterus is only a few millilitres per minute, whereas 600–800 millilitres of blood per minute must be delivered to the placenta at term. A reduced uteroplacental blood flow has been shown in pregnancies complicated by maternal hypertension[1].

Morphological adaptations of the uterine spiral arteries are an essential requirement to facilitate the increasing blood supply to the placenta as pregnancy advances. Over the past 20 years an increasing number of studies have described the physiological changes of uteroplacental vessels in normal pregnancy[2-4] and uterine vascular pathology in hypertensive pregnancy[5-7] and pregnancy complicated by intrauterine fetal growth retardation[8-11].

DEVELOPMENT OF THE ARTERIAL SUPPLY TO THE PLACENTA IN NORMAL PREGNANCY

Maternal blood reaches the intervillous space of the placenta through the spiral arteries, or coiled arteries, which are in turn, branches of the radial arteries (Figure 1). Basal arteries, which are smaller straight arteries also derived from the radial artery, supply the decidua and adjacent myometrium. The spiral arteries, in contrast to the basal arteries, undergo extensive morphological changes during normal pregnancy.

In the non-pregnant uterus the arteries exhibit an intimal lining of endothelium with underlying medial smooth muscle. In the myometrium the vessels have a prominent internal elastic lamina which becomes more tenuous as the arteries traverse the endometrium.

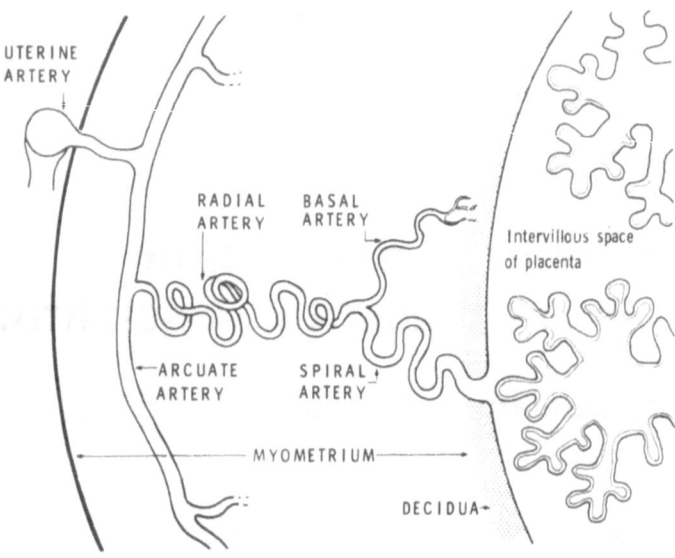

Figure 1   Diagram of the arterial supply of the human placenta

In early pregnancy the walls of the spiral arteries of the placental bed undergo a striking series of adaptations as the decidua is invaded by cytotrophoblast from the trophoblastic shell of the implanted blastocyst. Much of the endothelium of the decidual spiral arteries is replaced by cytotrophoblast which also infiltrates the media of the vessel walls. This is associated with a loss of elastic tissue and smooth muscle and the deposition of fibrinoid material, which has been shown by electron microscopy to contain fibrin[4]. It is believed that a second wave of endovascular trophoblast invasion occurs between the 16th and 20th week of gestation[12] as the myometrial segments of the uteroplacental spiral arteries undergo morphological changes. These structural alterations in the uteroplacental arteries have been termed 'physiological changes' of normal pregnancy[2] and as pregnancy advances progress into the deeper layers of the placental bed (Figure 2). They may even involve the distal segments of the radial artery in the myometrium.

The effect of the invasion of endovascular cytotrophoblast is to convert the uteroplacental spiral arteries into tortuous, distended, funnel-shaped vessels emptying into the intervillous space of the placenta. The loss of musculoelastic tissue renders the vessels incapable of responding to vasomotor influences. The physiological changes are associated with a reduction in vascular resistance[13] allowing a greater blood flow into the intervillous space of the placenta.

UTEROPLACENTAL ARTERIES IN HYPERTENSIVE PREGNANCY

The term 'acute atherosis' was introduced by Zeek and Asali[14] to describe lesions of decidual spiral arteries in pre-eclampsia, following the observation by Hertig[15] of predominantly lipid-containing lesions in hypertensive preg-

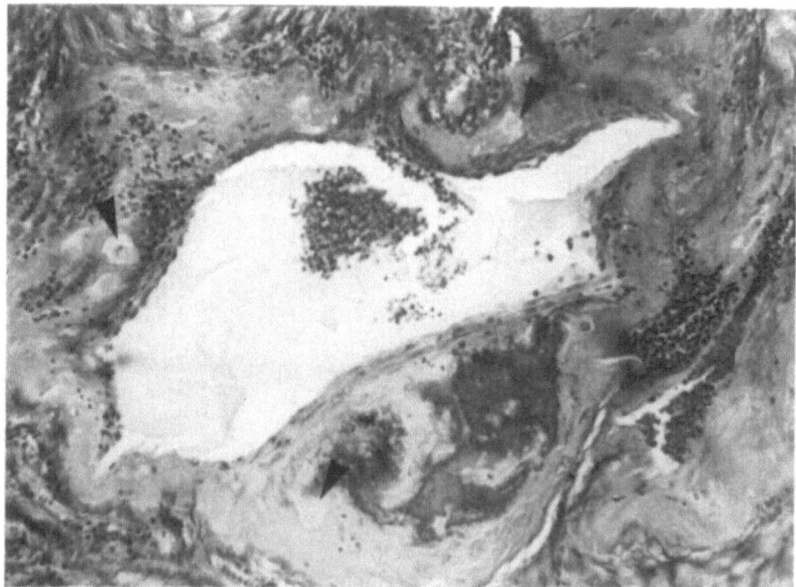

Figure 2 Myometrial spiral in late normal pregnancy. Trophoblast cells (arrows) surrounded by a fibrinous matrix are seen in the modified media of the vessel wall

nancies. The lesions are characterized by fibrinoid necrosis with accumulation of lipid-laden cells, in the intima and media of the vessel walls. It was later suggested that this lesion only occurred in pre-eclampsia[2] and that the physiological changes of spiral arteries extended 'without exception', only to the decidual myometrial junction in the placental bed[16].

In our own studies, however, we have found that in pre-eclampsia where the birth weight of the infant is appropriate for gestational age, although some myometrial segments of uteroplacental spiral arteries may show occlusive atheromatous-like lesions, the physiological changes of pregnancy are clearly visible in other segments of myometrial spiral arteries (Figure 3). These results suggest that a failure of physiological adaptations of myometrial spiral arteries is not a prerequisite for the occurrence of the lesion 'acute atherosis'.

Where the pre-eclampsia is superimposed on essential hypertension the restrictions of the physiological adaptations are similar to those observed in spiral arteries of the myometrium from patients with pre-eclampsia alone; however, in many of these cases myometrial uteroplacental arteries exhibit hyperplastic arteriosclerotic lesions. In patients with essential hypertension who do not develop pre-eclampsia, the myometrial spiral arteries show the physiological changes of pregnancy. However myo-intimal smooth muscle hyperplasia has been reported in myometrial placental bed spiral arteries which have not undergone physiological changes of pregnancy, and still retain a prominent internal elastic lamina in essential hypertension where the pregnancy has resulted in the delivery of a growth-retarded infant[11]

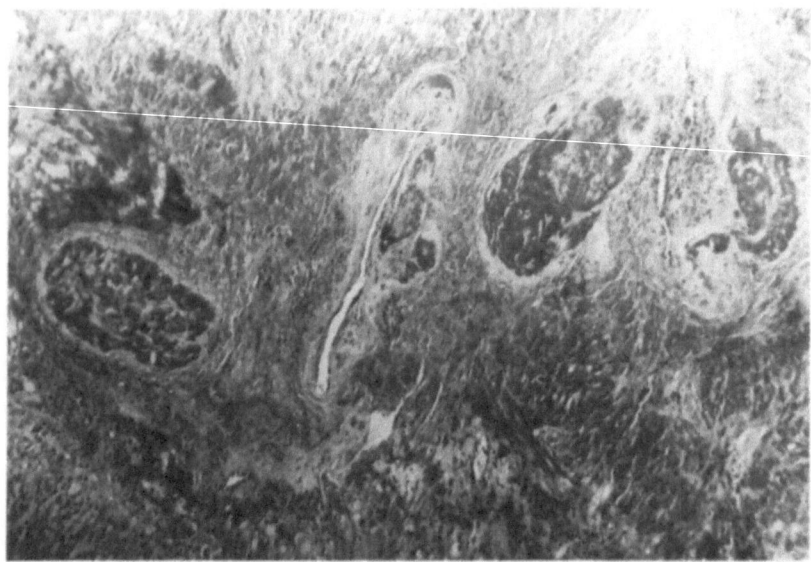

Figure 3 Myometrial spiral artery in a pregnancy complicated by pre-eclampsia where the birth weight of the baby was appropriate for gestational age. The vessel shows the morphological adaptations of pregnancy whereas three adjacent segments of the same artery are occluded with fibrin and lipid laden cells – typical of the lesion acute atherosis

VASCULAR PATHOLOGY IN INTRAUTERINE FETAL GROWTH RETARDATION

Recently there has been considerable disagreement about the relationship between uteroplacental vascular pathology, hypertensive pregnancy and intrauterine growth retardation. In a small series of 15 well-documented cases of severe intrauterine growth retardation of mixed aetiology we described atheromatous-like lesions in decidual spiral arteries, similar to those reported in pre-eclampsia, coupled with a failure of physiological adaptations in the myometrial spiral arteries[8]. In a retrospective study Brosens *et al.*[9] confirmed our findings in respect of physiological changes, but could only find lesions in intrauterine fetal growth retardation with pre-eclampsia and suggested that the lesion we described was perhaps analogous too, but not identical with, 'acute atherosis'.

We subsequently confirmed our original findings in a larger study by both light and electron microscopy[11]. We found vascular lesions exhibiting fibrin deposition and the accumulation of lipid-laden cells in pregnancy complicated by intrauterine growth retardation, whether maternal hypertension was present or not. These lesions are found in the uteroplacental spiral arteries of the basal decidua and to a lesser extent in the spiral arteries of the placental bed and myometrium (Figure 4). As the lesions showed identical morphological features to those described in pre-eclampsia, we concluded that the lesion 'acute atherosis' was not pathognomonic for pre-eclampsia. However other features, such as the number and size of the vessels supplying the placenta,

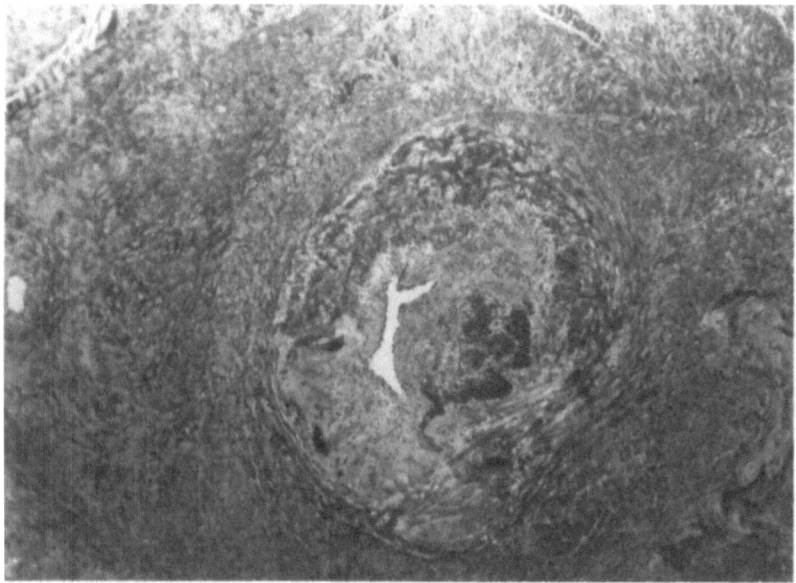

Figure 4 Spiral artery at the myometrial – decidual junction in a normotensive pregnancy complicated by severe intrauterine fetal growth retardation. Fibrin and lipid laden cells are evident in the vessel wall which has not undergone the physiological adaptations of pregnancy

may also be involved in pregnancy complicated by fetal growth retardation. Further studies are required on the complex uterine vascular changes in these pregnancies where the otherwise healthy fetus suffers impairment of growth or even death *in utero*.

CONCLUSION

In normal pregnancy the uteroplacental arteries undergo extensive morphological adaptations necessary to supply adequate blood flow to the intervillous space of the placenta to meet the demands of the growing fetus. In both normotensive and hypertensive pregnancy complicated by severe intrauterine growth retardation these physiological changes of pregnancy frequently do not extend beyond the decidual segments of the uteroplacental arteries. In preeclampsia, where the fetus is appropriate for gestational age, the physiological changes often extend into the myometrial segments of the placental bed vessels.

Atheromatous-like lesions are found in uteroplacental vessels in preeclampsia. However lesions exhibiting a similar morphology are found in spiral arteries of the placental bed in intrauterine growth retardation where the pregnancy has remained normotensive throughout. Until we understand more of the pathogenesis of these vascular lesions in uteroplacental vessels in normotensive pregnancy with intrauterine growth retardation we must assume there is no arteriopathy specific for pregnancy complicated by pre-eclampsia.

ACKNOWLEDGEMENTS

Part of this study was supported by the Friends of the Rotunda Hospital, Dublin.

References

1. Browne, J. C. M. and Veall, N. (1953). The maternal placental blood flow in normotensive and hypertensive women. *J. Obstet. Gynaecol. Br. Emp.*, **60**, 141–7
2. Brosens, I., Robertson, W. B. and Dixon, H. G. (1967). The physiological response to the vessels of the placental bed to normal pregnancy. *J. Pathol. Bacteriol.*, **93**, 569–79
3. De Wolf, F., De Wolf-Peeters, C. and Brosens I (1973). Ultrastructure of the spiral arteries in the placental bed at the end of normal pregnancy. *Am. J. Obstet. Gynecol.*, **117**, 833–47
4. Sheppard, B. L. and Bonnar, J. (1974). The ultrastructure of the arterial supply of the human placenta in early and late pregnancy. *J. Obstet. Gynaecol. Br. Commonw.*, **81**, 497–511
5. Robertson, W. B., Brosens, I. and Dixon, H. G. (1967). The pathological response of the vessels of the placental bed in hypertensive pregnancy. *J. Pathol. Bacteriol.*, **93**, 581–91
6. Robertson, W. B., Brosens, I. and Dixon, H. G. (1975). Uteroplacental vascular pathology. *Eur. J. Obstet. Gynaecol. Reprod. Biol.*, **5**, 47–65
7. Sheppard, B. L. and Bonnar, J. (1980). Uteroplacental arteries and hypertensive pregnancy. In Bonnar J., MacGillivray I. and Symonds, E. (eds.) *Pregnancy Hypertension*: Proceedings of the First Congress of the Society for the Study of Hypertension in Pregnancy, pp. 213–19. (Lancaster: MTP Press)
8. Sheppard, B. L. and Bonnar, J. (1976). The ultrastructure of the arterial supply of the human placenta in pregnancy complicated by intrauterine growth retardation. *Br. J. Obstet. Gynaecol.*, **83**, 948–59
9. Brosens, I., Dixon, H. G. and Robertson, W. B. (1977). Fetal growth retardation and the arteries of the placental bed. *Br. J. Obstet. Gynaecol.*, **84**, 656–63
10. De Wolf, F., Brosens, I. and Renaer, M. (1980). Fetal growth retardation and the maternal arterial supply of the human placenta in the absence of sustained hypertension. *Br. J. Obstet. Gynaecol.*, **87**, 678–85
11. Sheppard, B. L. and Bonnar, J. (1981). An ultrastructural study of the uteroplacental spiral arteries in hypertensive and normotensive pregnancy and fetal growth retardation. *Br. J. Obstet. Gynaecol.*, **88**, 695–705
12. Pijnenborg, R., Dixon, G., Robertson, W. B. and Brosens, I. (1980). Trophoblastic invasion of human decidua from 8–18 weeks of pregnancy. *Placenta*, **1**, 3–20
13 Moll, W., Kunzel, W. and Herberger, J. (1975). Hemodynamc implications of hemochorial placentation. *Eur. J. Obstet. Gynaecol. Reprod. Biol.*, **5**, 67–74
14. Zeek, Z. M. and Assali, N. S. (1950). Vascular changes in the decidua associated with eclamptogenic toxemia of pregnancy. *Am. J. Clin. Pathol.*, **20**, 1099–109
15. Hertig, A. T. (1945). Vascular pathology in hypertensive albuminuric toxemias of pregnancy. *Clinics*, **4**, 602–14
16. Brosens, I., Robertson, W. B. and Dixon, H. G. (1972). The role of spiral arteries in the pathogenesis of pre-eclampsia. In Wynn, R. M. (ed.) *Obstetrics and Gynaecological Annual*, pp. 177–91 (New York: Appleton-Century-Crofts)

20

A critical appraisal

J. A. McGarry

In every generation obstetricians have been faced by the clinical challenge of hypertension found in pregnancy or developing in response to pregnancy. Maternal safety and perinatal mortality rates have been used as the indicators of the effectiveness of regimens of management and drug therapy. In the past 20 years the obstetrician of scholarly or scientific disposition has sought to bring the investigation of the causes and mechanisms of pregnancy hypertension into the mainstream of fundamental investigation of hypertension in the non-pregnant, with success and much benefit.

The part played by fluid retention and sodium metabolism was defined, the role and limited success of anticonvulsants explored, coagulation changes and disseminated intravascular coagulation and then renin–angiotensin were followed by the immunological contribution labelled gestosis. The role of prostaglandins was studied and the significance of the capacity of the spiral arteries elucidated. New antihypertensive agents were tried and praised and criticized.

In spite of all this progress in elucidating the mechanisms of hypertension in pregnancy it remains very difficult to make clear statements which can give general guidance. It may be, as Redman has shown, that 'moderate' hypertension does not need antihypertensive treatment. The problem remains for the clinician who finds 'moderate' hypertension in a patient at the antenatal clinic. What are the criteria for admission to hospital? What investigations are useful and predictive?

Much of the improvement in maternal safety, and the lower perinatal mortality now achieved in pregnancies complicated by hypertension, may be less due to drug treatment than to premature delivery by caesarean section under epidural anaesthesia with all its benefits, delivering a baby in good condition to skilled and increasingly successful neonatal pediatricians.

29

A clinical appraisal

J.A. McGarry

21

Conservative management of pre-eclampsia: maternal risk

P. E. Treffers and M. E. Smorenberg-Schoorl

In recent years there have been challenging publications[1,2] concerning the threat caused by pre-eclampsia to the life and health of the mother, and the necessity of terminating the pregnancy in the interest of the mother irrespective of gestational age.

In the department of obstetrics at the University of Amsterdam the treatment of pregnancy hypertension and pre-eclampsia has been standardized to a large extent over a period of more than 15 years. Treatment has been relatively conservative, and we would like to report on maternal mortality and serious morbidity.

In our department patients are hospitalized when the diastolic blood pressure (BP) is 100 mmHg or more, or when proteinuria is 1 g/24 h or more. After hospitalization they are treated with bed rest, salt restriction, if necessary sedatives (phenobarbitone), and only when the diastolic BP exceeds 115 mmHg are hypotensive drugs (methyldopa) given. A number of maternal and fetal parameters are carefully monitored, as shown in the case histories. In pregnancies at or near term, labour is induced if the cervix is favourable, caesarean section is performed on the indication of (impending) fetal distress (as measured by oestrogen excretion in 24 h urine, non-stress CTG and echoscopy). Termination of pregnancy on maternal indication only is rarely performed. We use no diuretics, no heparin and only occasionally are thrombocytes and antithrombin III (AT-III)-concentrate given as a preparation for operative delivery when clotting disturbances need correction.

Over a 7-year period, 1977–83, we treated and monitored 385 patients with a diastolic BP of ≥100 mmHg in the third trimester. Thrombocytopenia (platelets $<100\times10^9$/l) occurred in 38 (10%) of these patients and in 78 cases (20%) liver enzymes were elevated (SGOT and/or SGPT >20 U/l). These symptoms are, according to recent literature, especially indicative of danger for the mother. Since we never terminated a pregnancy because of these symptoms, we could study the course of the disease during our treatment.

The caesarean section rate in this group of patients was 24%. In patients treated for pregnancy hypertension in our department major maternal complications were two cases of eclampsia occurring after admission. Some patients were referred to us because of complications: three cases of eclampsia and two patients with intra-abdominal bleeding from a subcapsular haematoma of the liver. One of these two patients died; this was the only case of maternal mortality associated with pregnancy hypertension in this 7-year period, and also over the past 15 years (± 25 000 deliveries). There were no cases of cerebral haemorrhage during these 15 years; the last case of cerebral haemorrhage observed in our department occurred in 1968.

Besides these maternal complications occurring before delivery, we observed nine cases of serious bleeding postpartum, especially haematomas in the abdominal wall following caesarean section. One patient with a haematoma of the abdominal wall was referred to us after a caesarean section elsewhere, because of serious morbidity.

CASE HISTORIES

Patient A (1300/83), gravida II, para 0, 39 years, was referred to our department at a gestational age of 27²/₇ weeks from a hospital elsewhere because her obstetrician considered termination of pregnancy necessary on maternal indication. Despite treatment with antihypertensive drugs and diuretics her BP was 160/110 mmHg, she had severe oedema and proteinuria, and she complained of headaches. In Figure 1 a number of maternal parameters are shown graphically. We treated her according to our protocol without diuretics and antihypertensives; her diastolic BP remained 110–115; only during the last days of her pregnancy was she streated with methyldopa because the diastolic BP showed a tendency to increase to values $\geq$ 120 mmHg. The haematocrit rose to high values ($> 45\%$) as did the haemoglobin (> 9 mmol/l). Plasma creatinine increased to > 140 μmol/l, liver enzymes were not seriously elevated in this case. The platelet count was normal ($\pm 200 \times 10^9$/l), but AT-III plasma values were low (± 50 U/l). Proteinuria increased to > 20 g/24 h.

We delayed the termination of pregnancy for 2½ weeks. At a gestational age of 29⁵/₇ weeks signs of fetal distress were apparent on the CTG, an uncomplicated caesarean section was performed, and a girl of 1120 g was born in good condition. Unfortunately, this preterm infant died 1 week postpartum of septicaemia. The mother recovered well; 6 weeks postpartum her diastolic BP was 90 mmHg.

Patient B (1206/83), a gravida I, para 0, 26 years, had a history of mild hypertension. At 26²/₇ weeks of gestation she was referred to our department, her obstetrician in a hospital elsewhere considered termination of pregnancy indicated because of her condition: she had been treated with atenolol for some weeks, her BP had risen to 170/125, and she complained of epigastric pain and vomiting. Her BP and laboratory data are shown in Figure 2. According to our protocol we prescribed methyldopa instead of atenolol. After some days the diastolic BP decreased but remained at a level of 100–110 mmHg.

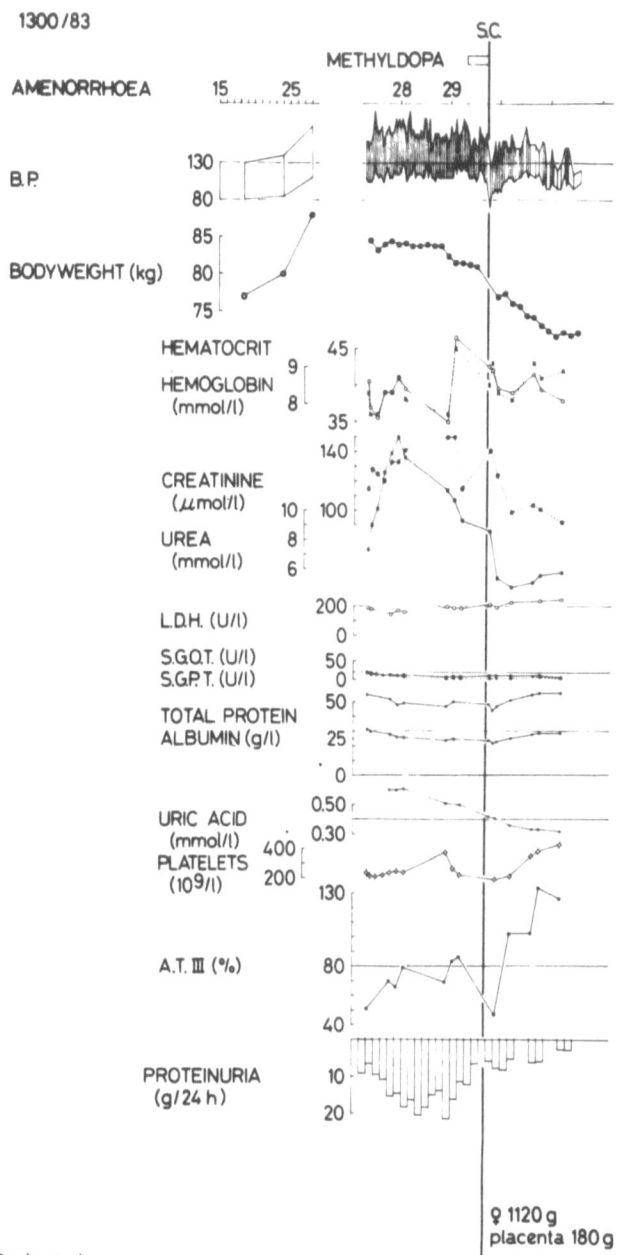

Figure 1 Patient A

Haemoglobin and haematocrit levels rose to high values, the plasma creatinine was only slightly elevated, but on admission liver enzyme levels were high: SGOT 302 U/l, SGPT 399 U/l, LDH 1147 U/l. Platelet count was low: 33 × 10⁹/l. Plasma AT-III levels were decreased: 70 U/l. Liver enzymes, thrombocytes

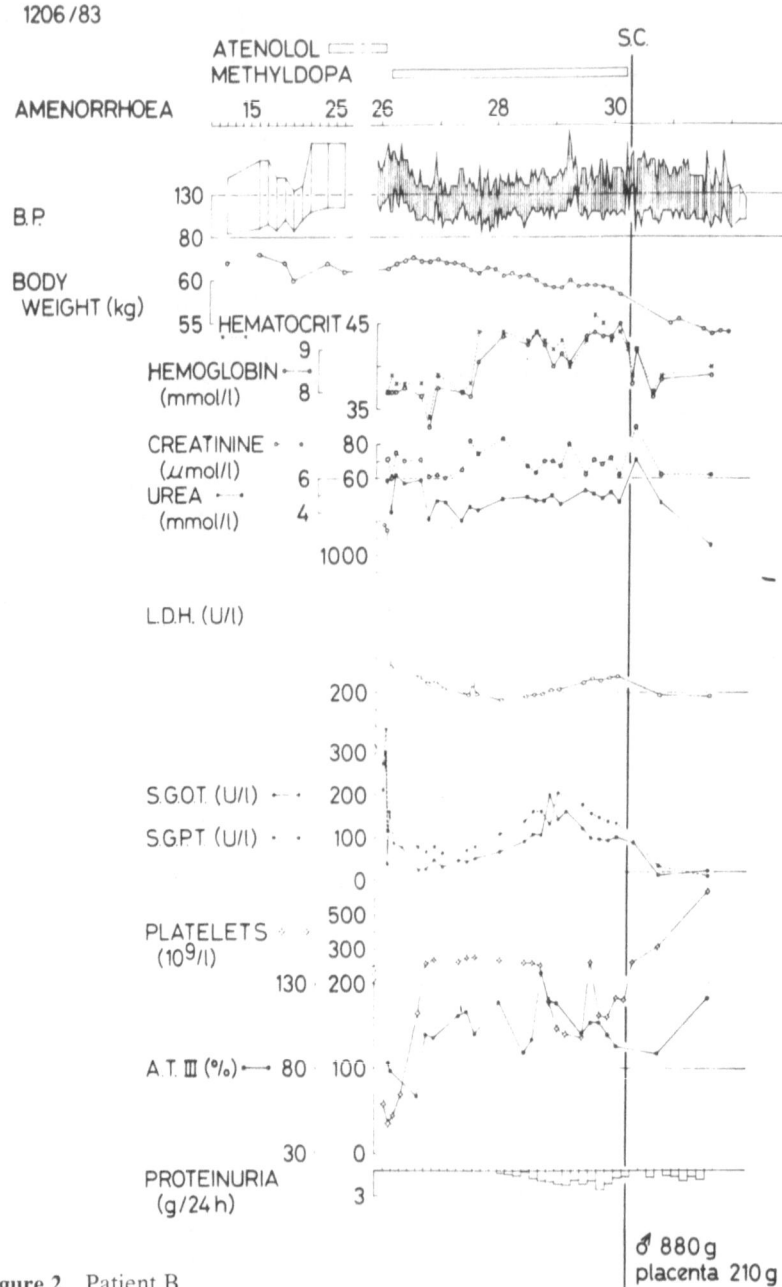

Figure 2   Patient B

and AT-III levels showed improvement after admission, but liver enzymes increased again after some weeks. Some proteinuria developed.

Using conservative therapy we succeeded in postponing the termination of pregnancy for more than 4 weeks. At 30²⁄₇ weeks gestation, signs of fetal distress were apparent, and an uncomplicated caesarean section was performed. A boy of 880 g was born, in good condition. The infant passed a favourable and relatively uncomplicated period in the neonatal intensive care unit, and was healthy 6 months after birth. Probably the life of this child was saved by the delay in the termination of pregnancy.

DISCUSSION

Our results show that a conservative, careful and consistent approach to pre-eclampsia is possible without undue risk to the mother. Obviously there remains a serious threat of fetal death. When overt signs of fetal distress are absent, especially early in the third trimester, there is often time for conservative management. Sometimes the condition of the mother improves during this treatment. Caesarean section is performed primarily in the interest of the fetus; it may even cause additional risk to the mother. In our opinion there is a place for conservative management, in the interest of both the fetus and the mother.

References

1. Killam, A. P., Dillard, S. H., Patton, R. C. and Pederson, P. R. (1975). Pregnancy-induced hypertension complicated by acute liver disease and disseminated intravascular coagulation. *Am. J. Obstet. Gynecol.*, **123**, 823–8
2. Weinstein, L. (1982). Syndrome of hemolysis, elevated liver enzymes, and low platelet count: a severe consequence of hypertension in pregnancy. *Am J. Obstet. Gynecol.*, **142**, 159–67

Section 6
Indication for
Caesarean Section

Chairman's introduction

M. Thiery

Little research has been done on the phenomenon of rising national caesarean-section trends in Europe. From what is known – mainly from international and hospital sources – this phenomenon seems to be recent, widespread, and self-perpetuating. The widely held assumption that (unduly) high caesarean-section rates are in the interest of both mother and child will be challenged in this workshop, and measures to curb caesarean-section rates without affecting the perinatal outcome will be assessed.

22

Trends and variations in the use of caesarean delivery

I. Chalmers

Caesarean deliveries have been increasing in almost every locality for which statistics are available. In some places this increase has been relatively modest, in others it could justifiably be characterized as an epidemic. These differing trends have led to a situation in which national rates of caesarean deliveries vary four-fold – from less than 5% of all deliveries in the Netherlands and Fiji to nearly 20% in Singapore, Canada and the United States (Figure 1). By no conceivable stretch of the imagination could this variation in practice be explained by differences in the characteristics of either the women who live in these different countries, or their fetuses.

The reasons for these trends and variations have been reviewed in Europe, North and South America and Australia[1-13]. The increase in the use of caesarean delivery has been attributed to a lowering of the threshold at which the operation is used in the management of dystocia, breech presentation, fetal distress and the delivery of small or preterm fetuses. An increased rate of primary caesarean delivery for these reasons has, in its turn led to an inevitable increase in the frequency of repeat operations. The dramatic difference between caesarean delivery rates in North America and in some European countries has been ascribed, in particular, to differences in the management of dystocia and of women who have had previous caesarean deliveries.

In addition to these 'obstetric' reasons for trends and variations in the use of caesarean delivery, there are also social determinants of the use of the operation[12]. In some settings, for example, women paying fees for maternity care are twice as likely as women with health insurance and three times more likely than indigent women to have a caesarean delivery[13]. Another social determinant of increased caesarean delivery rates is the fear of many obstetricians that they will face malpractice suits if a child whom they deliver vaginally subsequently shows any kind of disability. In spite of the lack of scientific evidence on which to base most of these claims[14-18] fear of litigation is the second most

145

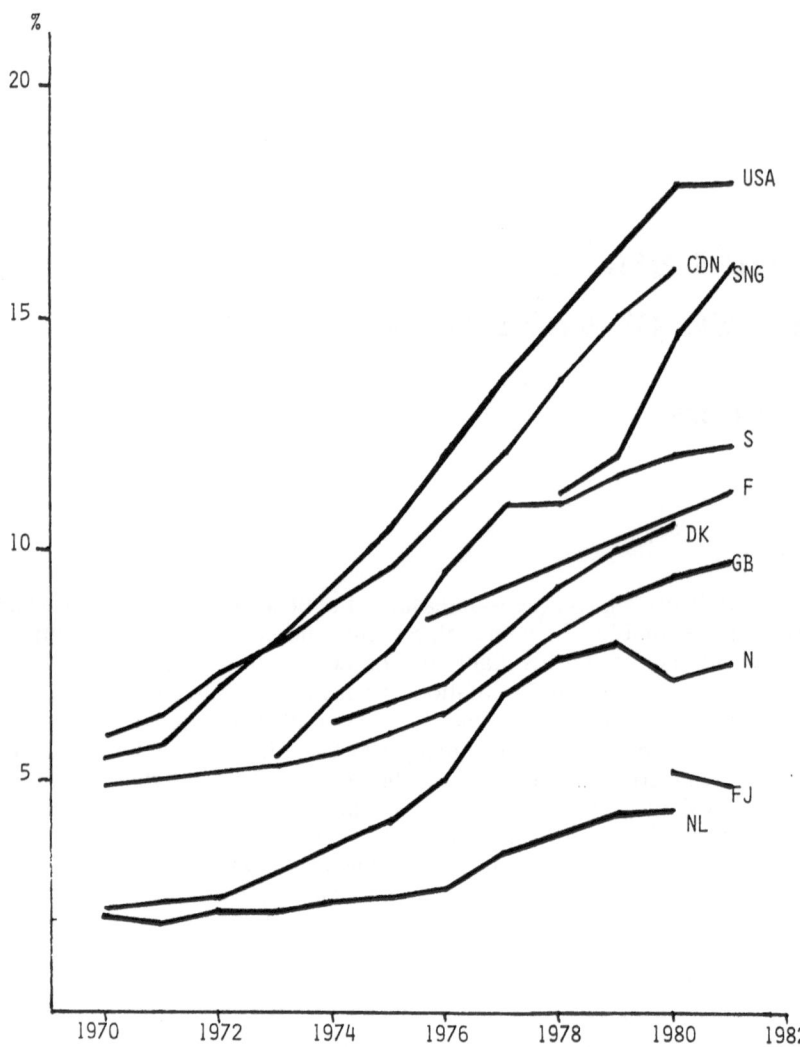

Figure 1   Trends in the rate of caesarean delivery, various countries, 1970–81[1]

common reason given by British obstetricians for their increased use of caesarean delivery[8].

Although difficult to quantitate, it would seem inevitable that this increased use of major surgery in obstetric practice will have led to an increase in both short-term and longer-term maternal morbidity. Indeed, analyses of maternal mortality statistics derived from the Reports on Confidential Enquiries into Maternal Deaths in England and Wales (Table 1) suggest that although the fatality rate associated with caesarean delivery has been falling as the use of the operation has been extended, the overall rate of maternal death associated with caesarean delivery has changed little during the past 20 years. Further-

Table 1 Fatality rate, incidence and overall rate of maternal death in association with caesarean section, England and Wales 1958/60 to 1976/78

	1958/60	1961/63	1964/66	1967/69	1970/72	1973/75	1976/78
Rate of maternal death per 1000 operations	2.3	1.9	1.6	1.2	1.1	0.8	0.8
Rate of caesarean section per 100 births	2.6	3.0	3.5	4.1	4.6	5.2	6.7
Rate of maternal deaths associated with caesarean section per million maternities	62.5	56.5	55.3	51.8	49.0	45.0	53.2

more, there is some suggestion that this rate may have risen somewhat during the 1970s; this may be part of the explanation for the unchanging overall risk of maternal mortality in England and Wales during the 1970s[19].

In addition to the costs of an increasing use of caesarean delivery in terms of maternal morbidity and possibly mortality, there are resource consequences to be considered. Five years ago[20] I estimated that if, in 1976, obstetricians in England and Wales had performed caesarean operations at the same rate as their American colleagues, an additional 35 000 women would have been subjected to this major surgical procedure at an additional cost to the health services of about £18 million. Similiar extrapolation using 1981 data suggests that there would have been an additional 115 000 operations in England and Wales at an additional cost of £88 million.

The costs of higher rates of caesarean delivery in terms of maternal mortality and morbidity, let alone the substantial resource consequences, could only be offset by scientifically strong evidence that fetal outcome is improved by more liberal use of the operation in particular clinical situations. There is no scientific evidence that a population caesarean delivery rate above 10% of all deliveries is justified. The available evidence suggests a variety of measures which could be used to contain the rate of caesarean deliveries below this level without compromising the health of either the fetus or the mother.

At one level, institutional changes are required:

1. Abolish differential fees and reimbursement rates for vaginal deliveries and caesarean deliveries.
2. Reduce pressure to practise defensive obstetrics by introducing 'no-fault' compensation for disability.
3. Institute regular, open, retrospective review of the justification for every caesarean operation performed.

At another level, there are clinical measures which can be taken to contain the rate of caesarean delivery:

1. Prevent and manage dystocia effectively, particularly in primigravidae.

2. Abolish policies of routine repeat caesarean section.
3. Only use continuous intrapartum fetal heart rate monitoring and diagnose fetal distress in conjunction with fetal acid–base assessment.
4. Manage breech presentation at term by external cephalic version under tocolysis.
5. Plan vaginal delivery for the frank breech presentation.

In addition, however, it is necessary to mount scientifically rigorous research to assess in what circumstances an extended use of the operation may be justified. The first research priority is to assess whether a policy of routine caesarean delivery offers any advantages to the immature or small fetus as compared with a more selective use of the operation. The published research in this field currently provides no scientifically sound evidence upon which to base clinical policies. Furthermore, such evidence will not be forthcoming unless clinical researchers abandon the observational approach and collaborate to mount clinical experiments which control for the selection biases which have plagued observational comparisons of caesarean and vaginal delivery for immature and small fetuses. As long as there is no evidence from randomized controlled trials upon which to base a more liberal use of caesarean delivery in these circumstances, obstetricians should resist the current pressures from neonatologists to subject mothers to what remains a major surgical procedure with the attendant risks to their well-being which this implies.

References

1. Chalmers, I. and Richards, M. P. M. (1977). Intervention and causal inference in obstetric practice. In Chard, T. and Richards, M. P. M. (eds.) *Benefits and Hazards of the New Obstetrics*, Clinics in Developmental Medicine, No. 64, pp. 34–61. (London: Spastics International Medical Publications/William Heinemann Medical Books)
2. Marieskind, H. I. (1979). An evaluation of caesarean section in the United States. (Washington DC: Department of Health, Education and Welfare)
3. Opit, L. J. and Selwood, T. S. (1979). Caesarean-section rates in Australia. *Med. J. Aust.*, **2**, 706–9
4. Francome, C. and Huntingford, P. J. (1980). Births by caesarean section in the United States of America and in Britain. *J. Biosoc. Sci.* **12**, 353–62
5. Bottoms, S. F., Rosen, M. G. and Sokol, R. J. (1980). The increase in the caesarean birth rate. *N. Engl. J. Med.*, **302**, 559–63
6. National Institutes of Health Consensus Development Task Force (1981). Statement on caesarean childbirth. *Am. J. Obstet. Gynecol.*, **139**, 902–9
7. Rosenberg, K., Hepburn, M. and McIlwaine, G. (1982). An audit of caesarean section in a maternity district. *Br. J. Obstet. Gynaecol.*, **89**, 787–92
8. Maternity Alliance (1983). One birth in nine: caesarean section trends since 1978. (Available from: Maternity Alliance, 309 Kentish Town Road, London NW5 2TJ, price £1.80, Telephone 01 267 3255)
9. O'Driscoll, K. and Foley, M. (1983). Correlation of decrease in perinatal mortality and increase in caesarean section rates. *Obstet. Gynecol.*, **61**, 1–5
10. Bergsjø, P., Schmidt, E. and Pusch, D. (1983). Differences in the reported frequencies of some obstetrical interventions in Europe. *Br. J. Obstet. Gynaecol.*, **90**, 628–32

11. Thiery, M. and Derom, R. (1984). Review of evaluative studies on caesarean section. Presented at the *EC Workshop on evaluative research in pre- peri- and post-natal care delivery systems*, 14–16 March, Brussels. (Publication details available from the authors at Department of Obstetrics, University of Gent, 9000-Gent, Belgium)
12. Guillemin, J. (1981). Babies by caesarean: who chooses, who controls? *Hastings Center Report*, **11**, 15–18
13. Janowitz, B., Nakamura, M. S., Lins, F. E., Brown, M. L. and Clopton, D. (1982). Caesarean section in Brazil. *Soc. Sci. Med.*, **16**, 19–25
14. Chalmers, I. and Macfarlane, J. A. (1979). Towards defensive obstetrics. *Lancet*, **1**, 53
15. Illingworth, R. S. (1979). Why blame the obstetrician? *Br. Med. J.*, **1**, 797–801
16. Mitchell, P. and Chalmers, I. (1980). Perinatal practice and compensation for handicap. *Br. Med. J.*, **2**, 868
17. Niswander, K. and Grant, A. (1982). Birth asphyxia and no-fault compensation. *Br. Med. J.*, **1**, 1555
18. Niswander, K., Henson, G., Elbourne, D., Chalmers, I., Redman, C., Macfarlane, J. A., and Tizard, P. (1984). Adverse outcome of pregnancy and the quality of obstetric care. *Lancet*, **2**, 827–31
19. Macfarlane, A. J. and Mugford, M. (1984). *Birth Counts: statistics of pregnancy and childbirth*. (London: HMSO)
20. Chalmers, I. (1979). The epidemiology of perinatal practice. *J. Maternal Child Health*, **4**, 435–6

23

Evolution of caesarean section in France

G. Breart

ABSTRACT

The surveys conducted in 1972, 1976 and 1981[1] by the epidemiological research unit on mother and child (INSERM, U149) on representative samples
of births, give data on the overall evolution of caesarean section rate in
France, as well as its variation by maternal and fetal characteristics.

OVERALL SECTION RATES BY PAST OBSTETRICAL HISTORY

Among singleton live births overall rate has increased: 6.2% in 1972, 8.7% in
1976 and 11.3% in 1981, and this increase is more important for section performed during labour.

The rate of intervention varies considerably according to past obstetrical
history. Among multiparas without previous section (group I) the rate is 4.5%
in 1981, it is 12.7% among primiparas (group II) and 72.5% among multiparas
with previous section (group III). The moment of the section varies as well,
since 83% of repeat sections are performed before labour compared to 41% of
sections performed among primiparas. Since the increase in section is
observed in the three groups, their distribution among women with section, is
very similar in 1972 and 1981: 49% of the women who had a section in 1981
were primiparous, 28% have had a section previously and 23% were multiparous (in 1972 the corresponding figures were 52%, 26% and 22%).

These figures suggest that, to decrease the overall section rate, one should
try first to lower the indications among primiparas since they represent half of
the sections. Such a policy would also result in a decrease of repeat section.

151

EVOLUTION OF SECTION RATES BY DIFFERENT CONDITIONS (Table 1)

Among primiparas, section rate before labour has increased mainly in case of non-cephalic presentation (+24%), hypertension (+10%), low birth weight (+8%) and preterm birth (+6%), whereas during labour it has increased mainly in case of fetal distress (+17%) and hypertension (+6%).

Table 1 Evolution, from 1972 to 1981, of caesarean section rate by past obstetrical history and conditions during the index pregnancy

| | Primiparas | | | Multiparas | | | | | |
| | | | | No. previous caesarean section | | | Previous caesarean section | | |
	1972	1981	p	1972	1981	p	1972	1981	p
Hypertension									
No. of cases	388	233		417	260		25	24	
Percentage of caesarean section									
before labour	2.3	12.4	<0.001	2.2	4.6	NS	40.0	79.2	<0.01
during labour	6.2	12.4	<0.01	1.9	3.5	NS	16.0	8.3	NS
Fetal distress									
No. of cases	524	268		473	205		25	10	
Percentage of caesarean section									
before labour	1.1	4.5	<0.01	0.6	6.8	<0.001	12.0	30.0	NS
during labour	7.6	24.6	<0.001	2.8	12.7	<0.001	24.0	40.0	NS
Malpresentation									
No. of cases	231	119		185	109		16	13	
Percentage of caesarean section									
before labour	13.8	37.8	<0.001	11.3	13.8	NS	62.5	76.9	NS
during labour	22.9	22.7	NS	13.0	22.0	<0.05	25.0	23.1	NS
Birthweight <2500 g									
No. of cases	263	104		250	91		10	11	
Percentage of caesarean section									
before labour	4.6	12.5	<0.01	3.2	15.4	<0.001	50.0	54.5	NS
during labour	3.0	5.8	NS	2.4	6.6	NS	0	27.3	NS
Gestational age ≤36 weeks									
No. of cases	287	105		426	132		12	15	
Percentage of caesarean section									
before labour	2.4	8.6	<0.01	2.1	8.3	<0.001	8.3	53.3	<0.05
during labour	2.8	4.8	NS	0.9	4.5	<0.01	16.7	20.0	NS
Overall									
No. of cases	4633	2211		5618	2913		265	219	
Percentage of caesarean section									
before labour	2.4	5.2	<0.001	1.4	2.2	<0.001	46.4	59.8	<0.01
during labour	4.8	7.5	<0.001	1.1	2.3	<0.001	17.0	12.8	NS

Among multiparas who never had a caesarean before, the section rate before labour has increased mainly in cases of low birth weight (+12%), preterm birth or fetal distress (+ 6%). During labour it has increased mainly in cases of fetal distress (+10%) and non-cephalic presentation (+9%).

These variations lead to an important modification in the pathologies which are mentioned when a section has been performed (Table 2) (it has not been possible to study dystocia). In 1981 fetal distress is the most cited pathology whereas in 1972 it was malpresentation.

Table 2 Percentage of mentioned pathologies among women with caesarean section

	Primiparas		Multiparas without previous caesarean section	
	1972 *(%)*	*1981* *(%)*	*1972* *(%)*	*1981* *(%)*
Fetal distress	14	29	12	31
Hypertension	10	21	12	16
Malpresentation	25	26	32	30
Birth weight <2500 g	6	7	10	15
Gestational age ≤36 weeks	4	5	9	13

Among multiparas with previous section, the above pathologies were responsible for only a limited number of sections, the increase appearing ascribable to systematic repeated caesareans.

Reference

1. Rumeau-Rouquette, C., Du Mazaubrun, C. and Rabarison, Y. (1984). *Naître en France, 10 ans d'évolution* (Paris: INSERM)

24

Caesarean section and perinatal mortality rates

K. O'Driscoll and P. Crowley

RECENT EXPERIENCE IN THE UNITED STATES

There have been few more dramatic changes across the whole range of medical practice than the explosive growth in caesarean section in recent times. With the incidence of caesarean section reaching 20% in the United States of America and 11% in the United Kingdom the problem can be justifiably regarded as a public health epidemic in the western world. The extent of change is best illustrated by the United States where the incidence increased from 5% of total births in 1970 to an estimated 20% in 1980: a 4-fold increase in 10 years. In numerical terms this represents 350 000 caesarean births, up from 150 000 to 600 000 per annum[1].

The precipitous fall in perinatal mortality rates that occurred during the same decade has been attributed to the increased use of caesarean section[2]. A special committee convened under the auspices of the National Institutes for Health to enquire into the escalating caesarean section rates, was impressed by the lack of evidence in support of this alleged cause-and-effect relationship[3]. However, evidence was not available as to the possible outcome in terms of perinatal mortality had the caesarean section birth rate been maintained at the previous level of 5%.

THE DUBLIN EXPERIENCE

The evidence sought by the National Institutes of Health task force is available from the National Maternity Hospital, Dublin, where the caesarean section rate has remained unchanged at 4.2% in 1970, 4.8% in 1980 and 4.4% in the first half of 1984. During the decade 1970–80 the perinatal mortality rate for infants over 500 grams fell from 36.5 per 1000 in 1970 to 16.8 per 1000 in 1980. This fall in perinatal mortality rates compares favourably with that experienced in United States centres with a 3–4-fold higher caesarean section rate[4]. Figure 1 represents that dramatic fall in perinatal mortality rate, juxtaposed against the static incidence of birth by caesarean section over the same period. Figure 2 represents the corresponding trends for the United States. Table 1 summarizes the most recent available statistics from the National Maternity Hospital, Dublin.

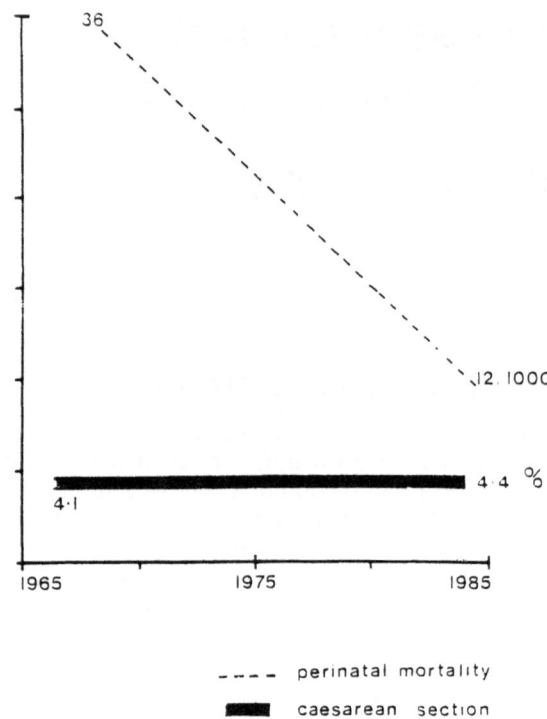

Figure 1 National Maternity Hospital

CLASSIFICATION OF CAESAREAN SECTION BY INDICATION

The National Institutes of Health consensus development statement contributed a useful diagnostic system for categorizing the indications for caesarean section[3]. Using this system, figures from the United States can be compared with figures from the National Maternity Hospital[5] (Table 2). In practice this classification can be simplified into three main groups, which in the United States in 1978 each accounted for 5% of all births. These three groups are: primary caesarean section for dystocia, repeat caesarean sections, and primary caesarean sections for breech presentation, fetal distress and other indications.

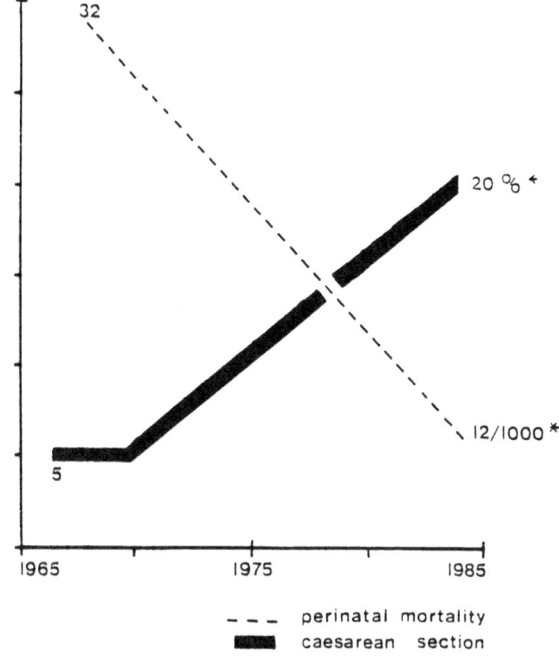

Figure 2   United States of America[4] (figures with asterisk are estimates)

DYSTOCIA

The seven-to-one differential between primary caesarean sections for dystocia in the United States compared with the National Maternity Hospital is striking. The low incidence of primary caesarean section for dystocia at the National Maternity Hospital has been achieved by early detection and prompt treatment of dystocia by non-surgical means[6]. A substantial reduction in the incidence of caesarean section for dystocia could be achieved in the United States by a new approach to the management of normal primigravid labour. The National Institutes of Health task force emphasized the need to review all aspects of the diagnostic category referred to as dystocia because of the nationwide prominence afforded to this indication for caesarean section.

REPEAT CAESAREAN SECTION

A further 5% of babies born in the United States are delivered by repeat caesarean section. There is a 4-fold differential between the United States and the National Maternity Hospital, with respect to this indication. This discrepancy stems partly from the fact that there are more primary caesarean sections in the United States, giving rise to repeat caesarean sections and partly because of the almost universal adherence to the precept 'once a caesarean section always a caesarean section'. A reduction in caesarean sections in this category

Table 1   National Maternity Hospital, Dublin, 1 January 1984–30 June 1984

Total births	3937
Caesarean section births	170 (4.4%)
Forceps deliveries	208 (5.4%)
Self deliveries	3659 (90.2%)
Perinatal deaths*	49 (12.4‰)
Lethal malformations	20 (5‰)
Corrected perinatal mortality rate	7.4‰

* Refers to all stillbirths of greater than 28 weeks or more than 1000 grams birthweight and neonatal deaths up to 7 days of age

is achievable firstly by reducing primary caesarean sections and secondly by aiming for vaginal delivery in a higher proportion of women with a previous caesarean section. In the National Maternity Hospital over two-thirds of women with a previous caesarean section are delivered vaginally.

Table 2   Frequency of caesarean deliveries according to diagnostic categories

	Indication	United States (1978)	National Maternity Hospital (1980)	Ratio US rate: National Maternity Hospital rate
Category 1	Dystocia	4.7	0.7	7
Category 2	Repeat section	4.7	1.1	4
Category 3	Breech	1.8 ⎫	0.6 ⎫	
	Fetal distress	0.8 ⎬ 5.8	0.5 ⎬ 3.0	2
	Others	3.2 ⎭	1.9 ⎭	

BREECH, FETAL DISTRESS AND OTHER INDICATIONS

The contrasts between the United States figures and the National Maternity Hospital are less stark with respect to the third category – caesarean section for breech presentation. Assuming that the incidence of breech presentation is similar in the two populations the 3-fold differential in caesarean section rate represents a reluctance to attempt vaginal delivery in the presence of a breech presentation, in the United States. The close similarity in the incidence of caesarean section for fetal distress between the two populations is surprising in view of the fact that the dramatic expansion in caesarean births in the United States was motivated almost exclusively out of concern for the welfare of the child.

The differential under the heading 'others' is comparatively small: less than two to one. The most likely explanation is that the indications for caesarean section least in dispute are included here, and that these represent a much larger proportion of the smaller number of operations performed in the National Maternity Hospital. Foremost of these complications is antepartum haemorrhage which competes with dystocia as the main indication for primary caesarean section in Dublin but no longer figures in the United States because it has been overtaken by increases elsewhere.

SUMMARY AND CONCLUSIONS

Experience at the National Maternity Hospital, Dublin, since 1970 shows that a substantial fall in perinatal mortality rates can be achieved without any increase in caesarean section rate. These results invalidate the hypothesis that the improved perinatal mortality rates experienced in the United States over the same period are attributable to the 3–4–fold increase in caesarean section rate over the same period. A comparison between United States caesarean sections and caesarean sections at the National Maternity Hospital shows that the most substantial savings in caesarean sections are to be made in the area of dystocia. Improved management of normal primigravid labour could achieve a reduction both directly, by reducing the number of primary caesarean sections, and indirectly, by reducing repeat caesarean sections. Further, smaller reductions could be made by allowing more women with a previous caesarean section and with breech presentation to deliver vaginally.

References

1. Rubin, G. L., Peterson, H. B. and Rochat, R. W. (1981). Maternal death after caesarean section in Georgia. *Am. J. Obstet. Gynecol.*, **139**, 681–5
2. Jones, O. H. (1976). Caesarean section in present-day obstetrics. *Am. J. Obstet. Gynecol.*, **126**, 521–5
3. National Institutes of Health Consensus Development Statement on caesarean childbirth. *Obstet. Gynecol.*, **57**, 537–41
4. Bottoms, S. F., Rosen, M. G. and Sokol, R. J. (1980). The increase in caesarean birth rate. *N. Engl. J. Med.*, **302**, 559–63
5. O'Driscoll, K. and Foley, M. (1980). Correlation of decrease in perinatal mortality and increase in caesarean section rates. *Obstet. Gynecol.*, **61**, 1–5
6. O'Driscoll, K., Jackson, R. J. and Gallagher, J. T. (1969). Prevention of prolonged labour. *Br. Med. J.*, **2**, 477–80

25

Situation in the German Federal Republic

F. Kubli

It is not possible to give a complete and reliable account on what is going on in terms of caesarean section in West Germany. However, some available data may serve as indicators and give some idea of the situation.

Table 1 Some data on caesarean section at the Department of Obstetrics and Gynaecology, University Hospitals, Heidelberg

1. *Incidence of caesarean section*
1973 → 1983: 9.2% → 20.0%

2. *Relationship intrapartum : antepartum caesarean section*
1977: 7.5 : 7.4%
1983: 5.8 : 14.2%

3. *Birth weight ≤2500 g*
1973: 13% of all caesarean sections (n = 20)
1983: 22% of all caesarean sections (n = 60)

4. *Breech presentation*
1973: percentage caesarean section: 55% (n = 38) = 25% of all caesarean sections
1983: percentage caesarean section: 87% (n = 90) = 33% of all caesarean sections

5. *Number of deliveries, percentage ≤2500 g and percentage breech presentation*

	n total	≤2500 g	Breech
1973	1605	8.5%	4.4%
1983	1337	11.7%	7.8%

CAESAREAN SECTION AT THE
DEPARTMENT OF OBSTETRICS AND GYNAECOLOGY,
UNIVERSITY OF HEIDELBERG

Some figures are given in Table 1. From 1973 to 1983 the incidence has more than doubled from 9.2% to 20%. This rise has been accompanied by an unchanged incidence of severe acidaemia (pH<7.10) in the umbilical artery and a slight but significant drop in perinatal mortality. It is felt, however, that the latter is primarily due to improved results of the neonatal intensive care unit and is the cause rather than the effect of the increase in abdominal deliveries. Compared to 1977, intrapartum caesarean section in 1983 had somewhat decreased, but the incidence of antepartum caesarean section had doubled. This reflects a growing attitude to decide for abdominal deliveries not on the basis of complications of labour, but of pre-existing pregnancy characteristics. Thus low birth weight infants accounted for 22% of all caesarean sections in 1983 against 13% in 1973. Breech presentations were delivered abdominally in 87% in 1983, compared to 55% in 1973, corresponding to one-quarter of all caesarean sections in 1973 and one-third in 1983. Finally, these figures also reflect an increased referral of risk pregnancies to the department, with an increase of low birth weight deliveries by 3% and an incidence of single breech deliveries in 1983 of 7.8%. More liberal use of abdominal deliveries with breech presentations, low and especially very low birth weight infants and more recently also with some viable malformations seem to be primarily responsible for the excessive caesarean section rate in this centre.

Table 2 Survey on management of breech presentation by questionnaire. List of participating hospitals as of September 1984

Univ. Clinic	Gent	(B)	Ziekenhuis	Breda	(NL)
Univ. Clinic	Brüssel	(B)	Ziekenhuis	Den Haag	(NL)
Kommunehospital	Aarhus	(D)	Ziekenhuis	Eindhoven	(NL)
Amts Sygehus	Glostrup	(D)	Ziekenhuis	Enschede	(NL)
Frauenklinik	Berlin-Neukölln	(GFR)	Hospital	Heerlen	(NL)
Univ. Frauenklinik	Bonn	(GFR)	Groot Ziekengasthuis	Hertogenbosch	(NL)
Univ. Frauenklinik	Mainz	(GFR)	Laurentiusziekenhuis	Roermond	(NL)
Univ. Frauenklinik	Würzburg	(GFR)	Canisius-Wilhelmina-Hospital	Nijmegen	(NL)
Univ. Frauenklinik	Heidelberg	(GFR)	Radbondziekenhuis	Nijmegen	(NL)
Univ. Frauenklinik	Halle	(GDR)	Sentralsykehuset	Nordbyhagen	(N)
Univ. Clinic	Helsinki	(SF)	Landesfrauenklinik	Linz	(A)
Univ. Clinic	Kuopio	(SF)	Univ. Frauenklinik	Wien I	(A)
Univ. Clinic	Oulu	(SF)	Univ. Frauenklinik	Wien II	(A)
Univ. Clinic	Tampere	(SF)	Regionsjukhuset	Ørebro	(S)
Clinique Gynecoloque	Lille	(F)	Karolinska sjukhuset	Stockholm	(S)
Service de Gynecologie	Suresnes	(F)	Academic Hospital	Uppsala	(S)
Service de Gynecologie	Strasbourg Cedex	(F)	Aker Hospital	Oslo	(S)
Hospital	Hull	(GB)	Univ. Frauenklinik	Lund	(S)
John Radcliffe Hospital	Oxford	(GB)	Univ. Frauenklinik	Lausanne	(Ch)
Queen Mother's Hospital	Glasgow	(GB)	Kantonspital	Münsterlingen	(Ch)
Istituto per l'Infanzia	Trieste	(I)	Univ. Clinico	Barcelona	(E)
Univ. Clinic	Trieste	(I)	Maternidad de 'la Paz'	Madrid	(E)
			Univ. School	Debrecen	(H)

CAESAREAN SECTION IN THE
BAVARIAN PERINATAL STUDY

The Bavarian Perinatal Study accumulates regionally based, non-selective data of almost 100 000 pregnancies per year and thus gives rather extensive and seemingly reliable data on about one-sixth of all deliveries in West Germany. The data therefore might be considered as representative for the situation in West Germany.

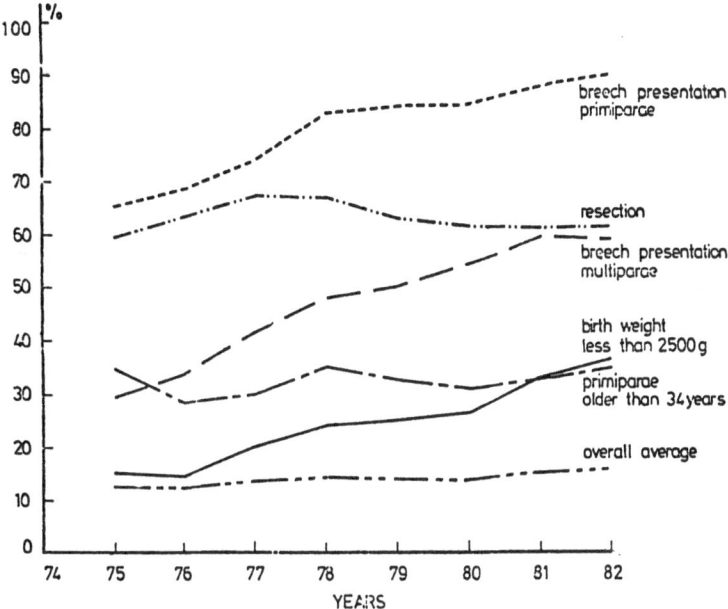

Figure 1   Bavarian Perinatal Study. Trends in caesarean section 1975–82. Data based on approximately 90 000 deliveries annually

The trends in incidence, overall and for specific indications, are given in Figure 1. Overall there was only a slight increase during the period 1975–82. In 1983 the incidence of abdominal deliveries was 13.7%. Over recent years there has been a parallel increase in caesarean section rates with breech presentation both for first pregnancies and multiparas, and a similar increase for abdominal deliveries with low birth weight infants, whereas repeat caesarean section as main or only indication has been decreasing. In 1983, 76% of all breech presentations were delivered abdominally.

INTERNATIONAL SURVEY ON MANAGEMENT
OF BREECH PRESENTATION

A questionnaire was sent to hospitals throughout Europe, as had been done previously in 1975. Up to September 1984, answers had been returned by about 40 hospitals listed in Table 2. The results will be published in detail later; but it is important to note that the question: 'Do you feel that systematic pre-labour caesarean section in all breech presentations irrespective of parity and gestational age is justified?' was virtually unanimously (43 out of 44 answers) answered by 'NO'. On the other hand, as is shown in Figure 2, a substantial increase in abdominal deliveries with breech presentation has occurred since 1975 in the majority of hospitals.

COMMENT

The rate of caesarean section in the German Federal Republic may be estimated – on the basis of the Bavarian Perinatal Study – to be around 13–15% and may, in some centres like the Heidelberg Department of Obstetrics and Gynaecology, run as high as 20%. These figures are high and certainly must give rise to concern and reflection to all those carrying responsibility.

On the other hand, caesarean section rates cannot be judged without taking into consideration results in terms of pregnancy outcome. Thus it can be noted (Figure 3), that perinatal mortality in Germany in the time period 1976–82 demonstrated an over-average fall compared to many other European countries. For the Bavarian Perinatal Study *uncorrected* perinatal mortality in 1983 was 5.9/1000 in babies weighing 1000 g and more, and 7.7/1000 in babies weighing 500 g and more.

Whereas it is probable that the high caesarean section rate may have contributed to what is felt to be very good results in perinatal outcome, the rise in abdominal deliveries may have been over-proportional and certainly all efforts should be made to prevent a further increase and if possible to lower the present rate. A more liberal approach to vaginal delivery with term breech presentation is certainly possible in our own department, but overall the caes-

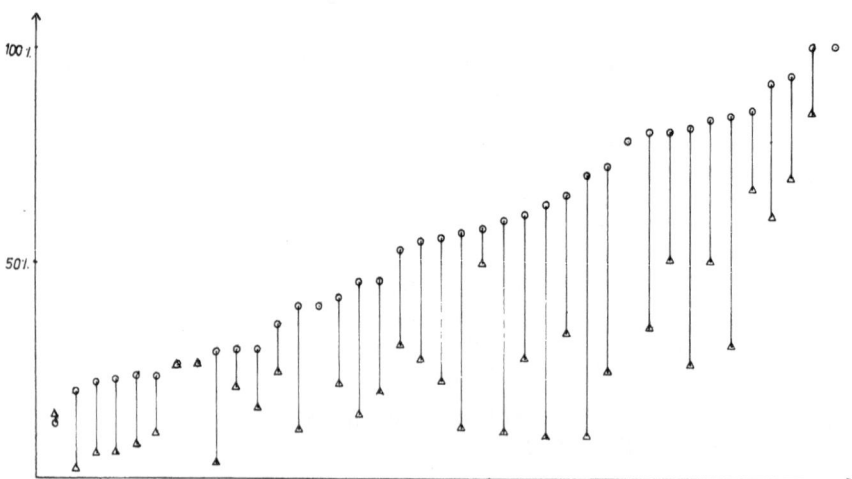

Figure 2 A survey by questionnaire on the management of breech presentation. Comparison of caesarean section rates 1975 and 1983 for 40 different hospitals throughout Europe (△ = 1975; ⊙ = 1983)

arean section rate with breech presentation will probably remain in the range of 60–70%. In a similar way, whereas excessive section rates with very low birth weight infants may be subject to correction, overall one would – with steadily increasing survivals in the neonatal intensive care units – not expect to see this figure drop substantially in the near future. What really is at the bottom of most high caesarean section rates is concern and possibly over-concern not so much of perinatal mortality, but of long-term infant morbidity. The best way to cope with the rising caesarean section rates will be to get better and more reliable data on the relationships between obstetrical man-agement and short-term as well as long-term infant morbidity and handicap.

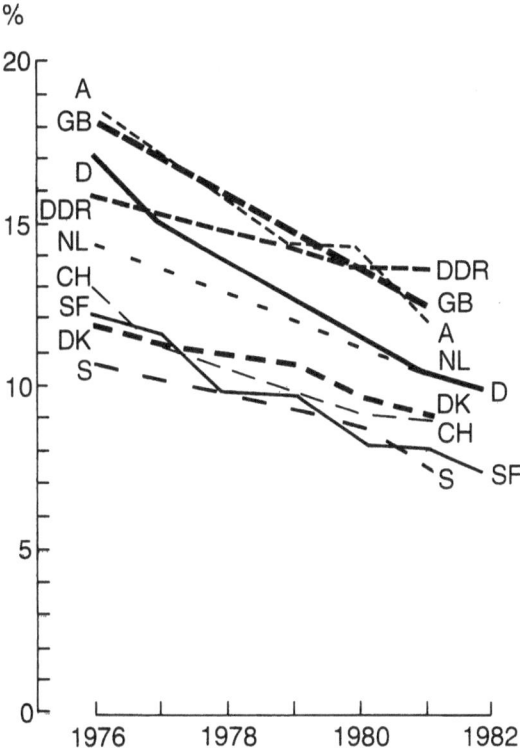

Figure 3 Perinatal mortality 1976–82 in different European countries. D = German Federal Republic (according to data by the Bayer. Statist. Landesamt.)

26

The European survey of obstetrical interventions

P. Bergsjø

The frequency of caesarean sections increased dramatically through the 1970s. The only way to get the true picture is through population-based statistics, in which all births in a defined area are counted; not only those from single hospitals.

It is impossible to draw meaningful conclusions without first knowing what really goes on. A perinatal study group of the WHO European Region collected information on existing perinatal rules and practices, in the years 1979–83. A detailed questionnaire was sent to all European member states, not through official government bodies, but to individuals with detailed knowledge of perinatology within the countries. Answers came in from 24 countries, and the full report has been presented elsewhere[1]. This is a brief summary. The questions on operative delivery concerned easily defined interventions, such as caesarean section, vacuum extraction and forceps delivery.

Among the 24 countries only 13, about half, had national data of some sort. Caesarean section figures from 1978 or 1979 showed large variations from 3.6% in the Netherlands to 11.7% in Sweden. The Eastern European countries which answered had 4% for Czechoslovakia, 5% for Poland and 8% for Hungary. For forceps the figures varied from 0.3% of all deliveries (Finland and Sweden) to about 13% in the United Kingdom. For vacuum extraction the situation was reversed. No figures were given for the United Kingdom, but they are thought to be approximately 0, while Sweden and Denmark were highest with 7–9%. The sums of operative deliveries varied from 6% in Poland and Czechoslovakia to 24% in Scotland. The Nordic countries were in the high range, with Finland and Norway as the lowest of the Nordic countries. Obviously the frequencies of caesarean section must be viewed in connection with the vaginal operative deliveries. However, associations are

167

not pre-evident. One possibility is that increasing use of caesarean section makes operative vaginal deliveries less necessary, and the other that our attitudes have changed, so that both types of operative intervention are used more frequently. The analysis does not give support to any of the two hypotheses, at least not for the 11 European countries for which data were available.

Concerning the connection between operative delivery and perinatal mortality there was a slight negative correlation. It is reasonable to assume that increased resort to operative deliveries will lower perinatal mortality, but other factors may be equally or more important. For example, in the Netherlands with a perinatal mortality of 12 per 1000 the frequency of operative delivery was 9%, against 20% in France, where the perinatal mortality was 16 per 1000.

It is impossible to base a meaningful discussion on the figures that emerged from the European survey. They represent a single year, and many pertinent factors are left out. It is surprising how little the official bodies know about medical practice in this field. We of the medical profession have a tendency to say that everything we do is medically indicated, but when medical indications are so elastic as this survey reveals, the intelligent layman can easily rebut our arguments. I believe that critical analysis is necessary. In this process statistical surveillance of important perinatal events is a necessary step.

Reference

1. Bergsjø, P., Schmidt, E. and Pusch, D. (1983). Differences in the reported frequencies of some obstetrical interventions in Europe. *Br. J. Obstet. Gynaecol.*, **90**, 628–32

Chairman's summary

M. Thiery

In most of the developed countries caesarean section (CS) rates have risen steadily during the past decade and some of these rates have now reached figures which can no longer be considered to be in the interest of the child[1].

Unduly high caesarean birth rates must be curbed, mainly on behalf of the mother. Dr Chalmers has suggested that one of the reasons for our inability to reduce maternal mortality rates significantly is the increased use of abdominal delivery.

However, it remains a moot question how to reduce CS rates without affecting the perinatal outcome, mainly because the factors responsible for the increased CS rates differ so widely between countries and hospitals. Besides the specific (obstetric) factors there are a number of general factors which are difficult to assess and interpret but which encouraged obstetricians, once surgical mortality had declined, to resort more and more often to the abdominal route of delivery.

Measures to curb rising CS rates must be aetiologic in nature, i.e. must be directed at the factors responsible for the phenomenon, and several speakers have put forward examples. To cite but two: the active management of nulliparous labour (Professor O'Driscoll) and the introduction of local or even regional audits on abdominal delivery (Dr Chalmers).

Notwithstanding the countless unanswered questions, there can be no doubt that progress has recently been made. This is reflected by (1) the professional and public concern about increasing surgical rates, (2) the assessment of alternative obstetric solutions on the basis of random studies, and (3) the collection of reliable national or at least regional data on surgical delivery and perinatal/maternal mortality/morbidity rates.

Reference

1. Thiery, M. and Derom, R. (1985). Review of evaluative studies on caesarean section. Medical aspects. In *Proceedings E.C. Workshop on Pre-, Peri-, and Postnatal Care Delivery Systems*. (Berlin: Springer Verlag; in press)

Section 7
Persistent
Fetal Circulation

27

Physiological control
of the pulmonary circulation

A. Wilkinson

Pulmonary blood flow in the fetus is dependent on pulmonary vascular resistance. This is high, primarily because the small pulmonary arterioles are constricted in response to the low arterial oxygen saturation. Only 7% of combined ventricular output usually flows to the lungs. The major branches of the pulmonary arterial tree are complete halfway through gestation and the preacinar arteries have a well-developed muscular layer. Late in gestation pulmonary vascular resistance decreases as the cross-sectional area of the vessels increases, but this change has not occurred in preterm babies.

Developmental steps are essential in the reflex control of the circulation and immaturity may give rise to paradoxical or inadequate responses. Sympathetic and parasympathetic nerve endings are present in the fetal myocardium and a baro reflex is found in lambs in late gestation. Aortic and carotid chemoreceptors are present and respond to hypoxia, acidosis and hypotension. The pulmonary vasculature is extremely reactive and a rise in oxygen or decrease in carbon dioxide tension leads to vasodilatation. Vasoactive agents such as bradykinin and isoprenaline have similar effects. The significance of hormonal effects such as vasoconstriction produced by adrenaline is not known in the human fetus, but recent work has shown the important modulating effect that prostaglandins have on the vessel tone and hence blood flow. Prostaglandins of the E series and prostacyclin inhibit calcium metabolism at cell membranes, thus encouraging vasodilatation. An opposing effect is mediated by the prostaglandins of the F series and thromboxane. The pulmonary vasculature is extremely sensitive to changes in oxygen tension. Postnatally, as breathing is established, systemic resistance increases and pulmonary vascular resistance decreases markedly with expansion of the lungs and the rapid increase in oxygen tension. This is accompanied by a 7–10-fold increase in pulmonary blood flow and, when the ductus arteriosus constricts, a decrease in pulmonary arterial pressure[1]. Maximal dilatation of the ductus arteriosus *in utero* by

prostaglandins has been shown by experiments in which perfusion of prostaglandins did not lead to further dilatation but an inhibitor of prostaglandin synthesis, indomethacin, caused significant constriction[2]. The use of inhibitors of
prostaglandin synthesis to delay parturition may be associated with constriction of the ductus arteriosis and postnatal pulmonary hypertension with severe
hypoxaemia[3].

An abnormally high pulmonary vascular resistance may be maintained after
birth as a result of various factors (see Table 1).

Table 1   Factors that may lead to elevated pulmonary vascular resistance
postnatally

---

1. *Normal pulmonary vessel development*
Pulmonary vasoconstriction due to hypoxaemia and metabolic acidosis or
elevated haematocrit

2. *Abnormal pulmonary vascular smooth muscle development*
Chronic fetal growth retardation with hypoxaemia
Prenatal constriction of ductus arteriosus
Congenital heart disease

3. *Decreased cross-sectional area of pulmonary vascular bed*
Abnormal development of chest wall
Diaphragmatic hernia
Adenomatous lung malformation
Maternal ingestion of prostaglandin synthetase inhibitors
Congenital heart disease

After normal development the response of the pulmonary circulation to
hypoxaemia and metabolic acidosis involves major adaptive changes including
a decrease in heart rate, a rise in blood pressure and a decrease in cardiac
output. Regional blood flow is redistributed predominantly to the heart and
the brain at the expense of blood flow to the limbs, lungs and kidneys. The organization of this response through the chemoreflexes and hormonal mechanisms is not fully elucidated. Changes in regional blood flow after an asphyxial
insult lead to the lungs, which have an oxygen consumption of 5.4% of the
total fetal oxygen consumption, receiving a lower blood flow of more poorly
oxygenated blood. The effect of this on surfactant synthesis may be responsible for the adverse affect that asphyxia, particularly during labour, has on
lung function immediately after birth[4].

Similar effects may be seen when there is an increased pulmonary vascular
smooth muscle layer, as is seen after chronic fetal hypoxia and congenital
heart disease (particularly with a raised haematocrit level). Finally, the cross-
sectional area of the pulmonary vascular bed may be decreased as a result of
maldevelopment of the lungs, resulting from thoracic wall deformities, diaphragmatic hernia or adenomatous malformation. Drugs such as prostaglandins synthetase inhibitors (e.g. indomethacin, aspirin, naproxen), taken
throughout pregnancy have been implicated in changes in pulmonary vascular
development[5].

Conclusions

The pathophysiology of the postnatal control of the pulmonary circulation is complex and several factors may coexist and interact. Therapeutic measures must be applied cautiously in the light of this knowledge to avoid paradoxically adverse effects[6].

References

1. Rudolph, A. M. (1977). Fetal and neonatal pulmonary circulation. *Am. Rev. Resp. Dis.*, **115**, 11
2. Friedman, W. F., Printz, M. P., Kirkpatrick, S. E. and Hoskins, E. J. (1983). The vasoactivity of the fetal lamb ductus arteriosus studied in utero. *Pediatr. Res.*, **17**, 331–74
3. Wilkinson, A. R., Aynsley-Green, A. and Mitchell, M. D. (1979). Persistent pulmonary hypertension and abnormal prostaglandin E levels in preterm infants after maternal treatment with naproxen. *Arch. Dis. Child.*, **12**, 942–5
4. Hallman, M. and Kankaanpaa, K. (1980). Evidence of surfactant deficiency in persistence of the fetal circulation. *Eur. J. Paediatr.*, **134**, 129–34
5. Levin, D. L., Filxler, D. E., Morriss, F. C. and Tyson, J. (1978). Morphological analysis of the pulmonary vascular bed in infants exposed in utero to prostaglandin synthetase inhibitors. *J. Pediatr.*, **92**, 478–83
6. Drummond, W. H. and Lock, J. E. (1984). Neonatal pulmonary vasodilator drugs: current status. *Dev. Pharmacol. Ther.*, **7**, 1–20

28

Persistent fetal circulation – aetiology

R. Cooke

Persistent pulmonary hypertension may be a contributing factor to many pulmonary diseases in the newborn; but the diagnosis persistent fetal circulation is usually reserved for those infants in whom the pulmonary hypertension is accompanied by minimal or no lung disease. The infants are usually at or near term and show clinical signs of cyanosis (even with oxygen therapy), a variable degree of respiratory distress and clinical signs of right ventricular strain (parasternal heave and active precordium). X-ray appearances are very variable. Characteristically clear lung fields indicative of under-perfusion are seen, but frequently the lung fields are abnormal and the appearances nonspecific. The cardiac outline is usually normal.

The principal differential diagnoses are between respiratory distress syndrome and congenital heart disease. The former condition almost invariably improves with oxygen administration and appropriate ventilator therapy, and is accompanied by a greater degree of respiratory distress. Transposition of the great vessels, total anomalous pulmonary venous drainage, severe pulmonary stenosis, and Ebstein's anomaly are the forms of cardiac disease most likely to provide diagnostic problems. The ECG is frequently normal in persistent fetal circulation although in infants who have experienced considerable asphyxia around the time of birth depression of ST segment in the ECG may be observed. In transposition of the great vessels the ECG is often normal or shows right ventricular hypertrophy and right atrial hypertrophy. Total anomalous pulmonary venous drainage is characterized by right atrial and ventricular hypertrophy often together with right axis deviation. Pulmonary stenosis usually shows right ventricular hypertrophy, particularly when severe. Ebstein's anomaly shows right bundle branch block with Wolff–Parkinson–White anomaly and right atrial hypertrophy.

Echocardiography, preferably using two-dimensional real-time scanning, is the most useful method of differential diagnosis. The demonstration of four normal chambers with normal arterial and venous connection makes the diagnosis of persistent fetal circulation almost certain. Using M-mode echocardiography, systolic time intervals may be determined. When pulmonary hypertension is present the ratio between the pre-ejection and ejection time of the pulmonary valve is increased, from a normal of about 0.25 to as high as 0.6 or 0.7. These findings are unfortunately not specific to persistent fetal circulation, and are often seen in severe hyaline membrane disease and some forms of congenital heart disease. Theoretically the systolic time intervals could be used for following the response to therapy, but in practice more easily measured variables such as the arterial oxygen tension are more directly useful.

The treatment of infants with persistent fetal circulation is directed to general supportive measures, and attempts at vasodilatation of the pulmonary vascular bed. Oxygenation and support of the circulation are the first priority. Correction of acidosis may improve cardiac output which may be poor following a postnatal or intrauterine hypoxia. When using mechanical ventilation it should be remembered that high pressures are unlikely to improve the right to left shunt that exists, but may well increase the risk of barotrauma to the lungs.

The general aim should be to produce moderate hypocarbia in order to encourage pulmonary vasodilatation. If the mean arterial blood pressure is low the use of isoprenaline or dopamine infusions in conjunction with moderate volume expansion with blood or plasma may be very helpful. Pulmonary vasodilatation with various agents may only be safely attempted with a normal blood pressure. Continuous blood pressure monitoring and blood or plasma for infusion should be to hand. All vasodilators to date are non-specific, and so dilatation of the pulmonary vasculature is accompanied by systemic vasodilatation also. If the latter is as great as, or greater than, that of the pulmonary circulation, the net effect is to worsen the problem.

Tolazoline is the widest-used vasodilator, but complications due to hypotension are frequent.[1] There is still no controlled evidence to suggest that its use alters the eventual outcome of the disorder. Prostaglandin E2 is frequently used now to maintain patency of the ductus arteriosus in the presence of ductus-dependent congenital heart disease. It is also a vasodilator, and has been used successfully in the treatment of persistent fetal circulation. Prostacyclin (epoprostenol, PGI_2) is a newer, more potent prostenoid, with a powerful vasodilator action. It has the advantage of a short half-life so that if systemic hypotension occurs, discontinuation of the infusion results in rapid return of the systemic blood pressure. Unfortunately, it is at present extremely expensive.

The mortality of infants with isolated persistent fetal circulation is high and despite therapy is usually quoted as about 50%. Those infants likely to recover usually show some improvement soon after the institution of therapy, although final recovery may take 7–10 days or more.

The aetiology of primary persistent fetal circulation is obscure. Recent work has shown that the lung lavage fluids of infants with persistent fetal circulation contained leukotrienes C4 and D4, in contrast to other ventilated infants in whom no leukotrienes could be detected[2]. Leukotrienes are known to be potent vasoconstrictors and cause other symptoms of persistent fetal circulation such as poor cardiac output, hypotension and an increase in capillary vascular permeability. Although it was not possible to determine whether the leukotrienes were causative or secondary to the persistent fetal circulation, their absence in other ventilated infants suggests the former explanation. The use of other prostanoids with a counter-action would seem a logical approach to therapy. The aetiology of the high levels of leukotrienes is unknown.

Histological studies of the pulmonary vasculature of infants dying of persistent fetal circulation has shown that the characteristic lesion is medial hypertrophy of the pulmonary vessels[3]. In the normal full-term newborn infant muscularization of the pulmonary vessels extends as far down the vascular tree as the level of the terminal bronchiole, but does not extend into the ascinus. In infants with persistent fetal circulation muscularization extended strikingly into all arteries in the wall of the alveoli or alveolar ducts. Perhaps more notably the extent of this muscularization caused a marked increase in the medial thickness of normally non-muscular arteries causing severe narrowing of the lumen. This observation has two important implications. Firstly, animal experiments suggest that such a degree of hypertrophy may take as many as 4 weeks to develop under the influence of hypoxia, indicating that the condition is likely to be the result of chronic intrauterine hypoxia rather than peripartum events. Secondly, since the lesion is causing increased pulmonary vascular resistance by its obstructive nature (likened to hypertrophic obstructive cardiomyopathy) it is not likely to be easily amenable to vasodilator therapy in many cases. The aetiology of medial hypertrophy is thought to be primarily hypoxic and the mechanism suggested to be mediated through the effect of angiotensin II. Although some infants with persistent fetal circulation are clearly growth-retarded and show signs of an adverse intrauterine environment, the majority are normally grown. This has led to the suggestion that the condition may arise secondarily to an abnormally sensitive pulmonary vascular bed rather than to severe chronic intrauterine hypoxia. If this is so it may make antepartum diagnosis of many affected individuals difficult or impossible with current techniques.

An alternative hypothesis, that fetal systemic hypertension, or early constriction of the ductus arteriosus, occurs *in utero*, has some support from an animal model in the sheep[4].

References

1. Drummond, W. H., Gregory, G. A., Heymann, M. A. and Phibbs, R. A. (1981). The independent effects of hyperventilation, tolazoline and dopamine on infants with persistent pulmonary hypertension. *J. Pediatr.*, **98**, 603–11
2. Stenmark, K. R., James, S. L., Voelkel, N. F., Toews, W. H., Reeves, J. T. and Murphy, R. C. (1983). Leukotriene C4 + D4 in neonates with hypoxaemia and pulmonary hypertension. *N. Engl. J. Med.*, **309**, 77–80
3. Murphy, J. D., Rabinovitch, M., Golstein, J. D. and Reid, L. M. (1981). The structural basis of persistent pulmonary hypertension in the newborn infant. *J. Pediatr.*,

98, 962–7

4. Levin, D. L., Hyman, A. I., Heymann, M. A. and Rudolph, A. M. (1978). Fetal hypertension and the development of increased pulmonary vascular smooth muscle: a possible mechanism for persistent pulmonary hypertension of the newborn infant. *J. Pediatr.*, **92**, 265–9

29

Persistent fetal circulation complicating other neonatal lung disorders – definition and diagnosis

N. R. C. Roberton

It was recognized 20 years ago[1,2] that the hypoxia in babies with respiratory distress syndrome (RDS) is due to right to left shunting. The sites at which right to left shunting can occur are shown in Table 1. Of these, only R–L shunts through a patent ductus arteriosus (PDA) or a patent foramen ovale (PFO) will be influenced by pulmonary artery pressure. However, using dye dilution curves in infants with RDS, the amount of shunt through the PFO has been shown to be very small. Other workers have shown that less than 10% of the total R–L shunt took place through a PDA[3,4].

Table 1   Sites for right to left shunting in neonatal lung disease

---

1. Cardiac veins draining into the left side of the heart; bronchopulmonary anastomoses
2. Blood passing through the lung without passing the ventilated alveolus. The true intrapulmonary shunt; with $\dot{V}_A/\dot{Q}_C$ of 0
3. Intrapulmonary shunting past partially ventilated alveoli with $\dot{V}_A/\dot{Q}_C > 0$ but < 1. This can be abolished by breathing pure oxygen for 15–20 minutes
4. Ductus arteriosus and foramen ovale

In the late 1960s a subgroup of babies with RDS were described in whom the blood gas changes were suggestive of cyanotic congenital heart disease (CHD), with a normal pH and $PaCO_2$, but marked hypoxia, yet cardiac catheterization showed only a large R–L shunt through the PFO and the PDA – the syndrome of persistence of the fetal circulation (PFC). In some neonates this occurred apparently as an isolated phenomenon[5,6]. Others described an identical clinical picture as a secondary phenomenon in infants with primary neonatal lung disease, and this has been recognized with increasing frequency in recent years in many other varieties of neonatal lung disease (Table 2).

Table 2 Diseases in which PFC may arise as a complication

1. Respiratory distress syndrome
2. Meconium aspiration
3. Pulmonary hypoplasia (especially diaphragmatic hernia)
4. Group B streptococcal sepsis
5. Pulmonary air leak (especially pulmonary interstitial emphysema)
6. Intracerebral lesions increasing intracranial pressure
7. Ischaemic myocardial injury

In some American units PFC could now be said to have reached epidemic proportions (Table 3), being the commonest cause of death in normally formed infants > 1.0 kg[8], yet many European units rarely see a case, never mind a fatality. The different incidence may be nothing more than a matter of

Table 3 Neonatal mortality, Boston, 1981[8] (approximately 10 000 live births)

Cause of Death	Number
Extreme prematurity	62
Malformations (>1.00 kg)	44
Meconium aspiration	24
Asphyxia	24
Persistent fetal circulation	24
Infection	12
RDS	6
Other	4

definition, but I think that this explanation is unlikely. I think it is more likely that we will find some pathophysiological explanation not only for why the condition occurs in the first place, but also for the different incidence figures, by considering conditions which might affect the pulmonary vasculature and pulmonary perfusion (Table 4).

A rise in intracerebral pressure in some as yet unclear way reduces pulmonary perfusion and lowers the PaO_2. Serious lung disease, by causing hypoxia, will also reduce pulmonary perfusion, as will lung hypoplasia. Acidaemia has a

Table 4 Factors influencing PFC

Cerebral injury
Parenchymal lung disease
Lung hypoplasia
Acidaemia
Hypotension
Overventilation
Hyperviscosity
Hypoglycaemia
Previous *in-utero* hypoxia
Drug exposure
Mild surfactant deficiency

major effect on pulmonary perfusion particularly in the presence of concomitant hypoxia (Figure 1)[9].

Hypotension from hypovolaemia or myocardial injury, by making the systemic pressure lower than the pulmonary pressure, allows a R–L shunt. Overventilating the lungs can also have deleterious effects (Figure 2), since if mean airway pressure exceeds mean pulmonary perfusion pressure, blood will be forced from the right side of the heart through a PDA or a PFO. Furthermore with very high inflating pressures, or if there is severe interstitial emphysema, the myocardium is splinted by the overdistended lungs, causing a further fall in

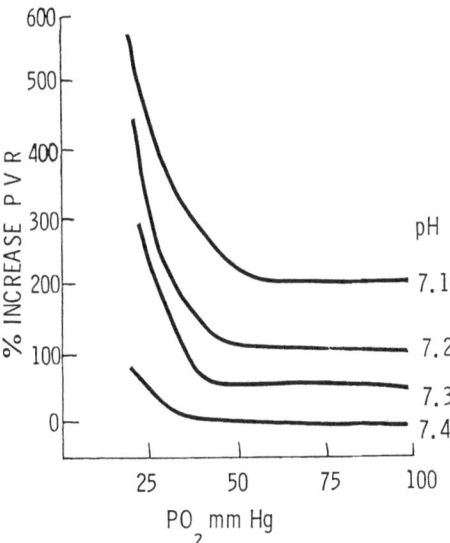

Figure 1 Percentage increase in pulmonary vascular resistance in newborn calves at different PaO_2 and pH values (data from ref. 9)

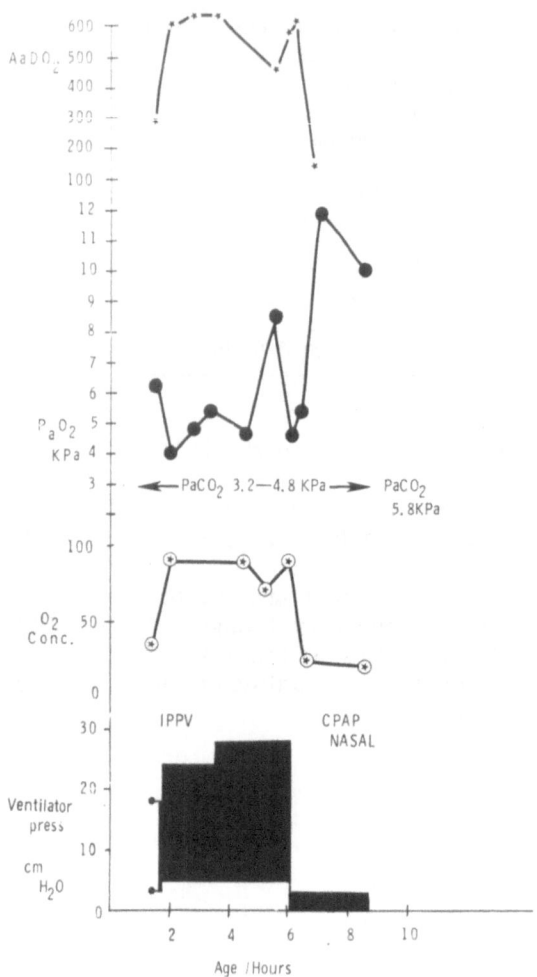

Figure 2 Baby who developed severe hypoxaemia (very high alveolar–arterial oxygen difference, A–aDO$_2$ and low PaO$_2$) due to overventilation. Note low PaCO$_2$ values during period of IPPV in 90–100% O$_2$. When IPPV discontinued at 6 hours of age and nasal CPAP started, A–aDO$_2$ and oxygen requirements fell markedly, and PaO$_2$ rose

cardiac output. Other factors which are purported to increase the likelihood of PFC are hyperviscosity, hypoglycaemia[10], and prenatal exposure to prostaglandin synthetase inhibitors[11].

However, the data at the heart of the problem show that babies who die of PFC in association with meconium aspiration, have pulmonary artery musculature which extends far out into the acinus, whereas in full-term babies who die from malformations but with normal lungs, the pulmonary musculature ends at the pre-acinar level (Figure 3)[12]. This degree of muscular hypertrophy

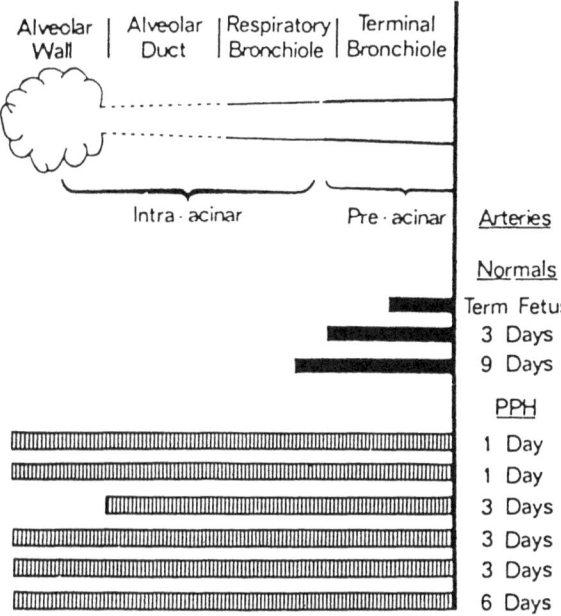

Figure 3 Diagrammatic location of muscle in the walls of the intra-acinar arteries. In normal infants less than 1 week of age no muscular arteries are found within the acinus. All the patients with PPH had extension of muscle into the small intra-acinar arteries (from reference 12, with permission)

could only be explained if the neonates had been exposed to hypoxia for considerably longer than their postnatal survival, implying that they must have suffered some hypoxic insult *pre*-delivery.

Reviewing all these data it seems likely, therefore, that PFC will develop in infants whose pulmonary vessel musculature is 'primed' and hypertrophied by prenatal events, and who then suffer peri- or postnatal insults such as acidaemia, hypoxia or rises in intracranial pressure likely to cause pulmonary arterial constriction. The nature of the prenatal events which 'prime' the pulmonary artery musculature must remain speculative, but drugs and smoking are obvious candidates. Another factor could be the increasing willingness of obstetricians to deliver by caesarean section women who are very ill with, for example, severe pre-eclampsia, whose babies would otherwise have died *in utero*. Even nowadays, these babies are likely to have suffered recurrent episodes of hypoxia *in utero* pre-delivery, causing hypertrophy of the pulmonary arterial musculature.

The variations in the incidence of PFC may thus reflect local variations in the incidence of those perinatal events which are likely to influence pulmonary perfusion, such as the incidence of meconium aspiration, the use of bicarbonate in acidaemic infants and the vigour of neonatal resuscitation. Meconium aspiration syndrome seems to be more common in North America (4/1000 live births)[8] than in Europe (1/1000 live births)[13]. If this is combined with what I believe has been over-reaction against the use of bicarbonate just because some papers[14,15] suggested (most unconvincingly) that giving too much bicarbonate might cause intracerebral haemorrhage, we may now be seeing many more babies being left acidaemic and at risk from pulmonary vasoconstriction than we did 15–20 years ago. With the increasingly aggressive approach to low birth weight babies in the delivery room, and their resuscitation and continuing care with IPPV we may also be generating iatrogenic PFC by overventilating them (Figure 2).

All these suggestions are, of course, sheer speculation, and much more work needs to be done to unravel this mysterious, and in Britain at least, comparatively rare complication of neonatal parenchymal lung disease.

References

1. Strang, L. B. and McLeish, M. H. (1961). Ventilatory failure and right to left shunt in newborn infants with respiratory distress. *Pediatrics*, **28**, 17–27
2. Warley, M. A. and Gairdner, D. (1962). Respiratory distress syndrome of the newborn – principles in treatment. *Arch. Dis. Child.*, **37**, 455–65
3. Stahlman, M. (1964). Treatment of cardiovascular disorders of the newborn. *Pediatr. Clin. N. Am.*, **11**, 363–400
4. Roberton, N. R. C. and Dahlenburg, G. W. (1969). Ductus arteriosus shunts in the respiratory distress syndrome. *Pediatr. Res.*, **3**, 149–59
5. Gersony, W. M., Duc, G. V. and Sinclair, J. C. (1969). PFC syndrome (persistence of the fetal circulation). *Circulation*, **39** (Suppl.), 87 (abstract)
6. Siassi, B., Goldberg, S. J., Emmanouilides, G. C., Higashino, S. M. and Lewis, E. (1971). Persistent pulmonary vascular obstruction in the neonate. *J. Pediatr.*, **78**, 610–15
7. Roberton, N. R. C., Hallidie-Smith, K. A. and Davis, J. A. (1967). Severe respiratory distress syndrome mimicking cyanotic heart disease in term babies. *Lancet*, **ii**, 1108–10
8. Avery, M. E. and Taeusch, H. W. (1984). *Schaffer's Diseases of the Newborn*, 5th Edn., p. 3. (Philadelphia: W. B. Saunders)
9. Rudolph, A. M. and Yuan, S. (1966). Response of the pulmonary vasculature to hypoxia and H^+ ion concentration changes. *J. Clin. Invest.*, **45**, 399–411
10. Emmanouilides, G. C. (1979). Persistence of the fetal circulation. In Thiebault, D. W. and Gregory, G. A. (eds.) *Neonatal Pulmonary Care*, pp. 277–95. (Menlo Park, California: Addison-Wesley)
11. Wilkinson, A. R., Aynsley-Green, A. and Mitchell, M. D. (1979). Persistent pulmonary hypertension and abnormal prostaglandin E levels in preterm infants after maternal treatment with naproxen. *Arch. Dis. Child.*, **54**, 942–5
12. Murphy, J. D., Rabinovitch, M., Goldstein, J. D. and Reid, L. M. (1981). The structural basis of persistent pulmonary hypertension of the newborn infant. *J. Pediatr.*, **98**, 962–7
13. Jones, R. A. K. and Roberton, N. R. C. (1984). Problems of the small for dates baby. *Clin. Obstet. Gynecol.*, **11**, 499–524
14. Simmons, M. A., Adcock, E. Q., Bard, H. and Battaglia, F. C. (1974). Hypernatremia and intracranial hemorrhage in neonates. *N. Engl. J. Med.*, **291**, 6–10

15. Wigglesworth, J. S., Keith, I. H., Girling, D. J. and Slade S. A. (1976). Hyaline membrane disease, alkali and intraventricular haemorrhage. *Arch. Dis. Child.*, **51**, 755–62

30

Treatment of persistent fetal circulation

V. Y. H. Yu

ABSTRACT

Factors which increase pulmonary vascular resistance should be avoided or promptly diagnosed and treated: hypoxia, hyperinflation/atelactasis, hypothermia, acidosis, polycythaemia, hypoglycaemia, hypocalcaemia, hypomagnesaemia. Mechanical ventilation is indicated if PaO_2 is < 80 mmHg in 80% oxygen or pH <7.3. The objective is to achieve a critical $PaCO_2$ (20–30 mmHg) at which PaO_2 improves. Rapid rates, low end-expiratory pressures and short inspiratory times should be used unless lung disease coexists. Weaning is done cautiously and slowly. When a trial of hyperventilation fails to sustain a PaO_2 >80 mmHg, vasodilator therapy is initiated. Treatment with tolazoline has a 60% response rate, 70% complication rate and 54% survival rate. Other vasodilators tried include chlorpromazine, nitroprusside, prostacyclin and tubocurarine. Prostaglandin D_2 shows promise as a selective pulmonary vasodilator. Maintenance of systemic artery pressure above pulmonary artery pressure is essential. Repeated blood transfusions and dopamine are effective. Hyperventilation and tolazoline/dopamine therapy combined has a better response than either alone. Neonates with pulmonary hypoplasia or pulmonary microthrombi syndrome are the most refractory to treatment. A clear understanding of the pathophysiology is required to optimize treatment.

After birth, the high fetal pulmonary vascular resistance (PVR) falls with expansion and oxygenation of the lungs. In persistent pulmonary hypertension (PPH) this reduction does not occur or the resistance subsequently increases. Pulmonary artery pressure become equal to or higher than systemic artery pressure[1]. As a result, right-to-left shunting of cardiac output occurs through the foramen ovale and ductus arteriosus, producing severe hypoxaemia.

PRINCIPLES OF TREATMENT

Treatment of PPH includes: (1) general stabilization of the neonate's condition, (2) efforts to decrease pulmonary artery pressure by ventilator and/or pharmacologic therapy and (3) efforts to maintain systemic artery pressure or to correct systemic hypotension. In PPH the balance between pulmonary and systemic artery pressures determines the direction of the shunt. The ratio of pulmonary artery to systemic artery pressure was found to average 1.14 in PPH[2]. This decreased to 0.98 following ventilator therapy with induced hyperventilation and to 0.87 following pharmacological therapy with tolazoline and dopamine. However the ratio was lowest at 0.70 following combined ventilator and pharmacological therapy. Hypoxaemia was reversed and oxygenation was satisfactory in all instances when the pulmonary to systemic pressure ratio was less than 1.0.

GENERAL STABILIZATION

There are a number of physiological factors which increase PVR in the neonate. The increased reactivity of the pulmonary vasculature in PPH to these physiological stimuli is reflected by the labile nature of pulmonary artery pressure with documented fluctuations up to 50 mmHg[1]. Therefore, supportive management of neonates with PPH includes the avoidance of such adverse factors or their treatment.

Hypoxia

It is unclear whether PVR increases as a result of alveolar or pulmonary vascular hypoxaemia. Hypoxaemia increased PVR[3] but it is also known that even small decreases in the inspired oxygen concentration often cause a rapid and severe fall in PaO_2, probably because the pulmonary vasculature is exquisitely sensitive to alveolar O_2. It was suggested that the extravascular (interstitial) PaO_2 is important in controlling pulmonary vascular tone[4]. Fluctuations in oxygenation in neonates with respiratory disease can be reduced by a policy of minimal handling[5], avoidance of routine endotracheal suctioning[6], reduction in environmental noise[7] and early use of continuous positive airway pressure in hyaline membrane disease[8].

Lung inflation

Both atelactasis[9] and hyperinflation[10] increase PVR. Since both result in hypercapnia, the degree of lung inflation should be assessed by chest X-ray when physical examination fails to determine whether higher or lower peak inflating pressures are required to provide the appropriate ventilation.

Hypothermia

Cooling of the neonate's skin increases PVR[11]. When the environmental temperature was reduced by 10 °C it was found that there was a 25% decrease in pulmonary blood flow[12]. This occurred despite a constant core temperature. Care should therefore be taken to nurse all neonates with respiratory distress in a thermoneutral environment.

Acidosis

In neonates with hyaline membrane disease, pulmonary blood flow improves after their acidosis is corrected[13]. A precipitous drop in PaO_2 may occur with metabolic or respiratory acidosis and in association with rapid blood transfusions. The arterial pH must be maintained above 7.25 in all neonates and above 7.30 in those with labile PaO_2.

Metabolic abnormalities

Hypoglycaemia, hypocalcaemia and hypomagnesaemia are predisposing factors for PPH. They should all be promptly diagnosed and treated.

Polycythaemia

Hyperviscosity increases PVR. When the central haematocrit exceeds 65% in neonates with respiratory distress, it should be corrected by partial exchange transfusion with fresh frozen plasma.

VENTILATOR THERAPY

Once PPH is diagnosed, mechanical ventilation should be considered earlier than uncomplicated pulmonary parenchymal disease. It should be initiated if 80% oxygen is required to maintain a PaO_2 of 80 mmHg or if the pH cannot be maintained above 7.30. As most neonates with PPH are relatively mature, it is advisable to maintain a moderately high PaO_2 of 80 mmHg. The objective of mechanical ventilation is to achieve a low 'critical $PaCO_2$' level at which PVR and pulmonary artery pressure falls, resulting in a reduction of right-to-left shunting and hypoxaemia. This critical $PaCO_2$ is usually between 20 and 30 mmHg, but in severe cases $PaCO_2$ has to be reduced below 20 mmHg before PaO_2 begins to improve. Its level is best determined with the hyperoxia-hyperventilation test in which the neonate is manually ventilated at 100–150 breaths per minute in 100% oxygen for 5–10 minutes[1]. During hyperventilation the $PaCO_2$ at which PaO_2 rises can be measured. Furthermore, with the test, a pressure manometer in line allows the peak inflating pressure and rate required on subsequent mechanical ventilation to be determined.

Guidelines for mechanical ventilation in PPH include rapid rates (up to 150 breaths per minute), low end-expiratory pressures (0–3 cmH_2O) unless pulmonary parenchymal disease coexists, and low inspiration–expiration ratios (1:2 to 1:6) to prevent air trapping at rapid rates. The critical $PaCO_2$ level should be maintained for several days until clinical stability and improvement herald the start of weaning. This should be carried out very slowly with 1–2% reductions in inspired oxygen and 1–2 cmH_2O reductions in peak inflating pressure at each step. This precaution is taken in view of the extreme sensitivity of pulmonary vessels in PPH to alveolar O_2 and acidosis. Transcutaneous oxygen monitoring is reliable even in neonates with PPH on vasodilator therapy[14], although severe hypotension does adversely affect correlation of transcutaneous and arterial PO_2.[15] By the time the neonate tolerates an inflating pressure of below 30 cmH$_2$O and an inspired oxygen concentration of below 60%, PPH would have resolved and the oxygen and ventilatory therapy can be weaned off more rapidly.

Muscle paralysis is indicated during the acute phase on mechanical ventilation because it increases chest wall compliance and eliminates struggling, both of which make ventilation more efficient. Pancuronium, 0.1 mg/kg i.m. q3–6 h, is commonly used. Tubocurarine 1–2 mg/kg i.m. q3–6 h is often used as it is also a histamine-releasing agent and acts as a vasodilator drug[16].

Table 1 Vasoactive drugs used in PPH

Tolazoline
  Loading dose 1–2 mg/kg i.v. over 10 min
  Infusion 1–2 mg kg^{-1} h^{-1} i.v. increasing to 10 mg kg^{-1} h^{-1}

Nitroprusside
  2 µg kg^{-1} min^{-1} i.v. infusion

Prostacyclin
  0.05–0.1 µg kg^{-1} min^{-1} i.v. infusion

Chlorpromazine
  0.1 mg kg^{-1} min^{-1} i.v. infusion

Tubocurarine
  1–2 mg/kg i.v. every 3–6 h

VASODILATOR THERAPY

When a trial of hyperventilation in 100% oxygen fails to sustain an improvement in PaO$_2$ to a level of 80 mmHg, vasodilator therapy is initiated (Table 1). The most widely used is tolazoline, an alpha-adrenergic antagonist with multiple actions as a cholinergic and histaminergic drug as well as being a direct vasodilator. Its pulmonary vascular effects can be abolished by continual blockage of H$_1$ and H$_2$ receptors[17]. A review of 21 clinical reports on the use of tolazoline in PPH, none of which were controlled randomized trails, shows that the published experience is variable[18]. Overall, 60% have an increase in PaO$_2$ after tolazoline administration, responses ranging from 40% to 90% in different series. Survival rates vary between 30% and 60%, the overall survival based on cumulative data being 54%. However, the incidence of complications was 70%, the major ones being systemic hypotension, oliguria and gastrointestinal bleeding. Other vasodilators tried in neonates with PPH include chlorpromazine[19], nitroprusside[20], prostacyclin[21] and tubocurarine[16]. Prostaglandin D$_2$ shows promise in selective pulmonary vasodilation but it has not been used in human neonates[22].

MAINTENANCE OF SYSTEMIC ARTERY PRESSURE

The limitation to the use of existing drugs is that they cause systemic hypotension as well as decrease pulmonary artery pressure. The maintenance of systemic artery pressure higher than pulmonary artery pressure is essential to reverse the right-to-left shunt and correct hypoxaemia. Repeated 10–20 ml/kg blood transfusions are necessary to fill the increased intravascular capacitance following vasodilation. In addition, dopamine is a useful agent for treating systemic hypotension[23]. Unlike isoprenaline, it produces very little tachycardia and increases renal blood flow and dilates mesenteric vessels[24,25]. It offers immediate inotropic support for the hypoxic failing myocardium and does not significantly alter PVR[26]. When used in conjunction with tolazoline, dopamine is ineffective in its normal dose of below 6 μg kg^{-1} min^{-1} and 20–125 μg kg^{-1} min^{-1} is required to increase systemic artery pressure or urine output[2]. Tolazoline may be an antagonist to dopamine, thus explaining the high doses of dopamine required.

FACTORS INFLUENCING RESPONSE TO TREATMENT

The clinical course of PPH is variable. Hypoxaemia may become extreme, and despite treatment, some neonates rapidly deteriorate and die. In survivors, improvement is usually seen within a week. A poor prognosis is suggested by an inability to reduce $PaCO_2$ with ventilation, requirement for a peak inflating pressure over 40 cmH$_2$O or a ventilator rate over 130 breaths/min, a critical $PaCO_2$ less than 20 mmHg and marked PaO_2 lability[27].

PPH is a disease which is caused by a variety of structural and physiological conditions (Table 2). It is usually associated with diseases of known aetiology during the course of which physiological factors such as pulmonary vasoconstriction or hyperviscosity result in an increase in PVR. The majority of neonates in this group has a satisfactory response to treatment.

A second group of neonates who are more refractory to treatment has structural pulmonary vascular changes. Some of these neonates have pulmonary arterial smooth muscle hypertrophy. Intrauterine hypoxaemia[28], fetal hypertension[29] or ductus arteriosus constriction due to maternal salicylate ingestion[30] have been reported to result in extension of smooth muscle into small pulmonary arteries which normally are non-muscular. This maldevelopment of the peripheral arterial bed occurs *in utero* and does not represent a failure of the fetal pattern to regress[31,32]. This structural abnormality results in the increased PVR as well as the increased reactivity and lability in PaO_2. Since PPH occurring in these neonates is not associated with clinically obvious lung disease, they were previously labelled as having 'idiopathic' PPH.

The second subgroup of neonates with structural pulmonary vascular changes who also respond poorly to treatment has decreased cross-sectional area of their pulmonary vascular bed. The increased PVR may be due to the small size of the lung[33] or to diseases affecting the small pulmonary arteries, such as peripheral pulmonary artery stenosis[34] and the pulmonary microthrombi syndrome[35]. The latter condition can result from inhalation of amniotic fluid which has thromboplastic effects and causes local aggregation of

Table 2 Conditions associated with PPH

Increased pulmonary vasoconstriction
   Perinatal asphyxia
   Meconium aspiration syndrome
   Hyaline membrane disease
   Pneumonia, especially group B streptococcus
   Upper airway obstruction
     Choanal atresia, micrognathia
   Neurological disorders causing hypoventilation
   Pulmonary microthrombi syndrome
     Amniotic fluid inhalation, non-bacterial endocardial thrombosis
   Severe hypoxaemia or acidosis from any cause
   Hypothermia
   Metabolic abnormalities
     Hypoglycaemia, hypocalcaemia, hypomagnesaemia

Hyperviscosity and polycythaemia
   Placental insufficiency
   Intrauterine growth retardation
   Maternal diabetes mellitus
   Beckwith–Wiedemann syndrome
   Twin-to-twin transfusion

Pulmonary arterial smooth muscle hypertrophy
   Chronic intrauterine hypoxia
     Placental insufficiency, postmaturity
   Fetal systemic hypertension
   Ductus arteriosus constriction
     Maternal salicylate or indomethacin ingestion
   Congenital heart disease

Decreased cross-sectional area of pulmonary vascular bed
   Primary pulmonary hypoplasia
   Diaphragmatic hernia
   Lung cysts, including congenital lobar emphysema
   Pulmonary microthrombi syndrome
   Peripheral pulmonary artery stenosis

---

platelets[36], or from non-bacterial endocardial thrombosis[37]. PPH in these neonates is caused not only by the physical effect of a decrease in cross-sectional area of the pulmonary vascular bed by platelet plugging of vessels, but also by the vasoconstrictive effect of prostaglandin $F_{2\alpha}$ and thromboxane A_2 released with platelet aggregation. Response to treatment is poor in pulmonary hypoplasia and unpredictable in the pulmonary microthrombi syndrome. There is no proven successful or safe therapy to prevent platelet aggregation, promote platelet disaggregation or block prostaglandin $F_{2\alpha}$ or thromboxane A_2 release.

PROGNOSIS

Present treatment has resulted in better survival for a condition which in the past was invariably fatal. Early diagnosis and prompt initiation of treatment prior to severe and prolonged hypoxaemia hold the key to improving outcome. Elevation of the systolic time interval ratios of both ventricles on M-mode echocardiography can now permit early identification of neonates with PPH several hours preceding clinical deterioration[38].

Cumulative data from the few studies on late outcome of PPH survivors [39-42] show that 85% of survivors had normal neurodevelopmental outcome. A clear understanding of the underlying pathophysiology is required in the treatment of PPH. This should only be undertaken in neonatal centres capable of intensive care monitoring and support, in order to minimize mortality and late sequelae.

References

1. Peckham, G. J. and Fox, W. W. (1978). Physiological factors affecting pulmonary artery pressure in infants with persistent pulmonary hypertension. *J. Pediatr.*, **93**, 1005
2. Drummond, W. H., Gregory, G. A., Heymann, M. A. and Phibbs, R. A. (1981). The independent effects of hyperventilation, tolazoline and dopamine on infants with persistent pulmonary hypertension. *J. Pediatr.*, **98**, 603
3. Rudolph, A. M. and Yuan, S. (1966). Response of the pulmonary vasculature to hypoxia and H$^+$ ion concentration changes. *J. Clin. Invest.*, **45**, 399
4. Fishman, A. P. (1976). Hypoxia on the pulmonary circulation. How and where it acts. *Circ. Res.*, **38**, 221
5. Danford, D. A., Miske, S., Headley, J. and Nelson, R. M. (1983). Effect of routine care procedures on transcutaneous oxygen in neonates: a quantitative approach. *Arch. Dis. Child.*, **58**, 20
6. Simbruner, G., Coradello, H., Fodor, M., Havelec, L., Lubec, G. and Pollak A. (1981). Effect of tracheal suction on oxygenation, circulation, and lung mechanics in newborn infants. *Arch. Dis. Child.*, **51**, 326
7. Long, J. G., Lucey, J. E. and Philip, A. G. S. (1980). Noise and hypoxemia in the intensive care nursery. *Pediatrics*, **65**, 143
8. Yu, V. Y. H. and Rolfe, P. (1977). Effects of continuous positive airways pressure breathing on cardiorespiratory function in infants with respiratory distress syndrome. *Acta Paediatr. Scand.*, **66**, 59
9. Hobbs, B. B., Hinchcliffe, W. A. and Greenspan, R. H. (1972). Effects of acute lobar atelactasis on pulmonary hemodynamics. *Invest. Radiol.*, **7**, 1
10. Nelson, R. M., Egan, E. A. and Eitzman, D. V. (1977). Increased hypoxemia in neonates secondary to the use of continuous positive airway pressure. *J. Pediatr.*, **91**, 87
11. Will, D. H., McMurty, I. F., Reeves, J. T. and Grover, A. (1978). Cold induced pulmonary hypertension. *J. Appl. Physiol.*, **45**, 469
12. Brady, J. P. and Rigatto, H. (1969). Pulmonary blood flow in infants. *Circulation*, suppl III, 50
13. Chu, J., Clements, J. A., Cotton, E., Klaus, M. H., Sweet, A. Y., Thomas, M. A. and Tooley, W. H. (1965). The pulmonary hypoperfusion syndrome. *Pediatrics*, **35**, 733
14. Boyle, R. J. and Oh, W. (1978). Transcutaneous PO$_2$ monitoring in infants with persistent fetal circulation who are receiving tolazoline therapy. *Pediatrics*, **62**, 605
15. Huch, R., Huch, A., Albani, M., Gabriel, M. Schulte, F. J., Wolf, H., Rupprath, G., Emmrich, P., Stechelle, U., Duc, G. and Bucher, H. (1976). Transcutaneous

PO$_2$ monitoring in routine management of infants and children with cardiorespiratory problems. *Pediatrics*, **57**, 681

16. Hutchison, A. A. and Yu, V. Y. H. (1980). Curare in the treatment of pulmonary hypertension as it occurs in the idiopathic respiratory distress syndrome. *Aust. Paediatr. J.*, **16**, 94

17. Goetzman, B. W. and Milstein, J. M. (1978). Pulmonary vasodilator action of tolazoline in the newborn. *Pediatr. Res.*, **13**, 942

18. Packham, G. J. (1982). Risk-benefit relationships of current therapeutic approaches. Proceedings of the 83rd Ross Conference on Cardiovascular Sequelae of Asphyxia in the Newborn, p. 110

19. Collins, D. L., Pomerance, J. J., Travis, K. W., Turner, S. W. and Pappelbaum, S. J. (1977). A new approach to congenital posterolateral diaphragmatic hernia. *J. Pediatr. Surg.*, **12**, 149

20. Abbott, T. R., Roes, G. J., Dickenson, D., Reynolds, G. and Lord, D. (1978). Sodium nitroprusside in idiopathic respiratory distress syndrome. *Br. Med. J.*, **1**, 1113

21. Lock, J. E., Olley, P. M., Coceani, F., Swyer, P. R. and Rowe, R. D. (1979). Use of prostacyclin in persistent fetal circulation. *Lancet*, **1**, 1343

22. Soifer, S. J., Morin, F. C. III, and Heymann, M. A. (1982). Prostaglandin D$_2$ reverses induced pulmonary hypertension in the newborn lamb. *J. Pediatr.*, **100**, 458

23. Fiddler, G., Chatrath, R, Williams, G. J., Walker, D. R. and Scott, O. (1980). Dopamine infusion for the treatment of myocardial dysfunction associated with a persistent transitional circulation. *Arch. Dis. Child.*, **55**, 194

24. Editorial (1977). Dopamine in cardiac failure and shock. *Br. Med. J.*, **2**, 1563

25. Editorial (1977). Intravenous dopamine. *Lancet*, **2**, 231

26. Holloway, E. L., Polumbo, R. A. and Harrison, D. C. (1975). Acute circulatory effects of dopamine in patients with pulmonary hypertension. *Br. Heart J.*, **37**, 482

27. Fox, W. W. and Duara, S. (1983). Persistent pulmonary hypertension in the neonate: diagnosis and management. *J. Pediatr.*, **103**, 505

28. Gersony, W. M., Morishima, H. O., Daniel, S. S., Kohl, S., Cohen, H., Brown, W. and James, L. S. (1976). The hemodynamic effects of intrauterine hypoxia: an experimental model in newborn lambs. *J. Pediatr.*, **89**, 631

29. Levin, D. L., Hyman, A. I., Heymann, M. A. and Rudolph, A. M. (1978). Fetal hypertension and the development of increased pulmonary vascular smooth muscle: a possible mechanism of persistent pulmonary hypertension of the newborn. *J. Pediatr.*, **92**, 265

30. Perkin, R., Levin, D. L. and Clark, R. (1980). Serum salicylate levels and right-to-left ductus shunts in newborn infants with persistent pulmonary hypertension. *J. Pediatr.*, **96**, 721

31. Murphy, J. D., Rabinovitch, M., Goldstein, J. D. and Reid, L. M. (1981). The structural basis of persistent pulmonary hypertension of the newborn infant. *J. Pediatr.*, **93**, 962

32. Haworth, S. G. and Reid, L. (1971). Persistent fetal circulation: newly recognised structural features. *J. Pediatr.*, **88**, 614

33. Swischuk, L. E., Richardson, C. J., Nichols, M. M. and Ingman, M. J. (1979). Primary pulmonary hypoplasia in the neonate. *J. Pediatr.*, **95**, 573

34. Salisbury, D. M. and Keeling, J. W. (1978). Peripheral pulmonary artery stenosis. *Arch. Dis. Child*, **53**, 428

35. Levin, D. L., Weinberg, A. G. and Perkin, R. M. (1983). Pulmonary microthrombi syndrome in newborn infants with unresponsive persistent pulmonary hypertension. *J. Pediatr.*, **102**, 299

36. Segall, M. L., Goetzman, B. W. and Schick, J. B. (1980). Thrombocytopenia and

pulmonary hypertension in the perinatal aspiration syndrome. *J. Pediatr.*, **96**, 727

37. Morrow, W. B., Haas, J. E. and Benjamin, D. R. (1982). Nonbacterial endocardial thrombosis in neonates: relationship to persistent fetal circulation. *J. Pediatr.*, **100**, 117

38. Valdes-Cruz, L. M., Dudell, G. G. and Ferrara, A. (1981). Utility of M-mode echocardiography for early identification of infants with persistent pulmonary hypertension of the newborn. *Pediatrics*, **68**, 515

39. Brett, C., Dekle, M., Leonard, C. H., Clark, C., Sniderman, S., Roth, R., Ballard, R. and Clyman, R. (1981). Developmental follow-up of hyperventilated neonates: preliminary observations. *Pediatrics*, **68**, 588

40. Bernbaum, J. C., Russell, P., Gewitz, M., Fox, W. W. and Peckham, G. J. (1981). Neurodevelopmental and cardiorespiratory follow-up of infants with persistent pulmonary hypertension of the newborn. *Pediatr. Res.*, **15**, 651

41. Cohen, R. S., Stevenson, D. K., Malachowski, N., Ariagno, R. L., Johnson, J. D. and Sunshine, P. (1980). Late morbidity among survivors of respiratory failure treated with tolazoline. *J. Pediatr.*, **97**, 644

42. Stevens, D. C., Schreiner, R. L., Bull, M. J., Bryson, C. Q., Lemons, J. A., Gresham, E. L., Grosfeld, J. L. and Weber, T. R. (1980). An analysis of tolazoline therapy in the critically-ill neonate. *J. Pediatr. Surg.*, **15**, 964

Chairman's summary

N. R. C. Roberton

After the formal presentations there was a vigorous and wide-ranging discussion about many aspects of the PFC syndrome. In general there was agreement about three aspects of the disease.

1. It seems very likely that babies who develop PFC have been 'primed' by prenatal events since at post-mortem they have muscle extending into their bronchiolar and acinar arteries[1]. This could only be due to hypoxic stresses which must have antedated delivery.

2. Although the condition needs to be more clearly defined (see below) it is clear that not only can it occur in babies with primary lung pathology (Chapter 29, Table 2) but it can occur as an isolated event, particularly if the myocardium has suffered some perinatal ischaemic insult.

3. The treatments currently available are unsatisfactory, unpredictable, and have a long list of undesirable side-effects. Only with tolazoline and hyperventilation has there been any widespread experience, and side-effects are common with both. Considerable anxiety was expressed over the potentially deleterious effects on cerebral blood flow of the hypocapnia and alkalaemia of hyperventilation.

Much of the discussion from the floor centred on the huge variation in the incidence of this condition in different parts of the world, in particular the high incidence in North America. The reasons for this remain obscure; socio-economic factors seem to be an unconvincing explanation for a disease without an obvious socioeconomic trend, and in a country with a high standard of living. Other more convincing, but unproven, suggestions were an as yet unidentified infection, a higher incidence of intrapartum asphyxia and meconium aspiration, and perhaps overvigorous resuscitation at birth with pulmonary overexpansion.

All of these, superimposed on a background of preceding intrauterine complications causing fetal pulmonary arterial muscular proliferation, could result in PFC.

In view of the fact that there was considerable debate about what actually constitutes PFC, the most valuable contribution which this workshop could make to the future would, I feel, be to establish diagnostic criteria for this condition. I would suggest the following:

A baby with:

1. PaO_2 < 40 mmHg (5.3 kPa) in F_IO_2 of 1.0 (with or without IPPV), despite a normal or low $PaCO_2$, and a normal pH.

2. $PaCO_2$ < 40 mmHg (5.3 kPa) if breathing spontaneously, or on IPPV with inspiratory pressures < 20 cmH$_2$O and a rate < 60/min; the $PaCO_2$ tending to drop further if ventilator pressures or rates are increased.

3. Absence of severe parenchymal lung disease assessed radiologically (i.e. CXR looking surprisingly radiolucent for severe hypoxaemia – the exception being babies with pulmonary hypoplasia) or assessed by other investigations (i.e. normal L : S ratios, and normal compliance measurements).

4. Normal ECG and echocardiogram – other than the changes of asphyxial myocardial injury.

5. These changes, irrespective of other precipitating factors; e.g. hypoglycaemia, acidaemia, polycythaemia which are not an integral part of the definition.

The diagnosis can be confirmed by pulmonary artery catheterization showing that the pulmonary artery pressure is higher than the aortic pressure, and the presence of a right to left shunt at the level of the ductus or the atria. Right to left shunting at these sites can also be demonstrated by contrast echocardiography.

In the absence of these sophisticated techniques, confirmation of the diagnosis can be made retrospectively

(a) at post-mortem – when no other lesions are found to explain profound hypoxia;

(b) if the infant survives with a normal cardiovascular system after treatment specifically designed to reduce pulmonary artery pressure.

Reference

1. Murphy, J. D., Rabinovitch, M., Goldstein, J. D. and Reid L. M. (1981). The structural basis of persistent pulmonary hypertension of the newborn infant. *J. Pediatr.*, **98**, 962–7

Section 8
Management of Breech Delivery

Chairman's introduction

J. Clinch

Vaginal breech delivery has always been more hazardous for the fetus than being born head first. Traditionally taught dangers such as cord prolapse, entrapment of the dead in the partially dilated cervix, and traumatic intracranial haemorrhage have resulted in a raised perinatal loss. At the Coombe Hospital during the early 1970s the perinatal mortality rate was 101/1000 for normally formed babies over 28 weeks gestation compared to the general hospital rate of 13.2/1000. To improve these results, increasing use has been made of caesarean section either electively at term or at the onset of labour. In our case this rose from 11% in 1971 to 50% at the end of decade. Distinction was always made between primigravidae and multiparous patients as it was thought that the baby of the former would be at greater risk. Such a distinction is not really valid as further analysis of perinatal mortality associated with breech births showed that most of the excess occurred in babies who were very small. The premature baby is more likely to present by the breech and many of its problems will be due to immaturity rather than the mode of delivery. It is important therefore to separate preterm and term breech management and the workshop was designed to do this.

In discussing premature breech presentation the available evidence implies that, in babies weighing less than 1500 g, caesarean section is preferable to vaginal delivery. Once over that weight the latter is satisfactory. However, most of the studies available are based on small numbers of babies and some of the others do not compare different types of management at the same time in the same institution but merely report how changes in practice have affected breech outcome in different periods of time. Nor has it been possible to assess, and then allow for, the various adverse factors other than the abnormal presentation which are so important to the outcome in preterm infants. It is only when this has been achieved that it will be possible to undertake prospective

203

studies to evaluate the best mode of delivery for the immature baby presenting by the breech.

The papers dealing with babies born after 37 weeks show that 45% of breeches require caesarean section. Twenty eight per cent of these are elective operations and 17% are performed during labour. Follow-up of these mature babies shows that there are inherent differences between normal vertex deliveries and breech babies whether the latter are delivered by caesarean section, either elective or emergency, or are born vaginally. These differences are physical, such as altered head shape and bodily configuration. They also involve cerebral function in that breech babies show altered verbal patterns at the age of 4 years. Such variations are more obvious in vaginal breeches than those born abdominally, but one can speculate as to whether this is due to the latter being significantly larger than the former. They emphasize the importance of careful follow-up for every breech baby no matter how well it appears at birth. They should also stimulate further study on the aetiology of the presentation in cases where there is no maternal factor.

31

The obstetric management of the premature breech

L. M. R. Westgren

It has long been recognized that the preterm infant presenting by the breech runs an increased risk compared to other presentations at vaginal delivery. Several authors have reported on a tendency of the aftercoming head to be entrapped in the incompletely dilated cervix, a greater likelihood of cord accidents and an increased risk for asphyxia. Concern about the high mortality rate associated with vaginal preterm breech delivery has caused many obstetricians to question whether the fetal outcome could be improved by alternative obstetric management and especially if caesarean section should be advocated or not.

A number of papers on preterm breech delivery have been published during the last decade[1-13]. Most of these authors have tried to evaluate benefits and hazards of abdominal delivery. However, it is difficult from these studies to evaluate the role of caesarean section, since all contain factors which can bias the results. All studies except those performed by Ingemarsson et al. (1978) and Bowes et al. (1979) were made retrospectively. Difficulties in retrospective studies are to evaluate the circumstance surrounding the decision to deliver by caesarean section or by the vaginal route. The two prospective studies also have limitations, since in the Ingemarsson paper one retrospective studied period is compared to another prospective studied period. The Bowes paper dealt with a rather limited number, and in neither of these studies are the patients matched or randomized. In a number of the investigations one time period is compared to another[2,7,9]. This factor can be expected to introduce a bias in favour of the latter period, often with the highest caesarean section rate since advances in neonatal care have not been taken into account. Furthermore, due to the limited number of patients the result is often presented as one group instead of in smaller weight or age groups[6,9,10,12]. Such a procedure often leads to a skew distribution in respect to birth weight and immaturity since many of the studies report more mature infants in the caesarean section group. Only in a few of the studies[2,3] has the patient been subjected to caesarean section solely due to breech presentation. In the other the caesarean sections were performed mostly due to other obstetric complications which could *per se* influence the outcome. In addition several of the papers lack detailed information on autopsy findings.

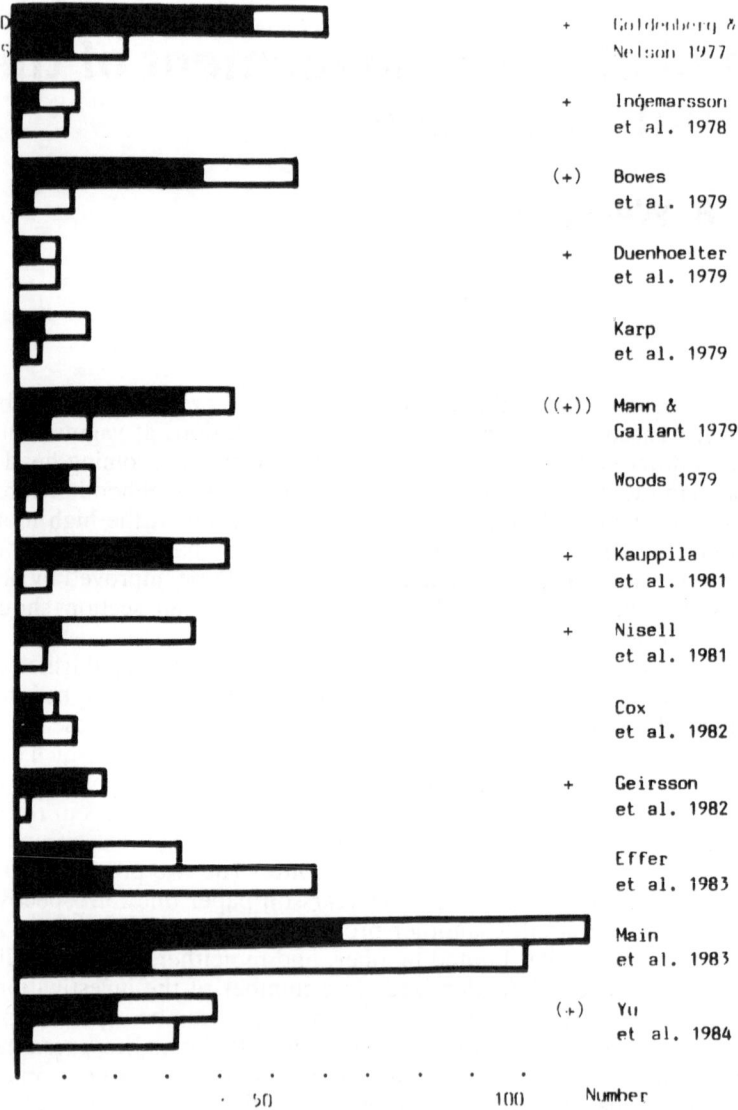

Figure 1 Vaginal delivery vs. caesarean section in infants weighing less than 1500 g. Vaginal delivery – upper bar, caesarean sections – lower bar. Filled part of the bar represents mortality. Plus sign indicates recommendation of caesarean section

In view of the limitations and difference between these studies it is surprising how well the results agree. Infants expected to weigh less than 1500 g or born before the 33rd week seem to survive more frequently after abdominal delivery than did those delivered vaginally. For infants weighing more than 1500 g there is no significant difference in survival rate between vaginally and abdominally delivered infants.

The outcomes for infants weighing less than 1500 g in the studies are presented in Figure 1. Most studies are of a rather limited number and only three[11-13] report more than 20 abdominally delivered infants. Moreover, in the most recently published studies no obvious difference between abdominally and vaginally delivered infants could be demonstrated. Despite the small size of the studies most authors conclude that caesarean section is the method of choice for delivery of the very low birth weight infant in breech presentation.

In conclusion, the studies bearing on the question of how preterm infants presenting by the breech should be delivered do not permit firm conclusions. The proof for the hypothesis that caesarean section represents the optimal made of delivery for these infants does not exist. There is still a need for a prospective randomized study and the author believes it would be ethically responsible to perform such a study.

ACKNOWLEDGEMENTS

Grants were obtained from the Research Foundation of Margaretahemmet and Allmänna BB. Swedish Medical Research Council grants no. B84–19X–04732–09A.

References

1. Goldenberg, R. L. and Nelson, K. G. (1977). The premature breech. *Am. J. Obstet. Gynecol.*, **127**, 240.
2. Ingemarsson, I. *et al.* (1978). Longterm follow-up of preterm infants in breech presentation delivered by caesarean section. A prospective study. *Lancet*, **2**, 172
3. Bowes, W. A. *et al.* (1979). Breech delivery: evaluation of the method of delivery on perinatal results and maternal morbidity. *Am. J. Obstet. Gynecol.*, **135**, 965
4. Karp, L. *et al.* (1979). The premature breech: trial of labor or cesarean section. *Obstet. Gynecol.*, **53**, 88
5. Mann, L. I. and Gallant, J. M. (1979). Modern management of the breech delivery. *Am. J. Obstet. Gynecol.*, **134**, 611
6. Woods, J. R. (1979). Effects of low-birth-weight breech delivery on neonatal mortality. *Obstet. Gynecol.*, **53**, 735
7. Kauppila, O. *et al.* (1981). Management of low birth weight breech delivery: should cesarean section be routine? *Obstet. Gynecol.*, **57**, 289
8. Nisell, H. *et al.* (1981). Preterm breech delivery, early and late complications. *Acta Obstet. Gynecol. Scand.*, **60**, 363
9. Cox, C. *et al.* (1982). Changed prognosis of breech-presenting low birth weight infants. *Br. J. Obstet. Gynaecol.*, **89**, 881
10. Geirsson, R. T. *et al.* (1982). Preterm singleton breech presentation: the impact of traumatic intracranial haemorrhage on neonatal mortality. *J. Obstet. Gynaecol.*, **2**, 219
11. Effer, S. B. *et al.* (1983). Effect of delivery method on outcomes in the very low-

birth weight breech infant: is the improved survival related to caesarean section or other perinatal care maneuvers. *Am. J. Obstet. Gynecol.*, **145**, 123

12. Main, D. *et al.* (1983). Cesarean section versus vaginal delivery for the breech fetus weighing less than 1500 grams. *Am. J. Obstet. Gynecol.*, **146**, 580

13. Yu, V. *et al.* (1984). Effect of mode of delivery on outcome of very-low-birthweight infants. *Br. J. Obstet. Gynaecol.*, **91**, 633

32

The pediatric approach to the premature breech

N. W. Svenningsen

INTRODUCTION

The special risks for preterm breech delivered infants are related to the vulnerability of the preterm baby as such, to occurrence of trauma in delivery, asphyxia intrapartum, and anaemia or haemorrhages. Congenital anomalies must also be taken into consideration.

Obviously there is a wide variation in the obstetrical management of the preterm breech-presenting fetus. Below 37 weeks of gestation and even more below 32 weeks of gestation the uncertainty of the approach to the mode of delivery becomes even larger. By and large the pediatric approach depends on the degree of immaturity at delivery. In a large Swedish survey it was shown that the preterm breech delivered infant is over-represented in infants with cerebral palsy (Table 1)[1].

Table 1 Fetal presentation of motor handicapped 266 of 89 500 children 4–16 years

	Vertex (%)	Breech (%)	Preterm/Term (%)
Cerebral palsy (243)	89	11	35/65
Meningocele (23)	74	26	3/97
0 motor handicap	97	3	5/95

South Swedish Region Survey[1]

PRETERM BREECH (30–36 WEEKS GESTATION)

The survival rate and the long-term outcome for breech-delivered infants after

30 weeks of gestation have both improved in recent years[2]. Some recent reports also suggest that the delivery of a least compromised infant who can benefit maximally from modern neonatal intensive care is best achieved with caesarean section in the breech infant expected to weigh 1000–1500 g. However, these hypotheses remain to be proved by randomized clinical trial[3].

VERY PRETERM BREECH (< 30 WEEKS GESTATION)

Regarding the long-term outcome after very early preterm delivery before the 30th week of gestation, whether vertex or breech, results published from different hospitals and different countries vary considerably. These differences are probably related not only to the technique in the birth process as such but also to the myriads of unknown or known variables operative in different materials under different conditions. In a very large study from Australia with long-term follow-up it was shown that in extremely low birthweight infants born in the 24th to 29th week of gestation the handicap rate was 65% for breech-delivered compared to 28% for vertex-delivered infants.[4] A similar tendency was found in a material of singleton preterm infants with a 2-year follow-up study in our own hospital (Table 2).

Table 2   Breech singleton preterm infants (born 1979–82, Lund University Hospital); 2-year-follow-up study. Multiple births, malformed and stillborn infants excluded

Gestational age (weeks)	N (CS)	Died 0–1 years	Handicap* rate in survivors	
			Breech	Vertex
24–29	12 (8)	3	30%	18%
30–32	20 (19)	2	5%	7%
33–36	36 (23)	0	2.8%	3%
Total	68 (50)	5	5/63	17/352
Rate	74%	7.4%	7.7%	4.8%

Total liveborn population: 12 280.
Singleton preterm <37 weeks gestational age: 420
CS = Caesarean section
* Cerebral palsy and/or psychomotor retardation >4 months according to Milani–Comparetti scale.

IMPACT OF INTENSIVE CARE FACILITIES

In a large series of infants born before the 32nd week of gestational age comprising 152 preterm babies we have analysed with computer multivariance analysis 65 variables in obstetrical care and neonatal care, and the relation to occurrence of intraventricular haemorrhage diagnosed by ultrasound. A statistically significant relationship was found to only 4 of the 65 variables, i.e.

low gestational age, low birth weight, asphyxia and occurrence of hyaline membrane disease. However, to understand the pathophysiological mechanisms of these variables and in order to really evaluate the impact of perinatal/neonatal intensive care facilities these mechanisms have to be defined in much more detail. It still remains to be clarified whether the decisive factor for survival or handicap for the very preterm baby (vertex or breech) is the mode of delivery (vaginal or abdominal) or adaptational imbalances, e.g. in circulation and blood pressure related to management in the delivery room or in the neonatal ward. These factors have not hitherto been quantified, but should be included in detail in any future investigations about the perinatal technique of delivery of the preterm breech infant.

CONCLUSIONS

As yet unidentified peri- and neonatal care manoeuvres may be more likely to affect the outcome in the very small preterm breech infant before the 32nd week of gestation than the mode of delivery as such. The peri- and postnatal management of these very preterm babies, both vertex- and breech-delivered, remains a unique challenge in perinatal medicine.

References

1. Lagergren, J. (1981). Children with motor handicaps. Epidemiological, medical and socio-paediatric aspects of motor handicapped children in a Swedish county. *Acta Paediatr. Scand.*, suppl. **289**, 24–31
2. Ingemarsson, I., Westgren, M. and Svenningsen, N. W. (1978). Long-term follow-up of preterm infants in breech presentation delivered by caesarean section. A prospective study. *Lancet*, **2**, 172–5
3. Yu, V. Y. H., Bajuk, B., Cutting, D., Orgill, A. A. and Astbury, J. (1984). Effect of mode of delivery on outcome of very-low-birthweight infants. *Br. J. Obstet. Gynaecol.*, **91**, 633–9
4. Kitchen, W. H., Yu, V. Y. H., Orgill, A.A., Ford, G., Rickards, A., Astbury, J., Ryan, M. M., Russo, W., Lissenden, J. V. and Bajuk, B. (1982). Infants born before 29 weeks gestation: survival and morbidity at 2 years of age. *Br. J. Obstet. Gynaecol.*, **89**, 887–91

33

The obstetric management of the mature breech

The Editors

(It was not possible for the presenter of the third paper in this session to produce a manuscript. However, as chairman of the session one of the editors had taken notes and with the aid of some of those who helped in the original study has produced this summary. We are grateful to all members of the hospital staff who contributed to the work.)

In the introduction to the workshop the Chairman stressed the importance of discussing preterm and term breech separately. During the 1970s it had become obvious that the raised perinatal mortality and morbidity associated with this abnormal presentation had been due more often to the high proportion of premature infants than to the mode of delivery and that increasing the incidence of caesarean section might not necessarily improve the outcome for breech babies. In 1977, in an attempt to rationalize this problem, a study of the management of the baby presenting by the breech at or after 37 weeks of pregnancy was commenced at the Coombe Hospital. The objects of the study were to examine the effect of breech presentation at term on the rate of cervical dilatation, to compare babies delivered by the breech with those who had a spontaneous vertex delivery and to look for differences between vaginally born breech infants and those who came to caesarean section either elective or emergency.

The criteria accepted for the management of breech labour were those which had obtained at the hospital for some years previously. A clinical estimate of the baby's weight was attempted. If it was felt to be larger than average, resort to elective caesarean section was likely, especially in a primigravid mother. If fetal size appeared to be compatible with safe vaginal delivery and if either ultrasound or abdominal X-ray showed the fetal head to be flexed an assessment was made of the maternal pelvis usually by means of a lateral X-ray. Provided this seemed adequate the spontaneous onset of labour was the aim with very few cases being induced or accelerated.

The study population consisted of 200 consecutive breech deliveries, 52 primigravidae and 148 multigravidae. All went into spontaneous labour at or later than 37 weeks gestation and all babies weighed 2500 g or over. Twins, malformations and intrauterine deaths prior to the onset of labour were excluded. Oxytocin stimulation and epidural analgesia were avoided. Control subjects were the next patient admitted in spontaneous labour with a cephalic presentation who fulfilled the same criteria as the study group and who underwent a spontaneous vertex delivery. The progress of labour was assessed every 2 hours in both groups by rectal or vaginal examination. All of the babies were delivered by doctors of registrar or consultant status. Breech extraction was not employed. Eighty-three per cent of cases had forceps applied to the after-head, the remainder being managed by spontaneous expulsion or the Mauriceau–Smellie–Veit manoeuvre. Immediate assessment of the baby was by means of a modified Apgar score, with a maximum count of 8 and excluding colour.

RESULTS

Table 1 summarizes the details of 450 term babies presenting by the breech during the study period. In a small number of cases labour was induced but these and the 40 patients in whom acceleration was used have been excluded from analysis. One hundred and twenty-six mothers were electively sectioned and the overall section rate was 45%.

Table 1   Breech presentation at term

	Number	Vaginal delivery	Caesarean section	Percentage
Spontaneous onset	261	200	61	23
Labour accelerated	40	26	14	35
Labour induced	23	18	5	22
Elective section	126	—	126	28

Cervical dilatation

Table 2 compares rates of cervical dilatation for breech babies with those of vertex presentations in both primigravid and multiparous patients. There is no difference in the rate of progress for primigravidae but the multiparous cervix dilated significantly more slowly with a breech presentation in both the early and latter parts of the first stage of labour. This difference did not persist into the second stage (Table 3).

The babies

Table 4 compares the 200 vaginally delivered breech babies with the 200 controls who had spontaneous vertex deliveries. In all parities the breeches

Table 2 Cervical dilatation (centimetres per hour)

	Primigravida		Multigravida	
Centimetres	Breech	Control	Breech	Control
1–5	1.3	1.3	1.8**	2.4
5–10	2.4	2.5	3.7***	5.7

** = 0.01; *** = 0.001

Table 3 Maturity and length of labour in 200 vaginally delivered breeches compared with spontaneous vertex controls

	Primigravida		Multigravida	
	Breech	Control	Breech	Control
Total babies	52	35	148	165
Weeks maturity	39.6	39.6	39.6	39.7
Hours 1st stage	6.5	5.3	4.6***	3.2
Minutes 2nd stage	29	28	16	14

*** = 0.001

Table 4 Baby weight, Apgar score and problems in neonatal period

	Primigravida		Multigravida	
	Breech	Control	Breech	Control
Birth weight (kg)	3.15	3.32	3.38**	3.53
1 min Apgar	6.6***	7.8	6.8***	7.5
5 min Apgar	7.7***	8.0	7.8***	8.0
Problems (%)	4	0	4	0

** = 0.01; *** = 0.001

weighed less than the controls. The Apgar scores were significantly lower for breech babies at both 1 and 5 minutes. There were no neonatal problems in the controls but eight of the breeches had complications in the first few hours of life. Four of these suffered mild cerebral irritation: one baby had a small sub-dural haemorrhage, another suffered a few hours of grunting respirations and one was slow to establish feeding. One infant died at 48 hours of life and post-mortem revealed spinal cord necrosis at the level of the seventh cervical vertebra. Antepartum X-ray had implied the presence of a spina bifida so even when labour appeared prolonged, caesarean section was not considered.

Table 5 Vaginally delivered breech babies compared with breech babies delivered by elective caesarean section

	Primigravida		Multigravida	
	Vaginal breech	Elective caesarean	Vaginal breech	Elective caesarean
Total babies	52	58	148	68
Birth weight (kg)	3.15**	3.41	3.38*	3.54
1 min Apgar	6.6***	7.6	6.8	7.1
5 min Apgar	7.7	7.9	7.8	7.9
Problems (%)	4	5	4	4

* = 0.05; ** = 0.01; *** = 0.001

Table 6 Vaginally delivered breech babies compared with breech babies delivered by emergency caesarean section

	Primigravida		Multigravida	
	Vaginal breech	Emergency caesarean	Vaginal breech	Emergency caesarean
Total babies	52	32	148	29
Hours 1st stage	6.5	8.3	4.5**	7.1
Birth weight (kg)	3.15**	3.38	3.38**	3.66
1 min Apgar	6.6	6.6	6.8	7.1
5 min Apgar	7.7	7.7	7.8	7.8
Problems (%)	4	3	4	7

** = 0.01

Elective caesarean section

Table 5 contrasts the 200 vaginally delivered breeches with the 126 who underwent elective caesarean section. The latter were significantly heavier than the former. The figures imply that it is worthwhile attempting an estimate of fetal size prior to deciding the mode of delivery. Many of these babies were sectioned because it was felt that they were larger than average. One minute Apgar scores (calculated out of 8) were significantly lower for vaginally delivered primigravid breeches but recovered by 5 minutes. Both groups in the multigravid patients had similar Apgar scores but it is of interest to note that the incidence of minor problems in the neonatal period was identical whatever the mode of delivery.

Emergency caesarean section

Of 261 breech presentations which went into spontaneous labour, 61 were delivered by caesarean section. Table 6 shows that the length of the first stage was longer in the latter patients and that the babies were significantly heavier in both primigravidae and multigravidae. There was, however, no difference in Apgar scores or in the incidence of neonatal problems.

DISCUSSION

The results of this study show that cervical dilatation after the spontaneous onset of labour was slower in multiparous patients with a breech presentation than when the baby was presenting head first. Presumably this was due to the babies of multiparous mothers having flexed legs which offered a less uniform surface to dilate up the cervix. There was no difference in the rate of dilatation in primigravid women and in neither group was the length of the second stage altered when compared to controls. Vaginally delivered breech babies had lower Apgar scores and slightly more neonatal problems than cephalically pre-senting controls. However, the only improvement brought about by resort to caesarean section occurred in the babies of electively sectioned primigravid mothers, whose 1 minute Apgar scores were significantly better than those who went on to vaginal delivery. Even so, this difference was not apparent at 5 minutes.

Attempts to estimate fetal weight prior to making a decision as to how a breech should be delivered appeared to be worthwhile. However, even if larger babies were not selected out before the onset of labour, their size often led to prolongation of the first stage of labour and subsequent caesarean section.

The findings presented here suggest that with careful selection the possibility of vaginal delivery should be entertained in 72% of term breeches with only 28% demonstrating factors which would normally lead to elective caesarean section. Of those who do go into spontaneous labour, approximately one-quarter will require emergency caesarean section. Vaginally delivered breech babies will have lower Apgar scores and more problems in the neonatal period than babies who are born head first. However, apart from 1 minute Apgar scores in electively sectioned primigravidae, abdominal delivery will not necessarily improve the outcome for the mature breech baby.

34

The term breech: subsequent growth and development

P. O'Connell and A. Keane

The management of breech presentation at term remains controversial. Aside from maternal considerations evaluation of methods of delivery is largely dependent on assessment of outcome in the infant. To this end a 4-year prospective longitudinal study of infants presenting as a breech at term was undertaken in the Coombe Lying-in Hospital. In addition to assessing outcome the study also aimed to determine whether term breeches have patterns of growth and development which differ from the norm. Results to 2 years of age are presented.

This study was initiated at the same time as a study of the obstetrical management of breech presentation was taking place in our hospital[1]. It differs from other similar studies in several respects[2-5]. Only infants whose gestational age was assessed at 37 weeks or over were included. Previous otherwise admirable studies have considered preterm and term breeches together. In our experience these are two different populations, with different characteristics, which should not be combined together for analysis. Also unlike some other studies, we have considered the term breech population as a whole irrespective of mode of delivery. Finally in addition to being prospective and longitudinal all breeches born during the study period were accounted for.

DATA OF STUDY GROUP

Study period: 9½ months
Deliveries ≥ 28 weeks: 5699
Singleton term breech presentation: 141
Incidence: 2.47%

Perinatal deaths (three with multiple anomalies): 5
Liveborn with severe anomalies: 2

219

Unable or unwilling to participate: 14
The remaining 120 formed the study group together with 63 control infants.

Admission criteria:

Study $n = 120$ Control $n = 63$
Breech presentation   Vertex presentation
Singleton pregnancy $\geq$ 37 weeks   Singleton pregnancy $\geq$ 37 weeks
                                       Absence of complications.
                                       Matched for parity and gestational age.

Basic data regarding the format of the study, assessment methods and details
of follow-up are available on request.

RESULTS

Maternal characteristics

Except in regard to parity, maternal characteristics were similar to those of the
general hospital population. Forty-five per cent of mothers were primipara
compared with 30% expected. Of the 66 multiparous mothers 12 had had a
previous breech delivery.

Mode of delivery

Breech group
  vaginal 56%
  caesarean section 44%
Sixty per cent of caesarean sections were elective; 59% of primiparas were sectioned.
  The control group were spontaneous vertex by definition.

Infant characteristics

Mean birth weight
  all breech 3.39 kg
  controls 3.44 kg
There was no significant difference in mean birth weight between study and
control groups, and these were in turn similar to the hospital norm.
  However, mean birth weight of the vaginally delivered breeches was 3.18 kg
compared with 3.41 kg for the elective section group and 3.65 kg for the non-
elective sections. As these data indicate, in general the smaller babies were delivered vaginally, whereas the larger babies came to section.

Male/female ratio

Analysis of the sex distribution in the breech group showed a greater proportion of females with a ratio of 1 : 1.3. A similar ratio was also present in the

total group of 141.

Congenital anomalies

There was a higher incidence than expected in the breech group. In addition to five infants with severe congenital abnormalities already noted there was an increased incidence of minor anomalies. Congenital dislocated hips and other anomalies of the lower limbs were more common, as were anomalies of the genitourinary tract.

Apgar score

Fourteen infants in the study group had an Apgar of less than 7 at 1 minute, and 4 less than 7 at 5 minutes; 6 required intubation. There was no significant difference between vaginal and caesarean section breeches.

Neonatal neurological assessment

There was a higher incidence of minor neuromotor dysfunction in the breech group. The breech group had a significantly lower Moro threshold ($p = 0.02^*$).

Of a total of 34 neurological items tested, only three showed a significant difference between breech and control groups.

Popliteal angle ($p = 0.001^*$)
Heel to ear test ($p = 0.001^*$)
Ventral suspension ($p = 0.02^*$)

The findings were significant both for vaginal and section breeches. These three items test tone in the trunk and lower limbs, and are an expression of maturity as well as of neurological function. It is possible that in the breeches this represents a more immature pattern of neurological development rather than neurological dysfunction. If so the question then arises as to whether this selective immaturity is causative to the persistence of breech presentation at term, or whether it is a consequence of immobilization of the breech in the pelvis.

Development assessment

Motor development

The breech group showed more immature patterns of trunk and lower limb development. At 32 week weight-bearing ($p = 0.01^*$), sitting pattern ($p = 0.05$) and overall gross motor development ($p = 0.01$) showed significant differences. Walking patterns at a year were later ($p = 0.02^*$), as was the age of independent walking ($p = 0.4^*$) Further analysis showed that the section breeches were later than the vaginal breeches.

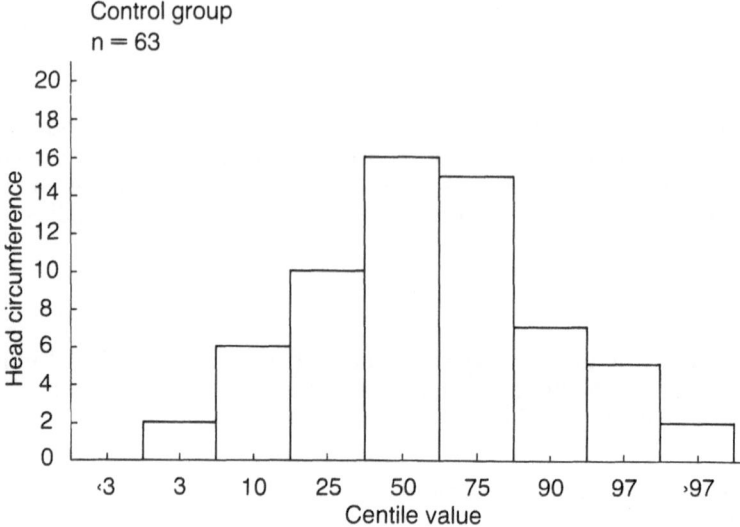

Figure 1   Control group: distribution of head circumference at birth (centile value; *n*=63)

Speech development

Some significant differences in aspects of speech development emerged at 12 months, 18 months and 2 years. Though minor they are interesting in the light of the psychological assessment at 4 years, when the breeches scored significantly lower in verbal testing.

It must be emphasized that though the developmental patterns are significantly different they are still well within the limits of normality

Anthropometric assessment

Some interesting features emerged from the study of growth differences between the breech and control groups.

Head circumference

There was no significant difference in mean head circumference between the two groups; however, the distribution curves were different. In the control group the curve is normal (Figure 1) whereas in the breech group the curve is skewed to the right (Figure 2). Forty infants, or one-third, had a head circumference on the 97th centile or greater. The importance of head size in the management and in the outcome of breech labour is shown by the fact that 75% of these came to caesarean section.

The distribution of head circumference at 2 years of age (Figure 3) showed a persistence of large head size, indicating that the findings at birth could not be

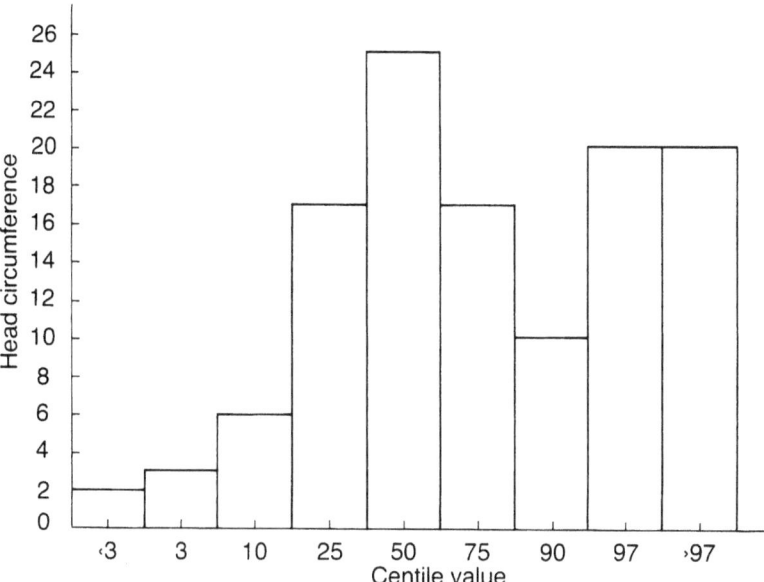

Figure 2 The term breech: distribution of head circumference at birth (centile value; $n=120$)

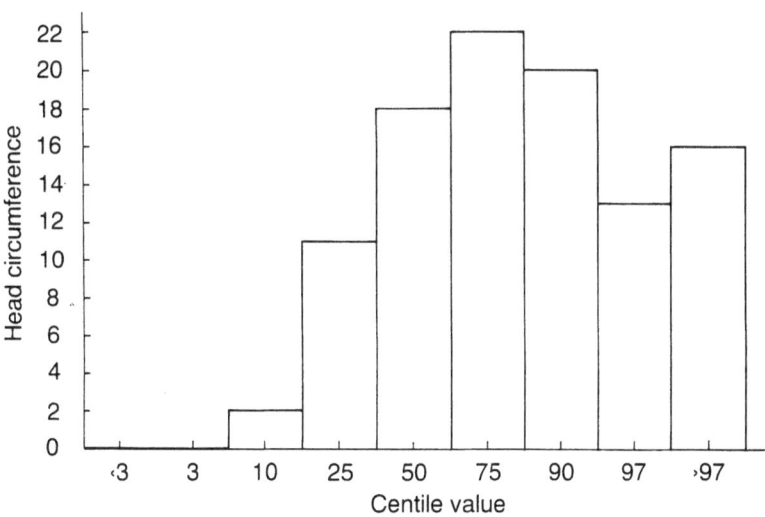

Figure 3 The term breech: head circumference at 2 years (centile value; $n=103$)

explained by lack of pelvic moulding in the later stages of pregnancy.

Data on height and weight at birth and 2 years of age were also presented, from which it would appear that many breeches have a body configuration which differs from the norm in that they tend to be shorter, heavier and with larger head size.

In summary, the term breech babies compared with a normal group showed

(a) a higher incidence of congenital anomalies;
(b) a higher incidence of minor neuromotor dysfunction;
(c) later patterns of motor development relating to the lower limbs;
(d) a greater number of babies with bodily configuration differing from the norm.

These findings were independent of the mode of delivery and would appear to be inherent in the breech baby.

Despite being an at-risk group the rate of morbidity noted was low. Also, as was emphasized, the development patterns observed in the breeches, though significantly later than in the controls, were still well within the limits of normality. It is possible that these differences have their origins in prenatal factors, either genetic or environmental, rather than in mode of delivery.

We consider that these results reflect good standards of obstetrical care and particularly the practice of opting for caesarean section to deliver not only the higher weight babies but also those with larger head circumferences. Moreover, it would appear that vaginal delivery of the term breech is a safe undertaking in controlled circumstances.

References

1. Duignan, N. M. (1982). The management of breech presentation. In Studd, J. (ed.) *Progress in Obstetrics and Gynaecology*, pp. 73–84. (London: Churchill Livingstone)
2. Bird, C. C. and McElin, T. W. (1974). A six-year prospective study of term breech deliveries utilizing the Zatuchni–Andros prognostic scoring index. *Am. J. Obstet. Gynecol.* **121**, 551–7
3. Neligan, G. A., Prudsham, D. and Steiner, H. (eds.) (1974). *The Formative Years. Birth, family and development in Newcastle-upon-Tyne.* (London: Oxford University Press)
4. Manzke, H. (1978). Morbidity among infants born in breech presentation. *J. Perinat. Med.* **6**, 127–38
5. Faber-Nijholt, R. (1981). *Breech Presentation and Neurological Morbidity. A Comparative Study.* (Rijksuniversiteit te Groningen)

35

The term breech: results of psychological assesment at 4 years of age

J. A. Connolly and A. Keane

This paper reports the results of intellectual assessment performed on a cohort of 183 4-year old subjects, comprising 120 successive term breech presentations (excluding those with major congenital anomalies) and a control group of 63 vertex deliveries. Subjects were matched for birth weight, gestation, parity and socioeconomic level. The study contributed to a longitudinal study of breech delivery in the Coombe Lying-In Hospital, reported elsewhere in this volume.

Subjects attended the hospital for examination as close to their fourth birthday as possible. Subjects were interviewed alone, with one or both parents next door. Testing usually took 1 hour and was carried out after the subject had settled down and relaxed. Ninety-nine of 120 breech subjects were traced, attended at 4 years, and had testing completed (82.5%). Fifty of 63 control subjects were also tested (79.4%).

The test instrument administered was the Wechsler Preschool and Primary Scale of Intelligence (WPPSI). It yields a full scale intelligence quotient (FSIQ), as well as a verbal intelligence quotient (VIQ) and non-verbal, or performance, intelligence quotient (PIQ). VIQ and PIQ scores are each obtained from a series of five constituent subtests. Thus, overall intellectual performance can be examined, as well as performance in specific areas.

The WPPSI has a VIQ test/retest reliability coefficient of 0.94; PIQ of 0.91; and FSIQ of 0.96. Each WPPSI subtest yields a scaled score, where 10 represents a mean or exactly average performance for any subject. An exactly average overall performance yields a mean FSIQ, VIQ and PIQ, all nominally valued at 100. The average range lies between 90 and 110 (SD = 15).

Mean VIQ score for the breech group was 103.9, and for controls 109.36. Mean PIQ score was 106.72 for breech, and 109.4 for control. Mean FSIQ for breech was 106.13, and for control, 110.4. The VIQ means for the groups show a statistically significant difference ($p < 0.05$). Neither PIQ nor FSIQ means are significantly different. Breech subjects fall into the upper quartile of average intellectual performance, and controls into the above-average range.

Figure 1 presents mean scaled scores for VIQ subtests, for both groups. On the information test, breech score 10.7, control 11.5. Vocabulary yields 9.5 for breech, 9.1 for control. Arithmetic yields a breech score of 11.8, control of 13.5 ($p < 0.001$). On similarities breech score 11.8, control 13.5 ($p < 0.01$). On

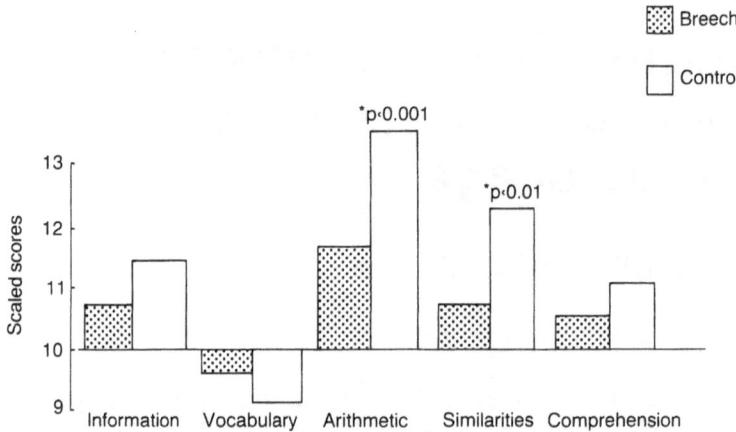

Figure 1   WPPSI: scale scores for verbal subtests, by delivery type

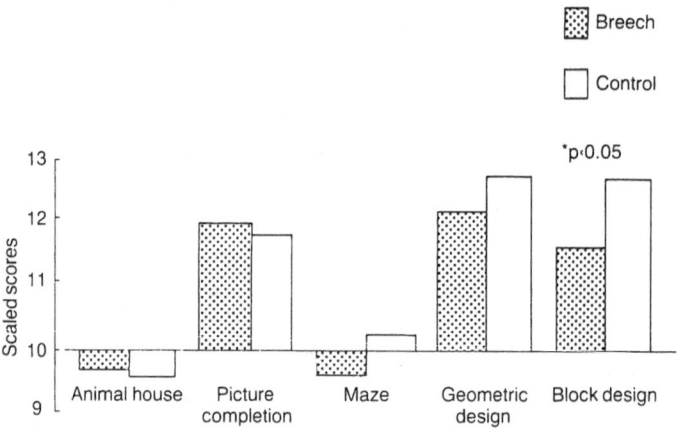

Figure 2   WPPSI: scale scores for performance subtests, by delivery type

the comprehension test, breech score 10.6, control 11. In general, scores favour the control group, with the exception of vocabulary where both fall below the mean, the controls more so.

Figure 2 presents the mean scaled scores for PIQ subtests, for both groups. On three tests both groups score well above the mean. Picture completion yields a score of 12 for breech, 11.8 for control. On geometric design, breech

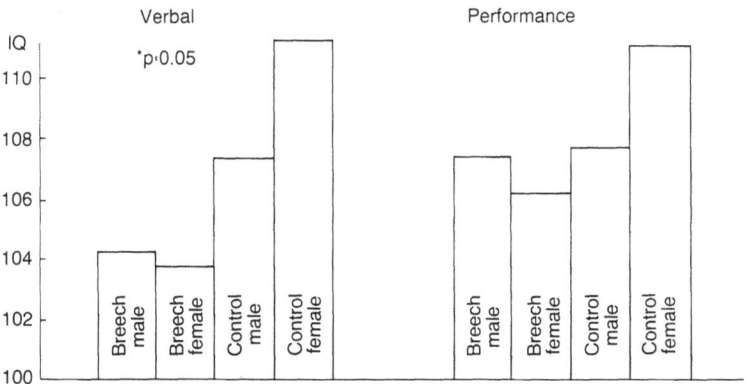

Figure 3 WPPSI: IQ scores Anova for sex, by delivery type interaction

score 12.2, control 12.8. On block design, breech score 11.6, control 12.7 ($p < 0.05$). On the maze test the breech group fall below the test mean with a score of 9.8, against the control group score of 10.2. On the animal house test both groups fall below the mean, breech with 9.7, control with 9.5.

Further analysis of variance (Anova) was carried out, examining the IQ/sex/delivery mode interactions. Figure 3 illustrates the VIQ and PIQ mean scores for both groups, with male and female scores separated out. In both sets, controls have higher scores. Mean VIQ scores are significantly different. With breeches, males have a higher VIQ than females, 104.2 compared to 103.7. This trend holds for PIQ scores also, with male mean at 107.4, female 106.2. Interestingly, this trend is reversed for the control group, which yields a male VIQ score of 107.3, female 111.4. With PIQ scores the control males average 107.7, females 111.1.

Although group differences are non-significant statistically, the trend holds for FSIQ scores. Breech males score 106.8, females 105.6. The pattern is again reversed among controls, with males scoring 108.4, females 112.3.

The trend for male breeches to be brighter than females can be explained by referring to breech type. Figure 4 illustrates the IQ scores for the elective caesarean section group.

Male VIQ is 109.5, female 102.3. Male PIQ is 114.9, female 104.3. FSIQ for males is 113.9, and for females, 103.6. This difference is significant ($p < 0.05$). Why such a major difference in IQ level should exist is unclear.

The mean FSIQ for the total group of elective caesarean sections is 108.3. For the non-elective sections it is 107.3, and for the full breech group, including sectioned breeches, it is 103.9. It can be seen that the brighter breech children at 4 years have a history of elective section; this is followed by non-elective section, and finally by vaginal breech.

In the case of the elective sections the significant effect on raised IQ levels is due directly to the male scores. The group displays a fairly symmetrical distribution of FSIQ scores; the four lowest are 81, 86, 91 and 92; the four highest, 124, 125, 127 and 129. These higher IQ scores are predominantly male.

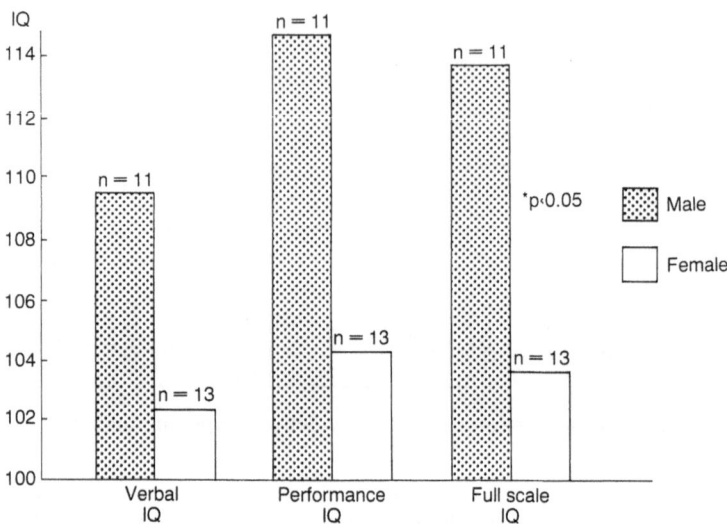

Figure 4   WPPSI: elective caesarean section IQ scores v. sex of subject

Elective caesarean sections differ further in that they were the only group to display significant correlations between head circumference at birth and IQ at 4 years. Male versus female associations are not as significant as those for the total group.

It is possible to question the method of sampling to obtain the cohort whose testing at 4 years is reported in this paper, in that not every live-born breech delivery was included. In addition, the matched pairing of control to breech subjects cannot be equated strictly with random sampling from a universe of possible control subjects. Nevertheless, these are two well-matched samples, and it appears valid to draw some conclusions from the data. The conclusions, based on the data obtained from the subjects following psychological test examination at 4 years, are as follows:

1. Both groups function above the test mean, and are intellectually in the high average range.
2. There is a trend for breech IQ scores to be lower than control IQ scores.
3. This difference is statistically significant for verbal IQ scores.
4. Breech males have higher IQ scores than breech females.
5. Control group female subjects reverse this pattern.
6. Elective caesarean section subjects are the brightest of the breech group subjects, and are not different from the control group in terms of IQ. Elective section females are notably less bright than elective section males, and the difference is statistically significant. This group differs more from other breech subjects than it does from controls.

Section 9
Perinatal Audit

36

Perinatal audit: an overview

M. J. N. C. Keirse

Although perinatal audit is a relatively new term, its history dates back far beyond that of the discipline of perinatology. From 1720 to 1750 England was swept by a gin epidemic as the government lifted the traditional restrictions on distilling in order to create new markets for grain. In 1726 the College of Physicians petitioned parliament calling gin 'a cause of weak, feeble and distempered children', and in 1736 a committee of the Middlesex sessions reported that '. . . children are born weak and sickly, and often look shrivel'd and old as though they had numbered many years'[1]. Applying the definition 'an official examination of accounts' listed in the Oxford dictionary[2], this must be a classical example of audit related to perinatology. Few examinations are more official than those of a parliamentary committee; the available accounts were certainly scrutinized; and supposedly the aim was some positive action for the improvement of perinatal health.

Such examples can be found throughout medical history, but this one is particularly instructive for three reasons. First, fetal growth retardation was not a recognized clinical entity at that time; yet the choice of words is remarkably similar to the classical description that would emanate two centuries later[3]. Second, medical textbooks of that era even lacked an appropriate frame of reference. Obstetric writings of such workers as Mauriceau (1637–1709) and Smellie (1697–1763) contained erroneously high birth weight estimates, and the first accurate measurements of size and weight at birth were only reported by Roederer in 1753[4]. Third, despite the fact that alcohol has been in use for centuries, and the evidence from the eighteenth century[1], the harmful effects of alcohol on fetal development needed to be rediscovered as a new syndrome at the end of the 1960s[5]. The lessons to be learnt are that audit may, as it has in the past, uncover significant deficiencies in perinatal care; that it may do so even in the absence of a satisfactory frame of reference; and that there is – unfortunately – no guarantee that its messages will be understood or remem-

231

bered by the providers of perinatal care.

Although essential, it is not easy to establish the true meaning of the term 'perinatal audit'. There are no universally agreed definitions of the words perinatal and audit. Perinatal should mean surrounding birth, but the definitions of WHO[6] and FIGO[7], distributed to the participants of the last three European Congresses of Perinatal Medicine, define birth as a weight of 500 g or more, and the perinatal period as starting from a fetal weight of 1000 g (about 28 weeks) and ending 7 days after birth. This certainly is too narrow a limit. For the purpose of audit it should probably start at, or pretty close to, conception and not end before the end of the entire neonatal period (28 days).

The word audit too has been variously defined. The Oxford dictionary defines it as 'an official examination of accounts'[2], but how official does it need to be? Where is the dividing line between an informal assessment, through study of case records and discussions with colleagues, and a formal gathering with edited minutes that are distributed for the benefit of the entire universe? Clearly this is a matter of judgment, but it is probably wise to avoid too narrow an interpretation and to concentrate on the nature rather than on the form of that examination.

When the words are combined, the question may arise whether the examination or the accounts need to be 'perinatal'. This is an important distinction and there is an excellent example of it. In the early 1950s at least three randomized controlled trials[8-10], looking at the then available accounts, showed diethylstilboestrol to have no beneficial effect whatsoever on the conditions for which it was being used in pregnancy. Yet it would take 20 years and another audit to show that this perinatal practice had not only been useless but also quite harmful for the development of the infants exposed to it[11,12]. Again, there are ample reasons for not putting too narrow a limit to what is understood as a meaningful perinatal audit. Dr Chalmers has defined perinatal audit as 'any evaluative process which explicitly aims to provide information which can lead to improvements in the care available to childbearing women and their families'[13]. It is not a definition that will satisfy those in want of appropriate cut-off points, but at least it accommodates the goals that are aimed at, and the diversity of ways in which they can be achieved.

There are many ways in which audit can and has been implemented. Perinatal mortality meetings and surveys are traditional examples. However, in its preoccupation with a minority of poor outcomes, that tradition has not infrequently neglected the large majority of births and the care provided for these mothers, fetuses and infants. Moreover, variation in the frequency of death – unadjusted for birth weight[14], congenital malformations[15] or pathological subgroups[16] – correlates poorly with variation in indices of perinatal care[17]. Probably because of their inherent tendency to decline, crude perinatal mortality rates have been relentlessly misused to support any view, trend or fashion[18]. While this is no reason to entirely disqualify them, it is a truism that they are often used in a manner which is the very antithesis of what perinatal audit should be about.

Some forms of audit are quite easy. Hospitals and departments collect countless items of data and these can easily be turned into useful tools for examining our practices. However, more time is usually spent in designing and

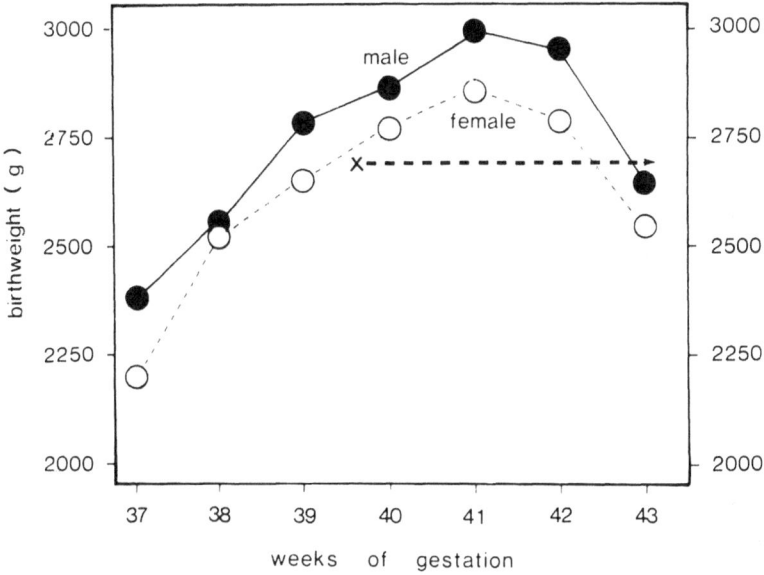

Figure 1 Tenth percentile of birth weight for gestation for male and female infants in the 1970 British Birth Survey[22]. Note that infant X, born at 39 weeks, would be considered as of low weight for gestation, but would be considered as appropriately grown (> 10th percentile) when born with the same weight 3 or 4 weeks later (adapted from *Clin. Obstet. Gynaecol.*[20])

completing the forms, than in examining what they may convey at the end of the year. Changes in policy, if noted, are not necessarily noticed and even less frequently subjected to proper evaluation. Various forms of intervention such as operative deliveries, episiotomies, and admission to special care baby units, are usually recorded in departmental reports, but how much time or effort is spent in examining whether their rates need to be as high as they are? Large data sets, which are available from many sources, can be useful tools if they are utilized with an understanding that – no matter how large it is – no large data set is more intelligent than the person using it. Our current use of fetal growth standards, a common misnomer for birth weight-for-gestational age standards, can easily illustrate that. For instance, the use of the criterion '2 SD below the mean weight for gestation' (a common criterion for retarded fetal growth) puts the cut-off points for retarded growth at 30 weeks of gestation at 300 g in Britain, at 640 g in Baltimore, and at 1023 g in Montreal[19]. This would seem to imply that a Montreal fetus, estimated to weigh 1000 g at 30 weeks, could be 'cured' from its growth retardation by intrauterine transport to London. Such measure would be effective even if the fetus loses two-thirds of its weight while crossing the Atlantic. Similarly, several respectable data sets show what is illustrated in Figure 1, i.e. that, at term, infants could be 'cured' from so-named fetal growth retardation merely by prolonging pregnancy for a few weeks[20]. Being evidently ridiculous, these proposals for effective treatment convey important messages. First, the proposals are based on respectable data sets and on weight-for-gestational age standards and definitions of growth retardation that are commonly used in perinatal medicine. If they are wrong – and they are – this can only be due to faulty interpretation[20,21] of the crude data consisting of weights and gestational ages. Second, how many measures and interventions have been introduced into perinatal medicine with a far lesser wealth of evidence to support them? Third, what evidence is there that other crude data (e.g. the outcome of preterm breech deliveries) have been interpreted with greater lucidity, before they were used to implement drastic changes in policy (such as routine caesarean section for the preterm breech)?

Some information is not always available in an easy and straightforward manner. It can be obtained, though, from those who use the perinatal services or from the numerous consumer groups that have sprung up in the past decade. While there is undoubtedly an element of fashion in the rise and success of these parties, most of what they voice should be an inbuilt part of any perinatal audit. Regrettably, there is a large discrepancy between the understanding shown for irrational fears and anxieties that women may have about the outcome of pregnancy, and the lack of understanding for any concern, rational or irrational, that they may have about the quality of the care or the providers thereof.

There are virtually no limits to the number and the nature of data that can be used for audits of perinatal practice. However, if perinatal audit is to become more than a fashionable concept, it will need to acquire the status of a self-perpetuating habit; but then, essentially a habit of continuously questioning medical customs, interventions and practices throughout the perinatal field.

References

1. Warner, R. H. and Rosett, H. L. (1975). The effect of drinking on offspring: an historical survey of the American and British literature. *J. Studies Alcohol.*, **36**, 1395–420
2. Sykes, J. B. (ed.) (1978). *The Concise Oxford Dictionary of Current English*, 6th edn, p. 61. (Oxford: Oxford University Press)
3. Clifford, S. H. (1954). Postmaturity with placental dysfunction: clinical syndrome and pathologic findings. *J. Pediatr.*, **44**, 1–13
4. Cone, T. E. (1961). De pondere infantum recens natorum. The history of weighing the newborn infant. *Pediatrics*, **28**, 490–8
5. Lemoine, P., Haronsseau, H., Borteyru, J. P. and Menuet, J. C. (1968). Les enfants de parents alcooliques; anomalies observées à propos de 127 cas. *Quest Med.*, **25**, 476–82
6. WHO (1977). Recommended definitions, terminology and format for statistical tables related to the perinatal period and use of a new certificate for cause of perinatal deaths. *Acta Obstet. Gynecol. Scand.*, **56**, 247–53
7. FIGO news (1976). Lists of gynaecologic and obstetrical terms and definitions. *Int. J. Gynaecol. Obstet.*, **14**, 570–6
8. Robinson, D. and Shettles, L. B. (1952). The use of diethylstilbestrol in threatened abortion. *Am. J. Obstet. Gynecol.*, **63**, 1330–3
9. Dieckmann, W. J., Davis, M. E., Rynkiewicz, L. M. and Pottinger, R. E. (1953). Does the administration of diethylstilbestrol during pregnancy have therapeutic value? *Am. J. Obstet. Gynecol.*, **66**, 1062–81

10. Ferguson, J. H. (1953). Effect of stilbestrol on pregnancy compared to the effect of a placebo. *Am. J. Obstet. Gynecol.*, **65**, 592–601
11. Herbst, A. L., Poskanzer, D. C., Robboy, S. J., Friedlander, L. and Scully, R. E. (1975). Prenatal exposure to stilbestrol: a prospective comparison of exposed female offspring with unexposed controls. *N. Engl. J. Med.*, **292**, 334–9
12. Brackbill, Y. and Berendes, H. W. (1978). Dangers of diethylstilbestrol: review of a 1953 paper. *Lancet*, **2**, 520
13. Chalmers, I. G. (1980). An introduction to perinatal audit and surveillance. In Chalmers, I. and McIlwaine, G. (eds.) *Perinatal Audit and Surveillance*, pp. 7–16. (London: Royal College of Obstetricians and Gynaecologists)
14. Lee, K., Paneth, N., Garter, L. M. and Pearlman, M. (1980). The very low-birthweight rate: principal predictor of neonatal mortality in industrialized population. *J. Pediatr.*, **97**, 759–64
15. Chalmers, I. and Macfarlane, A. (1980). Interpretation of perinatal statistics. In Wharton, B. (ed.) *Topics in Perinatal Medicine*, pp. 1–11. (London: Pitman Medical)
16. Wigglesworth, J. S. (1980). Monitoring perinatal mortality. A pathophysiological approach. *Lancet*, **2**, 684–6
17. Bakketeig, L. S., Hoffmann, H. and Sternthal, P. M. (1978). Obstetric service and perinatal mortality in Norway. *Acta Obstet. Gynecol. Scand.*, Suppl., **77**, 3–19
18. Keirse, M. J. N. C. (1984). Perinatal mortality rates do not contain what they purport to contain. *Lancet*, **1**, 1166–9
19. Keirse, M. J. N. C. (1981). Aetiology of intrauterine growth retardation. In Van Assche, F. A. and Robertson, W. B. (eds.) *Fetal Growth Retardation*, pp. 37–56. (Edinburgh: Churchill Livingstone)
20. Keirse, M. J. N. C. (1984). Epidemiology and aetiology of the growth retarded baby. *Clin. Obstet. Gynaecol.*, **11**, 415–36
21. Wilcox, A. J. (1981). Birth weight, gestation, and the fetal growth curve. *Am. J. Obstet. Gynecol.*, **139**, 863–7
22. British Births (1970). vol. 1, *The first week of life*, p. 80. (London: William Heinemann)

37

Use of routinely collected data for perinatal surveillance

P. Bergsjø

Data collection is not enough in itself. A wealth of information comes into special registries, only to be stored for later use, or, more often, is not used. By proper feedback such information can tell us the true state of affairs, and by periodic issuing of reports, the changes that occur. This can save us from guesswork, which for comfort is often labelled 'educated'. I shall give some examples of what we can do with routinely collected data on the national, international and local levels, drawing on Norwegian and Nordic experience.

NATIONAL LEVEL

In Norway, collection of medical information on births started in 1967. This was separated from the civil notification of births, and the Norwegian Medical Birth Registry was established at Bergen University in 1970. It covers every birth past 16 weeks of pregnancy, regardless of signs of life.

Monthly summary lists, based on the individual county, go to the county medical officer who sends them to the birth institutions. These cover numbers and rates of births, perinatal deaths, sex of child, birth order (first child), unmarried mothers, mothers below 20, low birth weight, maternal diseases, induced labours, operative deliveries, birth complications. In addition, the birth registry has a monitoring system for congenital malformations[1]. Deviations from expected incidence rates are automatically registered, and values beyond defined alarm limits investigated.

Data from the medical birth registry have been used to show temporal trends and regional differences, for example, in caesarean section rates. More sophisticated research has revealed a tendency for mothers to repeat birth performances in succeeding pregnancies[2,3]. This has been possible through the system of unique person identification numbers, through which there can be linkage of data from succeeding births.

In a country where nearly all births take place in institutions it is of interest to study the framework; that is, the number and size of the institutions, their staffing, equipment and care facilities. This is not on continuous record, but during the 1970s three surveys of Norwegian birth institutions were done[4-6]. The total number of birth institutions decreased by 40%, largely due to the closing of many small maternity homes. Nevertheless, the relative distribution of births by institution size has remained constant, due to the concomitant decline in birth rates. About 20% of all births in Norway take place in departments with less than 500 births per year (Table 1).

Table 1 Maternity institutions in Norway 1972–80 by annual number of births

Annual number of births	1972		1974		1980	
	Number of institutions	Percentage of births	Number of institutions	Percentage of births	Number of institutions	Percentage of births
<50	66	1.8	37	1.0	21	0.7
50– 499	51	17.4	58	21.6	46	20.9
500–1499	30	40.3	23	32.7	20	35.8
1500–2999	9	29.0	11	33.2	8	29.8
≥3000	2	10.3	2	10.8	2	12.8
Total	158	98.7	131	99.4	97	100.0

By combining information on personnel, equipment and availability into an 'obstetric score' for each county, we were able to show a slight but clear negative correlation to perinatal mortality in 1972[4], but not in 1980[6], at which time standards were generally improved.

INTERNATIONAL LEVEL

National data are fairly easy to obtain. International comparisons, on the other hand, run into numerous obstacles. However, the Nordic countries have a long tradition of co-operation, with geographic closeness (except for Iceland) and a common linguistic origin (except for most of Finland and some ethnic minority groups). Since 1970 a working party established by the Nordic Medical Statistical Committee has managed to agree on a common set of tables for births in the Nordic countries. Its first publication covered the year 1979[7], and key tables of more recent years have been incorporated in the book *Health Statistics in The Nordic Countries*[8].

One concern of the working party was that the lower limit of stillborn registration varied, being 16 weeks in Norway; 20 weeks in Iceland; and 28 in Denmark, Finland and Sweden. Such discrepancies will have clear implications for incidence rates of low birth weight and early pregnancy incidents, with the possibility of underreporting from the latter three countries. The solution with regard to presentation was that each relevant tabulation was given in two or three versions, viz.:

all notified cases,
birth weight less than 1000 g,
birth weight 1000 g or more.

By comparing these tabulations the error introduced by underreporting can be roughly estimated. An example is shown in Table 2, showing how the lower limit affects the stillbirth rates of births of less than 1000 g for Norway and Iceland. In Norway, however, the stillbirth rate for births of 1000 g or more is also substantially higher than in the other countries. This can only in part be explained by the cut-off effect, as the difference persists all through the weight range, as seen in Figure 1. Comparing perinatal and infant mortality rates between Denmark, Norway and Sweden the main difference lies in stillbirth rates. This calls for an explanation, which prompted a detailed case audit of every perinatal death in five Norwegian counties during 1 year[9].

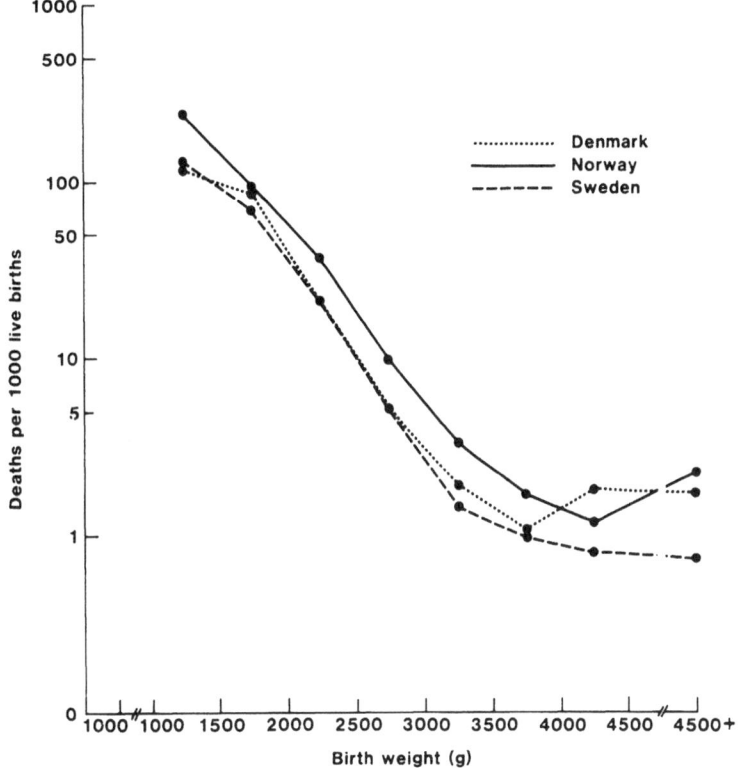

Figure 1 Birth weight specific stillbirth rates in Denmark, Norway and Sweden, 1979 (source: ref. 7)

The basic information of the Nordic tables is mainly hard data such as: age of mother, number of previous children, life or death, birth weight in grams, time in days, weeks or months. Producing these tables has been an elaborate

Table 2 Still births and live births in the Nordic countries 1979 reported to the Medical Birth Registration System, by birth weight of more or less than 1000 grams; weight-specific figures from Finland not available

| | Total | Births <1000 g | | Births ≥1000 g | | Still births per 1000 total births | |
Country	births	Still births	Live births	Still births	Live births	<1000 g	≥1000 g
Denmark	59 451	12	94	291	59 054	0.2	4.9
Iceland	4 477	9	6	18	4 444	2.0	4.0
Norway	51 941	253	97	334	51 257	4.9	6.4
Sweden	95 869	43	130	352	95 344	0.4	3.6

Source: ref. 7

task in itself, because of the need for common definitions and standardization. The next step, which is now well under way, is to compile and compare morbidity, habits of living, events and procedures during pregnancy, birth and the neonatal period.

In Britain a set of characteristics and tabulations for perinatal comparisons has been proposed, fairly similar to the Nordic set[10]. It is highly desirable that these are designed for international comparisons, which requires collaboration beyond adhering to FIGO/WHO standards.

LOCAL (DEPARTMENT) LEVEL

Finally, a few words about the use of hospital data for systematic surveillance of one's own activities. It is common experience that changes in medication, operative procedures or examination routines emerge gradually without a clear motive, or that they follow a quick decision based on limited experience. To detect changes in perinatal practice a model system for 'quality control' was designed, with monitoring of a few components of process and product variables (to use industrial terms). This was tested with quarterly checks in 1975 through 1978[11], but for various reasons it was not put into systematic use. Still, I think the idea is worth pursuing.

ENVOI

In conclusion, the value of routinely collected data depends on our care in collecting them and imagination in analysing and presenting them. Used wisely, they can be good tools in perinatal surveillance at national, international and local levels.

References

1. Bjerkedal, T. and Bakketeig, L. S. (1975). Surveillance of congenital malformations and other conditions of the newborn. *Int. J. Epidemiol.*, **4**, 31–6
2. Bakketeig, L. S., Hoffman, H. J. and Harley, E. E. (1979). The tendency to repeat gestational age and birth weight in successive births. *Am. J. Obstet. Gynecol.*, **135**, 1086–1103

3. Bakketeig, L. S. and Hoffman, H. J. (1981). Epidemiology of preterm birth: results from a longitudinal study of births in Norway. In Elder, M. G. and Hendricks, C. H. (eds.) *Preterm Labor*, pp. 17–46. (London: Butterworths)
4. Bjerkedal, T., Bakketeig, L. S. and Bergsjø, P. (1973). *Fødselshjelp i Norge pr. 1. januar 1972. Maternity services in Norway per 1 January 1972*. Institute of Hygiene and Social Medicine, University of Bergen
5. Bjerkedal, T., Bakketeig, L. S. and Bergsjø, P. (1975). *Fødeinstitusjoner i Norge pr. 1. juli 1974. Maternity Institutions in Norway per 1st July 1974*. Institute of Hygiene and Social Medicine, University of Bergen
6. Larssen, K. E., Bergsjø, P., Bakketeig, L. S. and Finne, P. H. (1981). *Perinatal service i Norge i 1970–årene. Perinatal service in Norway during the 1970s*. NIS-rapport 6/81, The Norwegian Institute for Hospital Research
7. NOMESKO (1982). *Fødsler i Norden. Medicinsk Fødselsregistrering. Births in the Nordic Countries. Registration of the Outcome of Pregnancy. 1979*. (Reykjavik: The Nordic Medico-Statistical Committee)
8. NOMESKO (1984). *Helsestatistikk i de nordiske land. Health statistics in the Nordic countries. 1982*. No. 19 (Københaven: The Nordic Medico-Statistical Committee)
9. Larssen, K. E., Bakketeig, L. S., Bergsjø, P., Finne, P. H., Laurini, R., Knoff, H., Holt, J., Vogt, H. and Hapnes, C. (1982). *Vurdering av perinatal service i Norge 1980. Perinatal audit in Norway 1980*. NIS-rapport 7/82, Norwegian Institute for Hospital Research
10. Mutch, L. and Elbourne, D. (1983). Standard national perinatal data: a suggested common core of tabulations. *Community Medicine*, **5**, 251–9
11. Bergsjø, P., Bakketeig, L. S. and Buhaug, L. S. (1980). Activities in an obstetrical department and outcome of labor evaluated by computer. In Sakamoto, S., Tojo, S. and Nakayama, T. (eds.) *Proceedings of the IX World Congress of Gynecology and Obstetrics*, Tokyo 25–31 October 1979, International Congress Series No. 512, Gynecology and Obstetrics, pp. 867–70. (Amsterdam: Excerpta Medica)

38

The use of tracer conditions to assess the quality of perinatal care

P. Buekens

Many investigators have attempted to simplify quality assessment by examining the care of a small group of representative health problems. Kessner has employed the term 'tracer diseases' for this purpose[1]. The method is based on the assumption that a properly selected set of health problems can serve as tracers for assessing the entire range of activities involved in the provision of health services to a specified population[2]. In this paper the tracer method has been used to assess the quality of perinatal care.

SELECTION OF THE TRACERS

Tracers are selected if they have the following characteristics[1-3]:

1. they should be well defined,
2. they should be highly prevalent,
3. they should have a definite impact on health,
4. the health outcome should be influenced by care.

In addition, as a group, the tracers should cover all the elements of the process of care, i.e. prevention, screening, diagnosis, management and follow-up. Tracers should also cover the three trimesters of pregnancy, delivery and the postpartum period. The method will be illustrated using two tracers: congenital rubella and urinary tract infection. Congenital rubella is addressed by screening during the first trimester and by prevention during the postpartum period. Urinary tract infection is addressed by screening, diagnosis, management and follow-up at all gestational ages.

SELECTION OF QUALITY CRITERIA

Explicit criteria[4] against which care could be evaluated can be derived from the literature or from a consensus among practitioners. For example, after a review of the literature, Mohide[5] concluded that immunization was efficacious in the protection of future pregnancies against rubella infection. The quality criteria derived were (1) that during the antepartum and postpartum period the rubella status of all patients should be documented and (2) that actions or arrangements for the immunization of the rubella-sensitive patients should also be documented.

Our study on urinary tract infection focused on screening using a nitrite strip test. There was no agreement on the value of this test in the literature[6,7]. We thus derived the criteria of quality from a questionnaire sent to the 122 gynaecologists in the hospitals associated with our university. Sixty-eight (56%) gynaecologists answered the questionnaire; 93% of them responded that a nitrite test should be performed at each antenatal visit and 88% said that a positive test should be followed by either urinary culture or treatment.

REVIEW OF MEDICAL RECORDS

Mohide[5] reviewed 128 obstetrical charts: 13 (10%) contained no prenatal record; of those with a record 14 (12%) had no rubella titre documented. Five of 12 (42%) rubella-susceptible patients were not vaccinated. A continuing medical education programme was then implemented in Mohide's hospital.

We reviewed prenatal records of nitrite-positive women in three hospitals. Patients were managed according to agreed criteria in 45 of 52 cases (87%) in hospital 1, in 20 of 25 cases (80%) in hospital 2 but only in four of 20 cases (20%) in hospital 3. The quality of care given by hospital 3 was significantly lower than that of the two others ($p<0.001$).

REPRESENTATIVENESS OF THE RESULTS

The validity of the hypothesis that tracers are representative of the process of care can be evaluated studying the relationship between quality assessments using different tracers.

In the same three hospitals we compared the quality of the management of nitrite-positive patients, the quality of screening for rhesus immunization in rhesus-negative women, and the quality of the screening programme applied to women who were not protected against toxoplasmosis[8]. Figure 1 shows that quality of hospital 3 was poor for all three tracers, indicating that the quality within each hospital was homogeneous across different tracers. This confirmed the results of Osborne[9], who studied the care provided by 166 physicians and found a significant correlation between the quality of care assessed using seven tracers.

DISCUSSION OF THE RESULTS

The interpretation of the results depends on the validity of the criteria used in the analysis. Consensus criteria are often not supported by scientifically valid studies. Moreover, even if the efficacy of a technique is well proven, its optimal level of utilization can vary according to the resources available. Never-

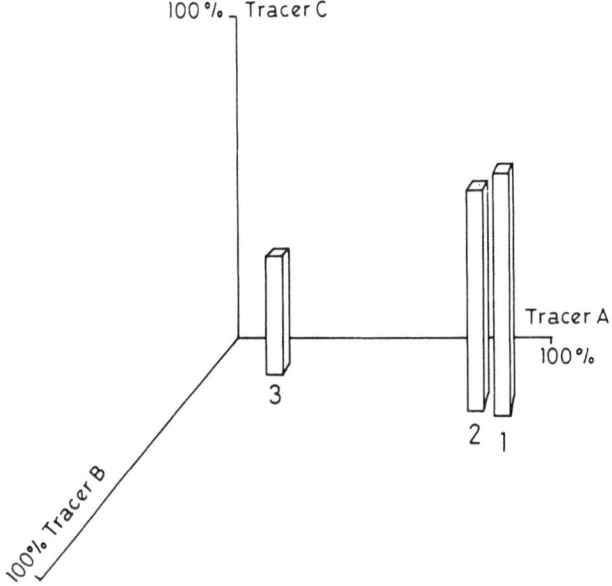

Figure 1 Quality (%) of three hospitals evaluated by three tracers: urinary tract infection (A), management of rhesus-negative pregnant women (B) and management of pregnant women not protected against toxoplasmosis (C)

theless, we believe that quality assessment can be a stimulating exercise for clinical staff. If the quality is found to be low, members of staff have to discuss the scientific validity of their criteria. If the criteria are valid, then performance has to be improved. If the criteria are not supported by well-designed studies, the necessity of such studies will appear clearly. This is indeed the main objective of quality assessment.

References

1. Kessner, D. M., Kalk, C. E. and Singer, J. (1973). Assessing health quality – the case for tracer. *N. Engl. J. Med.*, **288**, 189–94
2. Demlo, L. K. (1983). Assuring quality of health care. An overview. *Eval. Health Prof.*, **6**, 161–96
3. Shorr, G. I. and Nutting, P. A. (1977). A population-based assessment of the continuity of ambulatory care. *Med. Care*, **15**, 455–64
4. Donabedian, A. (1982). *The Criteria and Standards of Quality.* (Ann Arbor: Health Administration Press)
5. Mohide, P. T. (19833). Symposium: perinatal surveillance. *Annals RCPSC*, **16**, 51–2
6. Finnerty, F. A. and Johnson, A. C. (1968). A simplified accurate method for detecting bacteriuria. *Am. J. Obstet. Gynecol.*, **101**, 238–43
7. Lenke, R. R. and Van Dorsten, J. P. (1981). The efficacy of the nitrite test and microscopic urinalysis in predicting urine culture results. *Am. J. Obstet. Gynecol.*, **140**, 427–9

8. Buekens, P. (1984). Quality assessment of antenatal care by the tracer method. In
   v. Eimeren, W., Engelbrecht, R. and Flagle, Ch.D. (eds.) *Third International Conference on System Science in Health Care.* pp. 577–80. (Berlin/Heidelberg: Springer
   Verlag)
9. Osborne, Ch. E. (1977). Interdiagnosis relationships of physician recording in
   ambulatory child health care. *Med. Care,* **15**, 465–74

39

The role of collaborative clinical trials for auditing perinatal practice

A. Whitelaw

The history of perinatal medicine has been marred by a series of therapeutic interventions so obviously logical and beneficial that randomized controlled trials were not carried out before general use. Oxygen for preterm infants was the most famous example of these. Many thousands of preterm babies were blinded from retrolental fibroplasia before a collaborative trial demonstrated that use of high inspired oxygen concentration was linked to RLF[1]. Despite these bitter lessons from the past, the new generation of neonatologists may be tempted to grasp at new techniques of diagnosis, management, or therapy before the values and limitations of the new techniques have been rigorously and objectively tested.

One of the most important end-points of perinatal medicine is the survival of children without handicap. Put another way, death or handicap is the potential result of every serious problem the fetus and neonate may suffer. Trials that compare treatments of critically ill neonates are likely to be looking for significant reductions in death and/or handicap. Now that perinatal mortality is falling below 10 per 1000 in many regions of Europe and North America and cerebral palsy occurs in approximately 2 per 1000 births, very large populations are required to produce answers with the conventional statistical significance of less than 5%. The number of babies required may exceed those available in any one hospital attempting to conduct a randomized trial. This is exemplified in respiratory distress syndrome, periventricular haemorrhage, management of post-haemorrhagic ventricular dilatation and treatment of neonatal Gram-negative meningitis.

In 1981 Morley[2] published the results of a non-randomized trial in which artificial surfactant powder was blown down the endotracheal tube of 22 babies below 34 weeks gestation. During the 13-month period, 33 babies below 34 weeks gestation served as controls. All eight deaths were in the control group. Dr Morley has acknowledged that this first trial was not randomized and a col-

247

laborative trial involving at least 300 babies of less than 30 weeks gestation is planned. Babies over 30 weeks have been omitted because the mortality is extremely low with conventional treatment. Babies of 25–29 weeks gestation have a mortality of about 30% with the best conventional management[3]. With 300 babies there is a 63% chance of identifying a one-third reduction in mortality at the 5% level of significance. Increasing the sample size would give higher confidence or enable a smaller reduction in mortality to be confirmed. To enter 300 babies would take Cambridge Maternity Hospital almost 6 years. Clearly a multicentre trial is needed. The main question being asked is whether surfactant administered to babies of 25–29 weeks gestation is associated with a reduction in mortality. In addition to survival, IVH, pneumothorax and chronic lung disease are end-points being examined. An answer to the question should be available by the end of 1985.

Periventricular haemorrhage occurs in approximately half of all babies born at 30 weeks or less[4]. Since the condition could be diagnosed in life by real-time ultrasound there have been several approaches to its prevention. In 1981 Donn et al.[5] reported a statistically significant reduction in PVH with phenobarbitone prophylaxis in a randomized but non-blind trial on 60 babies below 1500 g birth weight. In 1982 Morgan et al.[6] reported no statistically significant difference in PVH in a randomized non-blind trial of phenobarbitone in 60 infants. In 1982 Bedard et al.[7] reported in a randomized non-blind study of 42 infants that phenobarbitone gave a statistically significant protection against large PVH.

In 1983 we published the results of our own randomized double-blind trial of phenobarbitone and concluded that there was no statistically significant difference in PVH between the two treatment groups[8]. Because our trial was double-blind we were able to look at adverse effects and documented respiratory depression in phenobarbitone-treated infants. Despite the conflicting results between the four trials for PVH overall, all four studies had fewer of the serious parenchymal haemorrhages among phenobarbitone-treated infants. Even with 284 babies enrolled, the reduction in parenchymal haemorrhages with phenobarbitone did not quite reach statistical significance. Thus after more than 4 years of work we are left with the possibility that in very low birth weight infants ventilated for respiratory distress, phenobarbitone may reduce parenchymal haemorrhage.

A major complication of large PVH is post-haemorrhagic ventricular dilatation which has a very high rate of major handicap. In many hospitals such babies are treated early after diagnosis with repeated lumbar punctures followed by ventricular shunt surgery[10]. No controlled trial of early lumbar punctures has ever been carried out. In other hospitals a more conservative approach is used with shunt surgery being reserved for those with excessive head growth. It has been suggested that repeated lumbar puncture may be beneficial[10] by controlling intracranial pressure and directly removing blood and protein from the cerebral spinal fluid pathways. Within each European regional neonatal intensive care unit these are no more than six cases annually.

In February 1984 a trial of early versus conservative management of PHVD, coordinated by the National Perinatal Epidemiology Unit in Oxford began, with the intention of enrolling 120 babies over 3 years. This sample size should give an 80% chance of detecting a statistically significant reduction in severe disability among survivors by half. A project developmental paediatrician will assess the outcome at 1 and 2 years without knowledge of the neonatal management. Ten neonatal intensive care units in Britain and Ireland have already entered cases and after 6 months 20 infants have been enrolled. Randomization is by telephone to the Oxford National Perinatal Epidemiology Unit, thus there is no possibility of manipulation by the clinician.

Neonatal meningitis remains a significant cause of death and handicap, particularly with Gram-negative organisms. In the late 1960s and early 1970s intrathecal gentamicin was advocated as a solution to Gram-negative meningitis with ampicillin-resistant organisms and the problem of poor CSF penetration by aminoglycosides. Because each hospital would have only a handful of cases, the first Neonatal Meningitis Cooperative Study was set up. McCracken and Mize reported the results in 1976[11]. Fifteen different centres in the USA, one in Mexico City and one in Colombia, entered babies. The 117 babies were randomized to receive either ampicillin and gentamicin i.v., or ampicillin and gentamicin 1 mg intrathecally daily for a minimum of 3 days. The results suggested that survival and morbidity at 12 months were almost identical in the two treatment groups. Logic had suggested that the failure of the intrathecal gentamicin might be due to the unidirectional flow of CSF from ventricle to subarachnoid space, and that intraventricular injection would achieve effective penetration throughout the CSF. Sixteen centres in the USA, and one each in Chile, Costa Rica, Mexico and Colombia, entered 52 cases with Gram-negative ventriculitis between 1976 and 1979; 42.9% of those receiving intraventricular gentamicin as well as i.v. ampicillin and gentamicin died, whereas only 12.5% of those receiving intravenous ampicillin and gentamicin only died ($p = 0.016$)[12]. The trial was terminated at this point. As a result of these two multicentre trials we have learned not to give intrathecal or intraventricular gentamicin.

It can be seen that rational conclusions about treatment of the most serious neonatal problems require larger numbers of affected babies than are available in any one neonatal unit. Small studies may be influenced by local fluctuations in population. They lack statistical power and so can miss real and worthwhile treatment effects. Multicentre trials are therefore necessary in neonatal intensive care, but are challenging to set up and maintain. The first problem is to identify a treatment dilemma that will interest not only oneself, but a considerable number of busy clinicians. If one can find a suitable question, many individuals have to agree entry criteria and treatment protocols. A very important step is to estimate target numbers to give adequate statistical power. A centre is needed where record-keeping and randomization can be carried out. All randomized trials and the question of parental consent to randomization have to be considered by the research ethics committee in each hospital. A number of ethics committees have taken the view that parental consent to randomization in neonatal intensive care causes unacceptable mental and physical distress and should be omitted when two accepted forms of treatment are being compared. When a new drug, or other treatment, is on trial, then parental consent must be obtained. The end-points of trial must be clear and unambiguous. Death (or survival) is widely used for this reason. In multicentre trials the participants may be hundreds or thousands of kilometres apart. Personal contact is thus time-consuming and expensive but must be encouraged for the sake of morale and uniformity. International congresses and learned-society meetings can act as convenient venues for the group collaborating in a multicentre trial. With greater collaboration between European centres in multicentre trials, many more of the therapeutic dilemmas facing us can be resolved in a more scientifically rigorous audit of our practice.

References

1. Kinsey, V. E. and Hemphill, F. M. (1955). Etiology of retrolental fibroplasia and preliminary report of collaborative trial. *Trans. Am. Acad. Ophthalmol. Otolaringol.*, **55**, 15–24
2. Morley, C. J., Bangham, A. D., Miller, N. and Davis, J. A. (1981). Dry artificial lung surfactant and its effect on very preterm babies. *Lancet*, **1**, 64–8.
3. Yu, V. Y. H., Orgill, A. A., Bajuk, B. and Astbury, J. (1984). Survival and 2 year outcome of extremely preterm infants. *Br. J. Obstet. Gynaecol*, **91**, 640–6
4. Levene, M. I., Fawer, C.-L. and Lamont, R. F. (1982). Risk factors in the development of intraventricular haemorrhage in the preterm neonate. *Arch. Dis. Child.*, **57**, 410–17
5. Donn, S., Roloff, D. W. and Goldstein, G. (1981). Prevention of intraventricular haemorrhage in preterm infants by phenobarbitone. *Lancet*, **2**, 215–17
6. Morgan, M. E. I., Massey, R. F. and Cooke, R. W. I. (1982). Does phenobarbitone prevent periventricular haemorrhage in VLBW infants? a controlled trial. *Pediatrics*, **70**, 186–9
7. Bedard, M., Shankaran, S., Slovis, T., Pantoja, A., Dayal, B. and Poland, R. (1982). Presented at the *Second Special Ross Conference in Perinatal Intracranial Haemorrhage*, December, Washington, DC
8. Whitelaw, A., Placzek. M., Dubowitz, L., Lary, S. and Levene, M. (1983). Phenobarbitone for prevention of PVH in VLBW infants. *Lancet*, **2**, 1168–70
9. Cooke, R. W. I. (1983). Early prognosis of low birth weight infants treated for progressive post-haemorrhagic hydrocephalus. *Arch. Dis. Child.*, **58**, 410–14
10. Papille, L. A., Burstein, J., Burstein, R., Koffler, H., Koops, B. L. and Johnson, J. D. (1980). Post-haemorrhagic hydrocephalus in low-birth-weight infants: Treatment by serial lumbar punctures. *J. Pediatr.*, **97**, 273–7
11. McCracken, G. H. and Mize, S. G. (1976). A controlled study of intrathecal antibiotic therapy in gram-negative enteric meningitis of infancy. *J. Pediatr.*, **89**, 66–72
12. McCracken, G. H., Mize, S. G. and Threlkeld, N. (1980). Intraventricular gentamicin therapy in gram-negative bacillary meningitis of infancy. *Lancet*, **1**, 787–91.

Chairman's summary

I. Chalmers

RESUMÉ OF CONCLUDING DISCUSSION

In response to a question about the input from clinicians to the design of the data form in Norway's perinatal information system, Professor Bergsjø said that, in contrast with the 1960s when the new medical birth registration system commenced, clinicians were now playing a more active role in deciding about the content of the form. He felt that there was considerable room for improvement on the question of providing regular feedback of useful information from the system to clinicians.

The relationship between perinatal mortality and morbidity was discussed. It was often stated that as perinatal mortality fell so did morbidity arising during this period. Dr Chalmers stated, however, that perinatal morbidity rates did not always reflect mortality rates. He pointed out that, while mortality rates had been falling world-wide, there was no evidence of similar trends in the incidence of cerebral palsy. In the most recent cohort in Professor Hagberg's population-based study in Sweden, the birth cohort prevalence of cerebral palsy was greater than in any of the previous cohorts. It was necessary to examine both mortality and morbidity. In the case of morbidity the most appropriate starting point was to monitor the incidence of cerebral palsy in birth cohorts using population-based studies.

Asked to give examples of clinical routines which had been altered as a result of randomized clinical trials (RCT), the panel cited the use of betamethasone prior to preterm delivery and the treatment of neonatal meningitis. When trials showed that particular interventions were not efficacious these were usually abandoned in the institutions where the research was conducted but often continued in use elsewhere. Dr Whitelaw felt that pediatricians were becoming more reluctant to embrace new treatments before evidence of their efficacy was available from RCTs. Professor Keirse expressed concern about

251

the number of new treatments which were still adopted without the support of RCTs. The 'fluidity' of the ethical decisions of clinicians was raised. The current situation whereby strict information requirements (i.e. informing patients about the possible benefits and hazards of treatments) were applied to RCTs but not to everyday clinical treatment was incongruous. Such double standards needed to be exposed.

In a multicentre RCT testing a specific intervention can one control for other aspects of care which may differ in the participating centres? Because the allocation of patients to treatment and control groups was done by randomization, the distribution of various confounding factors between the groups (including differences between centres in other aspects of treatment) was likely to be equal in large trials. It was important to ensure that the randomization could not be manipulated by participating clinicians, and this could be achieved by having a central randomization service. When possible, having the trial double-blind was a further safeguard.

What is an acceptable level of benefit in a RCT? One could not generalize about this. It was a question of deciding what level of benefit was considered to be clinically important. The smaller the level of benefit to be detected (for example, a reduction of 10% in a problem), the larger the trial would have to be. In a RCT the risks of obtaining a false-positive or false-negative result are minimized by having adequate numbers of subjects in the trial.

Section 10
Diabetes in Pregnancy

Chairman's introduction

A. Van Assche

The most striking thing about diabetes occurring during pregnancy is the fact that perfect diabetic control normalizes the intrauterine milieu. There is no doubt that this achievement is more important than sophisticated techniques for the evaluation of fetal growth and fetal well-being.

Since the most critical period of fetal life is situated early in pregnancy, efforts must be made to generalize preconceptional advice and treatment. Local and international health authorities must be convinced that this achievement is the only way to reduce the number of congenital anomalies in diabetes and pregnancy. There is also evidence that perfect diabetic control can prevent the development of diabetes in later life.

Chairman's introduction

A. Van Assche

40

Pregnancy in the clinical diabetic

M. I. Drury

The speaker presents a personal experience extending from 1951 to August 1984[1,2] The series, which is composed of 1013 pregnancies (1034 infants) in 504 women with *clinical* diabetes, is unique in that it represents the experience of one physician and is consecutive and unmodified. There was no maternal death and the perinatal mortality has improved consistently over the years. That part of the series which relates to the period 1979 to August 1984 will be discussed in detail, showing how a policy of strict control of diabetes permits uncomplicated cases to go to term or later with beneficial effects on neonatal morbidity and a high rate of spontaneous labour and vaginal delivery. In 270 viable infants delivered since 1979 the perinatal loss was 4% (corrected for malformations = 3%) and the overall caesarean section rate 26%

The author considers that the literature emphasizes unduly the need for intensive fetal monitoring, and that section rates in most published series are unnecessarily high.

References

1. Drury, M. I., Greene, A. T. and Stronge, J. M. (1977). Pregnancy complicated by clinical diabetes mellitus. A study of 600 pregnancies. *Obstet. Gynecol.*, **49**, 519–22
2. Drury, M. I., Stronge, J. M., Foley, M. E. and MacDonald, D. W. (1983). Pregnancy in the diabetic patient: timing and mode of delivery. *Ostet. Gynecol.*, **62**, 279–82

41

Tight metabolic control during early pregnancy prevents malformation in offspring of insulin-dependent diabetic women

K. Fuhrmann

This is a report on treatment in 620 insulin-dependent diabetic pregnant women*. The goal of our treatment was to achieve normal blood glucose levels as soon as possible prior to or during early pregnancy. Starting intensified conventional insulin therapy before conception, approximately 88% of all women achieved normal blood glucose levels during the first weeks of pregnancy. Without preconceptional treatment only about 20% of the pregnant women had normal blood glucose levels at the time of their first hospitalization after the 8th week of pregnancy. In 437 subjects who began intensive metabolic control after 8 weeks' gestation, there were 31 malformations, a rate of 7.1%. Of 185 infants delivered from insulin-dependent diabetic subjects with metabolic control started before conception and continued during the first critical weeks of pregnancy there were only two congenital malformations (1.1.%). The difference between the two groups is highly significant ($p < 0.001$).

Intensified insulin treatment during the preconceptional phase and during the first weeks of pregnancy prevents an excessive percentage of malformation in the population of offspring of diabetic women.

Until recently there have been no investigations of the influence of metabolic control of diabetic women during the important phase of embryogenesis. To answer the question whether or not meticulous metabolic control before conception and during the critical weeks of embryogenesis can significantly lower the high malformation rate in IDM, we started a prospective study in 1977. For this study the following tasks had to be accomplished: (1) diabetic women had to come to our pregnancy clinic before pregnancy, and (2) diabetologists, general practitioners, and gynaecologists had to be educated about the goals of this new management programme. A series of lectures on television and on radio, as well as special seminars for attending physicians and group talks with

* Zentralinstitut für Diabetes, DDR, 2201 Karlsburg

259

young diabetic women, was prepared. During 1977 we saw 10% of all delivered diabetic women in our prepregnancy clinic. During the next years the
number of patients who attended our prepregnancy clinic increased to 30%.
Seventy per cent were not willing to take part in a preconceptional treatment
programme. Our preconceptional programme consisted of three parts:

1. Patients were hospitalized for 5–7 days, depending on the degree of
   referred metabolic control. The goals of the first hospitalization were:

   (a) to normalize the blood glucose levels, and therefore insulin treatment
       had to be intensified in most cases;
   (b) to educate patients in blood glucose home-monitoring and in insulin
       self-adjustments;
   (c) to teach patients measuring of their basal body temperature in order to
       fix the date of conception and to estimate the time of delivery;
   (d) to motivate these women for meticulous metabolic control, especially
       during the first weeks of pregnancy;
   (e) to treat sequelae of diabetes such as retinopathy and urinary tract infec-
       tions before conception.

2. After the first hospitalization, patients attended a prepregnancy clinic once
   or twice a week. They measured blood glucose at home 2 or 3 days a week
   with seven to nine samples. During their visits to the prepregnancy clinic,
   insulin doses and diet were changed to effect optimal metabolic control
   (normal blood glucose levels).

3. Every 3 months, patients returned for 1–2 days to our hospital. This was
   mostly necessary because our patients lived in an area of about 500 square
   miles. During these short hospitalizations HbA_1 measurement and blood
   glucose day–night profiles were performed. The basal body temperature
   was observed and, if necessary, infertility was treated. We asked the
   patients to stop birth control only when metabolic control was stabilized
   and all necessary treatments were finished. If the basal body temperature
   remained high for more than 16 days, the patients were asked to come immediately to our hospital for the first metabolic control admission during
   early pregnancy. Normally we saw the patients from the beginning of pregnancy every month for 1–2 days in our hospital. If metabolic control was
   not managed in an optimal way at home, patients were immediately sent
   back to us. During hospitalization, blood glucose measuring was performed by our laboratory staff and by the patients to avoid mistakes in
   home monitoring. The HbA_1 was measured. The fetal development was
   observed by ultrasonography.

During early pregnancy, mid-pregnancy, and late pregnancy, an ophthalmolo-
gist did eye examinations, and, if necessary, treatment was started immediately. Routine gynaecological check-ups showed us abortus imminens or
preterm delivery tendencies in sufficient time. Routine alpha-fetoprotein
(AFP) screening during the 16th week and creatinine clearance during early
and late pregnancy or even more often, depending on the pregnancy status,
were also performed. Finally, we saw all patients during the 30th to the 32nd

week of pregnancy. Depending on the obstetrical conditions and the quality of metabolic control, patients were hospitalized between the 32nd and 36th week of pregnancy until delivery. This was usually necessary because of the long distance between home and hospital for many of our patients. Beginning with the 36th week of pregnancy, we performed routine fetal heart rate monitoring every day, and in some high-risk patients several times a day. In the case of contractions with shortening of the cervix, treatment with betamimetic agents was started, and, if necessary, corticosteroids were given for induction of fetal lung maturation. We delivered our diabetic women independently of the White classification, at term (completed 38th to 40th week). It should be noted that all diabetic women were given time off from their work for the duration of the pregnancy.

As a control group for these preconceptionally cared-for women, we used the diabetic women who came to our hospital for their first visit for metabolic control after the 8th week of pregnancy. These patients were hospitalized until the metabolic control was stabilized and blood glucose levels were normal. During this time these postconceptionally treated patients were educated in blood glucose home-monitoring and in self-treatment. From the first hospitalization until delivery, the late registered group had the same management programme as described in the prepregnancy group. After delivery all offspring were seen by one attending neonatologist. Routine examinations on the infant were performed several times during the first 21 days of life.

For comparison with non-diabetic women we formed a second control group. All newborn of non-diabetic mothers who were delivered at the same time as a diabetic delivery were checked by the neonatologist with the same criteria. The only difference in the offspring of diabetic mothers was the time period in the hospital for these babies. The newborn of diabetic mothers were in hospital until the 21st day of life, whereas babies from non-diabetic mothers remained only until the 5th day. From 1977 to 1981 we delivered 420 diabetic women compared to 420 non-diabetic women. These numbers were large enough to achieve statistical significance. From 1981 until 1983 we could subgroup the diabetic patients, depending on the beginning of management. According to White's classification, 123 of the diabetic subjects were Class B; 119 Class C; 148 Class D, and 30 Class R. One hundred and twenty-eight diabetic patients attended our prepregnancy programme; 292 came only after the 8th week of pregnancy, which formed our control group. In both groups of patients we tried to keep plasma glucose levels at 60–130 mg/dl from the beginning of management. We used various insulin and dietary programmes to achieve this goal. In most cases we used individually adapted injections of short-acting insulin four to six times a day. In others we used a method described by Jovanovic and Peterson[1] to tailor the initial dose to the weight of the patient. Total daily insulin dosage was calculated according to an initial dose of $0.7 \text{ U kg}^{-1} \text{ day}^{-1}$ with a division of the insulin into three injections of a combination of NPH and regular insulin. In a few patients, two injections of intermediate insulin were sufficient. Among the 420 infants of our diabetic patients there were 23 with malformations discovered during the first 21 days of life, corresponding to 5.5% of diabetic women. In 420 infants of non-diabetic women delivered at our hospital in the same time period, the malformation rate was 1.4%. The types of malformations in diabetic women are shown in Table 2. In 292 subjects who had intensive metabolic control after 8 weeks gestation, there were 22 malformations, a rate of 7.5% (Table 1). Of 128 infants delivered from insulin-dependent diabetic subjects with metabolic control started before conception and continued during the first critical weeks of pregnancy, there was only one congenital malformation (0.8%). The difference between the two groups is highly significant ($\chi^2 = 6.62$; $p < 0.01$). The distribution of congenital malformations among White's classes is also seen in Table 1. The malformation rate of 2.3% in Class B in the late registrants was significantly lower than that for infants of mothers in Classes C, D; and R ($\chi^2 = 3.86$; $p < 0.05$). There was no increase in rate of anomalies from Class C to R. There were no differences between the distribution of White classes in the early and late registrants. Among the 128 subjects with metabolic control started before conception, 49 (38.2%) were multiparas who had delivered 60 infants (Table 3). In this group there were 19 prior perinatal losses (31.7%) and eight congenital malformations (13.3%). In the group of 292 diabetic subjects who began metabolic control after the 8th week of gestation, 97 (33.2%) were multiparas who had delivered 180 infants. There were 25 prior perinatal losses in this group (13.9%), and 10 of the prior infants (5.6%) had congenital malformations. Prior reproductive failure may motivate diabetic women to participate in a prepregnancy management programme. In 420 infants from non-diabetic mothers we found six malformations, or 1.4%. The types of malformations in non-diabetic women are shown in Table 4. None of these malformations was fatal. In comparison, four of the 23 malformations in the diabetic group (17%) died during the first 17 days of life. Results of the control of glycaemia in the hospital during weeks 5–7 of gestation in the group of 128 women who registered and were educated before pregnancy are given in Table 5. These results are compared with mean daily glucose for the first weeks in the hospital in 111 women who registered at 8–14 weeks' gestation. In the prepregnancy group, mean daily plasma glucose was < 110 mg/dl in 88.3% of the subjects compared with only 20.7% of the later registrants ($\chi^2 = 110.6$; $p < 0.001$).

From this study we concluded that preconceptional intensified insulin treat-

Table 1 Congenital malformations related to White's classes and to the onset of strict metabolic control

White's class	Registered prepregnancy		Registered after 8 weeks gestation		Total	
	Anomalies	No anomalies	Anomalies	No anomalies	Anomalies	No anomalies
B	1	35	2 (2.3%)	85	3	120
C	0	35	9 (12.2%)	75	9	110
D	0	49	9 (9.1%)	90	9	139
R	0	8	2 (9.1%)	20	2	28
Total	1	127	22	270	23	397
	(0.8%)		(7.5%)		(5.5%)	

$\chi^2 = 7.84$, $p < 0.01$, for anomalies in group (all classes) with onset of metabolic control before conception compared with group (all classes) with onset of control after 8 weeks gestation

Table 2 Infants of diabetic mothers with congenital malformations listed according to the severity of malformations (Karlsburg 1977–81 series)

Malformations	IDM case no.	Diagnoses
Malformations incompatible with postnatal life	1,2*	Hypoplastic left heart (died on the 1st day of life)
	3	Hypoplastic right heart (died on the 1st day of life)
Severe malformations with bad prognosis for survival, further health, and social rehabilitation	4	Coarctation of the aorta (died on the 8th day of life)
	5	Ostium atrioventriculare commune
	6	Tetralogy of Fallot
	7	Ventricular septal defect, scoliosis of the thoracic spine, aplasia of the radius, club-hand, and agenesis of one kidney
	8	Coarctation of the aorta, hydronephrosis and megaureter on both sides associated with megacysti
	9	Robin's syndrome, scoliosis of the thoracic spine, aplasia and hypoplasia of several ribs, caudal regression syndrome, club-foot, ureter duplex, and ureter fissus (died after 17 days)
	10	Robin's syndrome, caudal regression syndrome, club-feet
Malformations with good prognosis for health and further social rehabilitation	11,12	Club-foot associated with hypoplasia of the lower leg muscles
	13	Scoliosis of the thoracic spine, aplasia and hypoplasia of several ribs
	14	Hypoplasia of the abdominal muscular cover, scoliosis of the spine associated with wringed position of the pelvis, and club-foot
	15	Cleft lip, maxilla, and palate
	16	Atresia of the duodenum
	17	Ventricular septal defect without haemodynamic disturbance
Minor congenital malformations	18,19	Club-foot, unilateral
	20	Funnel chest
	21,22	Supernumerary thumb and toe
	23	Ureter duplex, unilateral

* Metabolic control started before conception

Table 3   Prior pregnancies of mothers in early and late groups

	Early group	Late group
N	128	292
P$_1$	40	62 (21.2%)
P$_2$ or more	9 (31.2%)	35 (21.0%)
Total infants	60	180
Total losses	19 (31.7%)	25 (13.9%)
Anomalies	8 (13.3%)	10 (5.6%)

Table 4   Infants of non-diabetic mothers with congenital malformations listed according to the severity of malformations (Karlsburg 1977–81 series)

Malformations	Case no.	Diagnoses
Malformations incompatible with postnatal life	—	—
Severe malformations with bad prognosis for survival, further health and social rehabilitation	1 2	Exstrophy of the urinary bladder Cormonoventriculare et biatrále
Malformations with good prognosis for health and further social rehabilitation	3	Ventricular septal defect without haemodynamic disturbances in an infant with M. Langdon-Down
	4	Stenosis of the left main bronchus
Minor congenital malformations	5	Congenital coloboma on both sides
	6	Pes adductus congenitus on both sides

ment combined with education in blood glucose home monitoring and self-treatment lowers the incidence of malformation in babies of diabetic women to a range not significantly different from non-diabetic controls.

DEGREE OF NORMOGLYCAEMIA

The question remained of how good metabolic control had to be to totally preclude malformations in the offspring of diabetic women, and in what percentage of diabetic women can normoglycaemia be achieved. For this reason we counted all blood glucose readings during the time of conception and during the first 8 weeks of pregnancy in a series of 56 diabetic women who attended our prepregnancy programme between 1981 and 1983, and compared the results to all blood glucose readings from 144 diabetic women who came during the same time period but after the 8th week of pregnancy for a first visit. These

Table 5 Control of glycaemia during initial 3 week hospitalization of 239 diabetic women in the first trimester of pregnancy

Groups	Mean daily glucose (mg/dl)	Subjects educated before pregnancy and hospitalized during weeks 5–7 of gestation		Subjects hospitalized at weeks 8–14 of gestation	
		n	Percentage	n	Percentage
1	70–90	61	47.7	4	3.6
2	91–110	52	40.6	19	17.1
3	111–130	5	3.9	29	26.1
4	131–150	8	6.2	30	27.0
5	151–170	1	0.8	19	17.1
6	171–190	1	0.8	7	6.3
7	>190	0	—	3	2.7
Total		128	100.0	111	100.0

200 diabetic women gave birth to 202 babies. In the prepregnancy group with 56 women there were 57 babies, one of them with a heart malformation, a 1.7% malformation rate. The group registered after the 8th week of pregnancy gave birth to 145 babies, nine of them with malformations, a 6.2% malformation rate. In the 56 patients who were able to follow our advice before a planned pregnancy, insulin therapy was markedly intensified. Once instructed, these women achieved quite good adherence to and effectiveness in home blood glucose monitoring. In this group of patients a total of 271 weeks of early pregnancy were covered for the assessment of metabolic control by home blood glucose monitoring and by the records of hospitalization before the 8th week of gestation. In order to assess the degree of metabolic control, all blood glucose readings in the range between 45 and 140 mg/dl were evaluated. The readings deviating from this range were divided into the following classes: < 45; 141 to 160; 161 to 215, and > 215 mg/dl.

If the assumption that frequent blood glucose profiling gives information on metabolic control during the periods between the profiles is justified, the number of normoglycaemic values may be taken as a criterion of normoglycaemia achieved in the respective intervals. Thirty-nine patients of the early-treated group (70%) achieved the therapeutic goal, i.e. close approximation to normoglycaemia between 45 and 140 mg/dl in 1745 of a total of 2007 blood glucose readings (87%). Another nine patients (16%) had 77% of their blood glucose readings within this range. Eight patients (14%), however, failed to achieve sufficient metabolic control despite similar efforts. These eight patients presented the most unstable metabolic characteristics within the entire patient series: 309 out of a total of 514 of their blood glucose readings (60%) were within the range aimed at, 9% were < 45 mg/dl and 12% exceeded 215 mg/dl. The only malformed newborn from the early group belonged to a mother from the metabolically unstable group of eight patients who did not achieve optimum control. In 144 women admitted after 8 weeks of gestation, all blood glucose readings were evaluated from the first admission to our hospital until strict metabolic control was achieved. In only 14 (10%) of these women were more than 87% of their blood glucose values within the range of 45–140 mg/dl. Twenty-three patients (16%) had more than 70% of their readings within this range. However, 107 patients (74%) of this group did not achieve optimal metabolic control. Four hundred and eighty-four of their blood glucose readings, i.e., 8.3%, exceeded 215 mg/dl, 31% were between 141 and 215 mg/dl, and only 3403 values, i.e. 59.6% of a total of 5690, were within the range of 45–140 mg/dl. In this late registered group no malformations were seen in the 14 patients with optimal metabolic control at the beginning of treatment. From the results of 184 diabetic women who were controlled prior to conception as well as during early pregnancy until delivery, and 436 diabetic women with the first control after the 8th week of pregnancy, we conclude that optimal metabolic control (i.e. mean blood glucose < 110 mg/dl in more than 87% of all blood glucose readings between 45 and 140 mg/dl can be achieved in about 85% of all diabetic women during the time of embryogenesis if the patients are motivated to attend a prepregnancy programme. Diabetic women who start intensified treatment only after the 8th week of pregnancy have only a 20% chance of achieving nearly normal blood glucose levels from the beginning of treatment. The malformation rate in the prepregnancy group of 184 diabetic women was 1.1%. The malformation rate in 436 in the late registered group was 7%. From 33 malformed offspring, 31 mothers came to our hospital only after the 8th week of pregnancy for a first visit, and 32 mothers did not achieve optimal metabolic control during the critical weeks of embryogenesis.

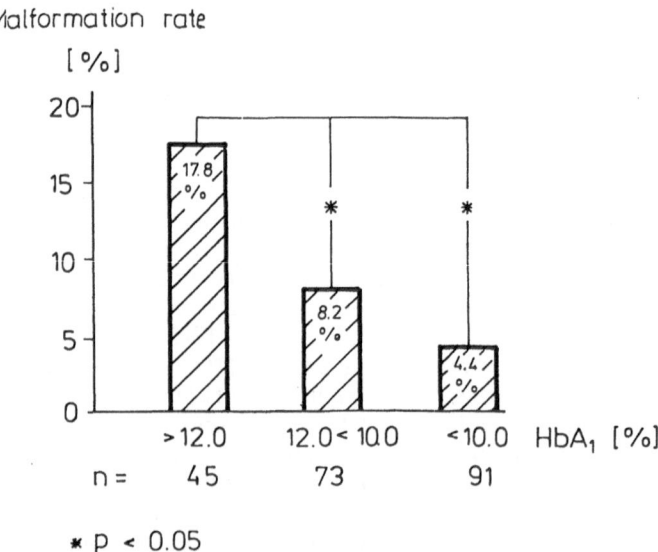

Figure 1   Malformation rate depending on the HbA_1 levels measured before the 13th week of pregnancy

HbA₁ SCREENING FOR MALFORMATIONS IN EARLY PREGNANCY?

Leslie and co-workers[2] observed that glycosylated haemoglobin levels were high early in pregnancy in a few diabetic women delivering babies with congenital anomalies. Miller and colleagues[3] also used haemoglobin A_{1C} as a retrospective index of diabetic control early in pregnancy. In a series of 116 insulin-dependent diabetic women seen in the first trimester, the incidence of major malformations was 22% in infants of 58 women with initial $HbA_{1C} >$ 8.5% compared with 3.3% in 58 infants of women with initial $HbA_{1C} < 8.5\%$ ($p < 0.01$).

In a prospective study we followed all women with HbA_1 levels performed before the 13th week of pregnancy. In the time period from 1981 to 1983 we managed 445 diabetic women during pregnancy. In 209 patients an initial HbA_1 level could be evaluated before the 13th week of pregnancy. The definition of normal HbA_1 by our laboratory was < 8.5%. The malformation rate in diabetic women with an initial HbA_1 of > 12.0% was 17.8%. At HbA_1 levels between 12.0% and 10.0%, 8.2% malformations occurred; diabetic women with an initial $HbA_1 < 10\%$ produced 4.4% malformations. The difference between the numbers of malformations in the three groups is statistically significant ($p < 0.05$) (Figure 1). HbA_1 values estimated before the 13th week of pregnancy indicate the risk of malformations in diabetic women.

References

1. Jovanovic, L. and Peterson, C. M. (1980). Management of the pregnant insulin-dependent diabetic woman. *Diabetes Care*, 3, 63–8
2. Leslie, R. D. G., Pyke, D. A., John, P. N. and White, J. M. (1978). Hemoglobin A₁ in diabetic pregnancy. *Lancet*, 2, 958–9
3. Miller, E., Hare, J. W., Cloherty, J. P., Dunn, P. J., Gleason, R. E., Soeldner, J. S. and Kitzmiller, J. L. (1981). Elevated maternal HbA₁C in early pregnancy and major congenital anomalies in infants of diabetic mothers. *N. Engl. J. Med.*, 304, 1331–4

42

Long term morbidity in infants of diabetic mothers

L. Aerts and F. A. Van Assche

With advances in medical and obstetrical care in diabetes and pregnancy, indices such as perinatal mortality and morbidity are no longer the best criteria for the evaluation of perfect metabolic and fetal control. Therefore it can be argued that the long-term consequences must also be considered. Diabetes of the mother involves an abnormal intrauterine milieu for the developing fetus[1]; the function and structure of the fetal endocrine pancreas is mostly affected. In the human as well as in animals morphological signs of B-cell hyperstimulation and increased insulin secretion have been noted[2-4]. Hyperstimulation of the fetal B cells in a diabetic milieu can induce changes which become manifest in later life.

Hultquist and Olding[5] have demonstrated an increased fibrosis and hyalinose in islets of neonates born to diabetic mothers. Farquhar[6] has shown that children of diabetic mothers have a higher incidence of diabetes than children of diabetic fathers. Furthermore the data of Pettit et al.[7] clearly show a higher incidence of diabetes in offspring when the mother had diabetes during pregnancy than when she developed diabetes after pregnancy. We recently documented B-cell degranulation as a sign of overstimulation in a human fetus from a severe diabetic mother[4].

In our experimental model of diabetes and pregnancy in the rat we have clearly shown that diabetes during pregnancy has an effect until the third-generation offspring; this transmission is not of genetic origin, but must be due to (over)stimulation of the B-cells during intrauterine life. Indeed an effect is only found when the mother of the second generation was born to a diabetic mother, and not when the father was born to a diabetic mother. Furthermore, these changes in the third-generation fetuses were induced in spite of the fact that the second-generation mothers showed a very mild hyperglycemia, indicating that gestational diabetes must be considered as a disorder of total fuel metabolism and the exposure of the fetal pancreas to this increase in 'mixed nutrients' might be at the origin of fetal B-cell overstimulation, inducing the long-term consequences.

References

1. Pedersen, J. and Molsted-Pedersen, L. (1971). Diabetes mellitus and pregnancy. The hyperglycemia–hyperinsulinemia theory and the weight of the newborn baby. In Rodrigues, R. R. and Vallance-Owen, J. (eds.). *Diabetes*, pp. 678–700. (Amsterdam: Excerpta Medica)
2. Kim, J. N., Runge, W., Wells, L. J. and Lazarow, A. (1960). Pancreatic islets and blood sugars in prenatal and postnatal offspring from diabetic rats: beta granulation and glycogen infiltration. *Anat. Rec.*, **138**, 239–60
3. Aerts, L. and Van Assche, F. A. (1977). Rat foetal endocrine pancreas in experimental diabetes. *J. Endocrinol.*, **73**, 339–46
4. Van Assche, F. A., Aerts, L. and De Prins, F. (1983). Degranulation of the insulin-producing beta cells in an infant of a diabetic mother. Case report. *Br. J. Obstet. Gynaecol.*, **90**, 182–5
5. Hultquist, G. T. and Olding, L. (1975). Pancreatic islet fibrosis in young infants of diabetic mothers. *Lancet*, **2**, 1015–16
6. Farquhar, J. W. (1969). Prognosis for babies born to diabetic mothers in Edinburgh. *Arch. Dis. Childh.*, **44**, 36–47
7. Pettit, D. J., Bavid, H. R., Aleck, K. A. and Knowler, W. C. (1983). Diabetes mellitus in children following maternal diabetes during gestation. *Diabetes*, **31**, suppl. 2, p. 66A

Section 11
Surfactant

Chairman's introduction

G. McClure

Over recent years the development of intensive care for sick newborn babies with respiratory distress syndrome has led to a gratifying reduction in the mortality rates of these babies. Intensive care is now widely available in most countries and we can now reasonably expect babies who are born immaturely to survive. However, we should not lose sight of the fact that intensive care is extremely difficult to do properly, and is stressful to the baby, to the parents and to the staff looking after them. It is totally invasive medicine and, although most children do survive it, some are handicapped permanently. How much better it would be if we could avoid the requirement for such intensive therapy.

Surfactant replacement therapy has been tried for some considerable time but until recently such efforts have met with failure. Recent studies indicate that we may be at the dawn of a new era and much recent work indicates that surfactant replacement is possible. We should not be precipitate, though, in our efforts to give all immature babies surfactant. The water is still extremely cloudy and almost all of the questions remain unanswered. This symposium has been significant in posing such questions. We do not yet know what type of surfactant to use, whether natural or artificial, we do not yet know how much to give and we do not know when to give it. It is still unclear how effective surfactant will be, and quite clearly we have no understanding of the long-term sequelae of this new drug therapy. However, none of these problems are insurmountable but we must wait patiently for the next few years while the story unfolds.

Chairman's Introduction

G. McClure

43

Human surfactant

D. V. Walters and A. C. Barber

Natural pulmonary surfactants are superior to synthetic surfactants in treating hyaline membrane disease in animals[1]. However, unmodified natural animal surfactants have not been used to treat hyaline membrane disease in humans because of the anxiety of provoking potentially serious immunological reactions to the protein contained in those surfactants. The use of natural *human* surfactant should minimize the immunological risk, and indeed surfactant obtained from human amniotic liquid has been used clinically with encouraging results in a pilot study by Hallman *et al.*[2]. We investigated an alternative source of human surfactant which should give a greater yield, namely cadaver lungs lavaged at post mortem. The right or left lungs of 14 cadavers were lavaged within 48 hours of death using cold isotonic buffer (Tris pH 7.3) containing calcium. The surfactant was isolated by a process of differential density centrifugation[3]. The average specific gravity of the surfactants harvested from a continuous density gradient, which is an important step in this procedure, was 1.073 ($\pm$0.002). Although bacterial and viral pathogens are unlikely to survive the isolation procedure, as a final precaution the surfactant was dialysed against 0.1% sodium azide solution. Further dialysis removed the bactericide. The surfactant was stored frozen as a suspension in sterile tubes.

Of the 14 lung lavages, it was immediately apparent that four contained little surfactant, but isolation was continued to obtain composition data on their lipoproteins. The other 10 lavages yielded a total of 1.242 g of phospholipid. This is twice as much as the yield from 38 isolations from amniotic liquid performed by Hallman *et al.*[2]. A comparison of the phospholipid compositions of the surfactants from the two sources is given in Table 1. Also included are other data on the surfactant obtained from lung lavage of dead infants[4]. The phospholipid compositions are very similar. However, our surfactant preparation contains considerably more protein (lipid/protein ratio 6.6) than that of Hallman *et al.* (lipid/protein ratio 15). This is most likely due to contamination by plasma proteins at the time of lavage because of leakage across the dead pulmonary epithelium. Certainly, the proteins in our surfactant react with anti-human plasma protein serum, albumin being the major component. However, also present is a non-plasma protein which on SDS gel electrophoresis has a molecular weight of about 70000. Under reducing conditions the molecular weight is about 35000, suggesting that it is a dimer at the larger molecular weight. This protein is probably the major surfactant apolipoprotein which has been isolated from whole minced human lung[5] and is similar to the surfactant apolipoproteins of other species[6]. The human apolipoprotein does not, in our hands, cross-react with antisera raised to dog, rat or sheep apolipoprotein, nor does antiserum raised to it cross-react with dog, rat, sheep or calf apolipoprotein.

Table 1 Phospholipid and protein composition of some human surfactants

Phospholipid	Ours (n = 14) (% total)	Hallman et al.[2] (n = 6) (% total)	Morley et al.[3] (n = 16) (% total)
Phosphatidyl choline (PC)	75.0	77.6	76.2
Saturated PC	52.3	51.2	51.6
Phosphatidyl glycerol	6.9	7.6	4.0
Phosphatidyl ethanolamine	4.8	5.0	5.6
Phosphatidyl serine and inositol	4.5	6.8	7.7
Lysophosphatidyl choline	1.3	0.6	1.9
Sphingomyelin	2.4	1.6	3.0
Unidentified	5.2	—	—

Our surfactant preparations adsorb rapidly to an air–liquid surface *in vitro* to give an equilibrium surface tension of about 25 dynes/cm and on compression of the surface give surface tension values below 10 dynes/cm. The effects of different handling procedures on the adsorption characteristics of the surfactants were investigated. Adsorption rates of small samples of surfactant (5–10 μl containing 50 μg phospholipid) which were injected onto the bottom of clean glass Petri dishes (64 cm^2 surface area) containing 35 ml of buffer (0.14 mol/l NaCl, 0.01 mol/l Hepes, 0.05 mol/l $CaCl_2$, pH 7.4) were measured with a platinum flag connected to a strain gauge with an output to a chart recorder. Care was taken not to contaminate the surface before or after the injection, and all measurements were performed at 37°C with 100% humidification. Stirring was not necessary because 1 to 2 seconds after the injection there was a definite deflection and a rapid fall in the surface tension record. Four or five measurements were performed on each sample and a control sample was always alternated with a test sample. Each observation was in fresh buffer in a clean dish. The adsorption curves for each sample were averaged and *t* tests performed at each time point. A synopsis of these data is given in Table 2.

Irradiation and sonication both adversely affected adsorption and furthermore equilibrium surface tensions similar to controls were not achieved even after 8 minutes. Freeze-drying also significantly affected adsorption rate but the surface tension was the same as control at 1 minute. It has been shown that

Table 2 The effects of sonication, irradiation and freeze-drying on adsorption time of natural human surfactant (data abstracted from curves: units are dynes/cm)

Time (s)	1	5	10	30	60	480
Sonication ($n = 4$)						
Sample	53*	45*	43*	41*	39*	33*
Control	43	35	34	31	29	28
Irradiation ($n = 4$)						
Sample	56	47	45*	42*	40*	30*
Control	49	35	30	26	25	25
Freeze-dried ($n = 5$)						
Sample	53	40*	36*	30*	25	24
Control	44	31	28	25	24	24

Sonication: 5 s in ice bath, 24 μm probe amplitude, 23 kHz
Irradiation: 0.25 megarads, suspension sealed under nitrogen
Freeze-dried: samples reconstituted to give original volume with distilled water. Measurement within 3 h of reconstitution
* Significantly different from control at least at $p < 0.05$. (figures rounded up for clarity)

calcium is necessary for the rapid adsorption of natural surfactant[7] and that tubular myelin figures (seen on electron microscopy) correlate with the presence of calcium. Sonication is used to solubilize proteins and to make liposomes in lipid suspensions; irradiation even at low doses can interfere with lipid protein binding[8]. The effects of irradiation, sonication and freeze-drying can be explained by proposing that they alter the physical state of surfactant lipoprotein in a way which is analogous to the effect of removing calcium ions. It is suggested, therefore, that natural surfactant preparations should be used in suspension with the minimum of interference. Irradiation is not a practical means of sterilizing natural surfactant since doses higher than 0.25 megarads (the dose we used) is required to kill viruses.

Studies are in progress to ensure that human surfactant from cadaver lungs is pathogen-free after its isolation procedure and also that it has biological activity in animal models of hyaline membrane disease before its use is contemplated in humans.

ACKNOWLEDGEMENT

This work is supported by the UK Medical Research Council.

References

1. Robertson, B. (1980). Surfactant substitution; experimental models and clinical applications. *Lung*, **158**, 57–68
2. Hallman, M., Merritt, T. A., Schneider, H., Epstein, B. L., Mannino, F., Edwards, D. K. and Gluck, L. (1983). Isolation of human surfactant from amniotic fluid and a pilot study of its efficacy in respiratory distress syndrome. *Pediatrics*, **71**, 473–82

3. King, R. J. and Clements, J. A. (1972). Surface active materials from dog lung. I. Method of isolation. *Am. J. Physiol.*, **223**, 707–14
4. Morley, C. J., Brown, B. D., Hill, C. M., Barron, A. J. and Davies, J. A. (1982). Surfactant abnormalities in babies dying from sudden infant death syndrome. *Lancet*, **1**, 1320–3
5. Shelley, S. A., Balis, J. U., Paciga, J. E., Espinoza, C. G. and Rickman, A. V. (1982). Biochemical composition of adult human lung surfactant. *Lung*, **160**, 195–206
6. Sueishi, K. and Benson, B. J. (1981). Isolation of a major apolipoprotein of canine and murine pulmonary surfactant. Biochemical and immunological characteristics. *Biochim. Biophys. Acta*, **665**, 442–53
7. Benson, B. J., Williams, M. C., Sueishi, K., Goerke, J. and Sargeant, T. (1984). Role of calcium ions in the structure and function of pulmonary surfactant. *Biochim. Biophys. Acta*, **793**, 18–27
8. Verma, S. P. and Wallach, D. F. (1982). Action of ionizing radiation on lipid-protein interaction. *Biochem. Biophys. Res. Commun.*, **105**, 105–9

44

The Cambridge experience of artificial surfactant

C. J. Morley

It is well known that premature babies have less surfactant than mature babies, its composition is different and the surface tension lowering properties are unsatisfactory. Replacing this with mature surfactant might improve the function of the immature lungs. Enhorning and Robertson[1], along with many others, have consistently shown that concentrated natural surfactant, when given to animals with immature lungs, produces a considerable improvement in their function. A number of groups have been encouraged to develop a surfactant treatment which would have similar effects on the lungs of premature human babies.

Although this seems an attractive idea there are other factors which also affect respiratory function. Premature babies have immaturity not only of their surfactant but also of almost all the other systems concerned with respiration, and it is not easy to single out which one is of greatest importance.

Among the many respiratory problems human premature babies have are:

1. very immature lung structure;
2. considerable difficulty clearing their lung fluid after birth;
3. problems with an immature pulmonary circulation and pulmonary hypertension;
4. shunting of blood from right to left and patent ductus arteriosus;
5. comparatively weak respiratory muscles and a chest wall which is so compliant that it cannot be stablized to enable the lungs to expand:
6. respiratory control and rhythms which are erratic;
7. proteinaceous exudation onto the alveolar surface which inhibits effective surfactant function;
8. surfactant with an ineffective composition which will mix with exogenously applied surfactant and may alter its function.

RDS is therefore a complex condition with many interrelating factors, most of which are compounded by hypoxia and acidosis. Immaturity of the surfactant system is only one of the factors, albeit a reasonably important one. Surfactant treatment is given to premature babies on the assumption that RDS is due to a deficiency of surfactant with an abnormal composition. However, if this is not correct or only partially correct then surfactant treatment may be ineffective or at best only partially effective.

Premature animals with respiratory problems have been used in acute experiments as models for surfactant treatment, but these are difficult to interpret because animals do not necessarily react in the same way as premature babies. In some lamb experiments the benefit of surfactant lasted for only a few hours and those lambs with respiratory problems similar to infants with RDS did not benefit at all.

In the face of such a complex problem we need to consider what effect can reasonably be expected from exogenous surfactant treatment in very premature babies. Will it abolish RDS altogether? This is highly desirable but probably quite unrealistic. Will it reduce the numbers of babies being ventilated, their time on ventilation or the ventilator pressures needed? Possibly, but by how much? When considering the need for ventilation one has to remember that a high proportion of very premature babies are ventilated from birth. Poor oxygenation and right to left shunting of blood is one of the major problems in RDS, and the studies so far have shown that this is one of the parameters which changes most after surfactant treatment. Will surfactant treatment enable babies to be treated with a reduced inspired oxygen concentration and what change in inspired oxygen can reasonably be expected and over what period: 1 hour, 6 hours or 1 day? Do we expect any improvement to be transient or will it be permanent?

If surfactant therapy improves RDS could one expect it to reduce the serious complications? It is possible that with improved lung expansion there might be an increase in pneumothoraces and patent ductus arteriosus, and these complications might reduce any benefit from the treatment. Surfactant might improve the condition of the babies sufficiently to stop them dying but leave them with chronic lung disease or handicap.

Lastly, will the same response occur when surfactant is given prophylactically at birth to babies who are at risk of RDS, as occurs with surfactant given several hours after birth when RDS is established?

Before we consider the results of clinical trials of surfactant therapy we also have to consider how many babies are needed in a trial to demonstrate with confidence the true differences produced by the new treatment.

There are two ways of studying the effect of surfactant therapy. Short-term 'physiological studies' of the acute effects before and after intervention do not require many babies, depending on the variability of the outcome measured. These studies depend on the surfactant being given to babies with established disease, and they rely on the idea that the short-term effects are the important ones to measure. Studies of longer-term effects such as time in oxygen, or ventilation, mortality and morbidity require larger numbers of babies.

Table 1 shows a simulation of a clinical trial Dr S. M. Gore produced to educate us about the problems of small trials and the need for large numbers. The facts stated are that 36% of the controls die compared with 24% of the treated

Table 1 Simulation of 10 randomized trials of surfactant treatment with 20 babies in each trial

Centre	Control deaths	Treated deaths
A	5	1
B	1	3
C	4	4
D	6	5
E	5	0
F	3	1
G	3	1
H	3	3
I	4	2
J	1	2
$\chi^2 = 4.15$	35%	22%

Power = 60%

The mortality of the controls is 36%. The mortality of the treated babies is reduced by 33% to 24%. Each trial would be unlikely to show the true result

babies. If a multicentre trial contained 200 babies with 10 centres randomizing 20 babies each, 10 treated and 10 controls, each centre would be unlikely to show the true result. Centre A would say that surfactant treatment was very good, Centre B would say that it was terrible, Centre C that it was useless, etc. Even with 200 babies only six of the 10 centres showed that the surfactant worked even when the truth of the study was a one-third reduction in mortality.

I would now like to consider what sort of surfactant should be used for clinical trials. There is good evidence that natural surfactant properly extracted and purified should be effective in the treatment of RDS. Unfortunately, it has to be obtained from either animal lungs or human sources, and this means that it is difficult to obtain in large quantities, hard to purify and sterilize and always contains a small amount of foreign protein. We decided to synthesize an artificial surfactant which would mimic the physical properties of natural surfactant yet was simple to make, non-toxic and easily delivered to the baby by resident neonatal staff anywhere, at any time. Dr Bangham, Mr Miller and I felt that we had succeeded in these aims with our artificial surfactant. This is a mixture of dipalmitoylphosphatidylcholine and unsaturated phosphatidylglycerol in a mixture of 7 : 3 w/w. Its physical properties *in vitro* are similar to those of natural surfactant when used in a crystalline state at 37 °C.

Surfactant can either be given prophylactically at birth or after birth to babies with established RDS. From the evidence of several researchers and our own ideas, we felt that it was best to give the surfactant at birth to try to reduce the severity of the disease.

Our first trial of 78 patients was published in the *Lancet* in January 1981[2]. This has been extended to 129 babies. It was a trial of the prophylactic use of surfactant at birth. Babies were entered into the trial if they were born in Cambridge at less than 35 weeks gestation and needed intubation for resuscitation at birth. All babies fulfilling these criteria born in the hospital during the time of the trial were entered into the trial. It was not a randomized trial because babies were treated with surfactant if either I or Dr Greenough attended the delivery, and became controls if we were unable to attend. The duty pediatric team were present to resuscitate and care for the baby. The treatment was one 25–50 mg dose of surfactant powder insufflated down the endotracheal tube at birth.

The basic results of this trial are that the surfactant only appears to benefit the babies below 30 weeks of gestation. These are the group who are at the highest risk of complications. The babies above 30 weeks have fewer complications and therefore large numbers are needed to show statistically significant differences.

There were 28 surfactant-treated babies and 35 controls of less than 30 weeks. The treatment required to maintain the babies' blood gas status in the normal range was recorded using a scoring system which we devised for the purpose. The inspired oxygen level, ventilator pressure and rate was scored for each baby for every hour during the first 2 days. A baby in air would score zero and a baby on maximum ventilation 24. By the end of the 48 hours the surfactant-treated babies had significantly lower scores than the controls. Interestingly, this effect was not apparent for the first few hours after the surfactant had been given at birth, but thereafter there was a slow and steady improvement.

One of the most striking differences was the improvement in mortality in the surfactant group. In the whole trial there was a 20% mortality in the control group and a 3% mortality in the treated group. The deaths were almost all in the group below 30 weeks gestation. Here 41% of the controls died and 7% of the treated babies. The median age at death for the controls was 21 hours compared with 80 for the surfactant-treated babies. There was also an increase in the number of surviving babies ventilated for less than 5 days from 61% to 83% and the incidence of pneumothoraces fell from 50% in the controls to 10%.

It is not possible to determine from this study whether one small dose of this artificial surfactant really has a beneficial effect because of the non-randomized nature of the study. However, these results encouraged us to set up a randomized controlled trial.

This trial was started in January 1982 with the help of Dr S. M. Gore (MRC statistician). It was planned that 360 babies with a gestation of less than 34 weeks would be needed to give an 80% chance of identifying a 30% reduction in the proportion of babies needing ventilation. Although our original trial showed a difference in mortality this trial only has a 50% chance of detecting a 50% improvement in mortality. The babies are randomly allocated to surfactant treatment or control by opening a sealed envelope just before delivery. All deliveries are attended by either Dr Greenough or myself. In this trial the surfactant is given to the babies as a dose of between 50 and 100 mg of powder suspended in 1 ml of cold saline. As long as the surfactant crystals are kept below their transition temperature of about 25 °C the surfactant maintains the properties of a crystalline solid and melts and spreads over the surface of the lungs as it warms up in the baby. The control substance is 1 ml of cold saline. All the babies in the trial are born in the hospital. The surfactant or saline is placed in the pharynx just after birth, if possible before the first breath, and as the baby breathes some of it is inhaled. If the baby does not breathe very well and is intubated for resuscitation a second dose is delivered down the endotracheal tube. If the baby is intubated at 1 hour and 24 hours third and fourth doses are given down the endotracheal tube.

This trial is still in progress; by August 1984, 200 babies had been entered from Cambridge and 52 from Nottingham. It is not appropriate therefore to disclose the full results of this trial until it has been completed but the results at this interim analysis are promising.

In conclusion, the Cambridge experience of surfactant therapy suggests that if the results we have obtained are sustained this artificial surfactant mixture given in this way may improve the outcome for babies with RDS by reducing the severity and complications of RDS.

References

1. Enhorning, G. and Robertson, B. (1972). Lung expansion in the premature rabbit fetus after tracheal deposition of surfactant. *Pediatrics*, **50**, 58–66
2. Morley, C. J., Miller, N., Bangham, A. and Davis, J. A. (1981). Dry artificial lung surfactant and its effect on very premature babies. *Lancet*, **1**, 64–8

45

Overview of surfactant replacement therapy

B. Robertson

The efficacy of surfactant replacement therapy has been documented extensively in various animal models of the neonatal respiratory distress syndrome (RDS) (for review, see ref. 1). In contrast, clinical studies have given conflicting results – especially concerning the value of synthetic surfactant substitutes. Most of these discrepancies are only apparent, reflecting variations in surfactant composition and study design. As will be discussed below, the efficacy of surfactant therapy is determined not only by the composition and the physical properties of the exogenous material, but also by the type and severity of the lung lesions in the recipient.

TIMING OF REPLACEMENT THERAPY IN RELATION TO PATHOLOGY OF RDS

The first phase of neonatal RDS is characterized morphologically by delayed resorption of fetal pulmonary fluid and desquamation of bronchiolar epithelium. Treatment with surfactant is probably more effective during this early stage than later on, when many bronchioles may have become plugged with hyaline membranes and large amounts of surfactant inhibitors have accumulated in the airspaces (see below).

Data from animal experiments point in the same direction. In general, prophylactic treatment at birth has a more impressive and long-standing effect on blood gases and lung compliance, than has administration of surfactant to animals who have developed epithelial lesions and respiratory failure[2]. However, strikingly improved lung function has been documented in premature newborn rabbits[3] and lambs[2,4,5] treated with natural surfactant during the early course of experimental RDS; a moderate therapeutic response was noted also with 'dry artificial surfactant', i.e. dipalmitoylphosphatidylcholine (DPPC) and phosphatidylglycerol (PG) mixed in proportions 7 : 3[6]. The dose of natural surfactant required for a therapeutic response is, in this type of experiments, 40–50 mg/kg[2-5].

PROTEIN LEAKAGE AND
SURFACTANT INHIBITORS

Immature lungs are leaky. This simple fact is particularly relevant to the pathogenesis of neonatal RDS, as at least one of the proteins that tend to enter the airspaces of immature lungs is a potent inhibitor of pulmonary surfactant. The inhibitor has a molecular weight of 110 000 dalton[7]; its activity has been demonstrated in the airspaces of immature lambs[4,7-9] and babies[10] with RDS. A leaking alveolar epithelium might also lead to a rapid 'wash-out' of surfactant material, instilled into the airspaces.

The inhibitory activity of proteins leaking into the airspaces can be quantified in alveolar wash samples by mixing different concentrations of the protein fraction with a fixed amount of isolated natural surfactant, and analysing the surface properties of the mixtures with pulsating bubble[10]. Inhibition of surfactant function is then reflected by elevated minimal surface tension during surface compression. The resistance of any particular surfactant substitute to isolated surfactant inhibitor can be determined with the same technique in an analogous manner.

Inhibitors flooding the airspaces of an immature lung tend to trigger a vicious circle, as any deterioration of the surfactant system implies a risk of further disruption of alveolar and bronchiolar epithelium, with increasing leakage of inhibitory proteins, etc. This vicious circle can be prevented by surfactant replacement: experiments on immature lambs have documented a significantly reduced transpulmonary leakage of proteins, including the specific surfactant inhibitor, in animals receiving tracheal instillation of surfactant at birth[9].

CLINICAL TRIALS OF SURFACTANT
REPLACEMENT

During the past 5 years, various preparations of natural surfactant have been tested in patients with neonatal RDS (Table 1). These include bovine surfactant enriched with DPPC and PG[11] or with tripalmitin and palmitic acid[17], lipids extracted from porcine[12,15] or bovine[14,16] crude surfactant, and surfactant isolated from human amniotic fluid[13]. All natural surfactant preparations listed in Table 1 contain protein, between 1 and 5%. The quantities of phospholipids applied vary from about 25 to 200 mg/kg body weight; these doses all represent an excess, compared to the amount of phospholipid molecules required to form a monolayer on the interior surface of the lung (about 6 mg/kg). Figures for survival and incidence of bronchopulmonary dysplasia are similar in the various studies referred to in Table 1.

Clinical trials of natural surfactant have shown that most patients with severe RDS respond to replacement therapy with a dramatic improvement of gas exchange, and that one large dose of surfactant is usually sufficient to reverse the clinical course. Some patients, however, show only a transient

Table 1 Published non-randomized clinical trials of natural surfactant replacement in neonatal RDS

Authors	No. of treated patients	Birth weight (g)	Phospho-lipid dose (mg/kg)	Survival	Incidence of broncho-pulmonary dysplasia
Fujiwara et al. 1980[11]	10	1150–2143	100	8/10	2/10
Kobayashi et al. 1981[12]	1	1226	25	1/1	0
Hallman et al. 1983[13]	5	850–1240	60	5/5	1/5
Smyth et al. 1983[14]	6	1180–1800	140	6/6	1/6
Nohara et al. 1983[15]	6	835–1850	25	4/6	1/6
Berggren et al. 1984[16]	4	795–1680	200	4/4	1/4

response. As mentioned above, this could be due to accumulation of surfactant inhibitors in the airspaces, or to 'wash-out' of the exogenous material from the alveoli. Both compromising mechanisms may operate in cases of severe RDS.

CLINICAL TRIALS OF SYNTHETIC SURFACTANTS

In general, trials of synthetic surfactants have been disappointing (Table 2). The exception is the current randomized Cambridge study[26], in which infants with low birth weight are treated prophylactically with a mixture of DPPC and PG (7:3), administered via the airways. Interim reports[21,26] from this study have revealed reduced oxygen dependency, improved lung–thorax compliance, and lower mortality rate in surfactant-treated babies, in comparison with controls. Wilkinson et al.[23] failed to confirm these results in a small randomized trial, and Milner et al.[25] found no beneficial effect of DPPC+PG in patients with manifest RDS. Details from the Cambridge trial are presented elsewhere in this volume (see chapter 44).

All synthetic surfactants so far used in clinical trials are based on DPPC; in recent studies other lipids have been added to facilitate spreading of the DPPC molecules in the air–liquid interface. Such 'fluidizers' need to be present in the surfactant system, as DPPC is solid at normal body temperature and, therefore, cannot be expected to be physiologically active by itself when administered via the airways. Mixtures of DPPC and PG spread rapidly in an air–liquid interface, provided that the material is administered in dry form[28], and the physiological activity of this type of 'dry artificial surfactant' has been documented by Morley et al.[6] in experiments on immature newborn rabbits. However, the general impression from other animal studies[8,29,30] is that preparations based on synthetic lipids only are clearly less effective than natural surfactant. In comparison with bovine material, a mixture of DPPC and PG (9 : 1) is also less resistant to surfactant inhibitor[8].

Even if administration of synthetic surfactants at birth does not lead to immediate improvement of lung function, it remains possible that the exogenous phospholipids exert a long-term beneficial effect by increasing the pool size of surfactant molecules, available for recycling and reprocessing by the alveolar epithelium. In the normal neonatal lung, about 95% of exogenous DPPC is reutilized[31]. No information has been presented on the recycling of surfactant phospholipids in the immature lung, nor on the capacity of this important mechanism in babies with RDS.

Table 2 Published trials of synthetic surfactants in neonatal RDS

Authors	No. of treated patients	Surfactant	Effective
Robillard et al. 1964[18]	11	DPPC*	?
Chu et al. 1967[19]	15	DPPC*	?
Ivey et al. 1977[20]	21	DPPC+DPPG*	yes
Morley et al. 1981[21]	22	DPPC+PG	yes
Friedman and Doody 1982[22]	3	DPPG+DOPC+ DOPG+Cholesterol	yes (?)
Wilkinson et al. 1982[23]	24	DPPC+PG	no
Pettenazzo et al. 1983[24]	3	DPPC+PG	yes (?)
Milner et al. 1983[25]	10	DPPC+PG	no
Morley et al. 1984[26]	58	DPPC+PG	yes
Halliday et al. 1984[27]	49	DPPC+HDL	no

* aerosol
DPPG: dipalmitoylphosphatidylglycerol
DOPC: dioleoylphosphatidylcholine
DOPG: dioleoylphophatidylglycerol
HOL: high-density lipoprotein

ROLE OF SURFACTANT APOPROTEINS

At least two apoproteins seem to be associated with natural surfactant (for review, see ref. 32). These proteins, which have molecular weights of about 35 000 and 10 000 daltons, may be essential for the formation of tubular myelin in the alveolar lining layer, and for the subsequent adsorption of the surface film[33]. Absence of apoproteins could explain why synthetic surfactants exhibit poor physiological activity in animal experiments and in most clinical trials.

Recent studies have shown that the *in vitro* surface adsorption of DPPC + PG is improved significantly by addition of the smaller apoprotein to the system[34]. A mixture of DPPC, dipalmitoylphosphatidylglycerol, and the smaller apoprotein is physiologically active also in experiments on immature newborn rabbits; tracheal instillation of this 'artificial surfactant' results in improved lung–thorax compliance[35] (Figure 1). Although the activity of the apoprotein-based artificial surfactant is still suboptimal, the *in vivo* effect is comparable to that obtained with natural surfactant in the same concentration. Additional efforts should be made to identify, if possible, more effective surfactant substitutes based on synthetic phospholipids and isolated apoproteins.

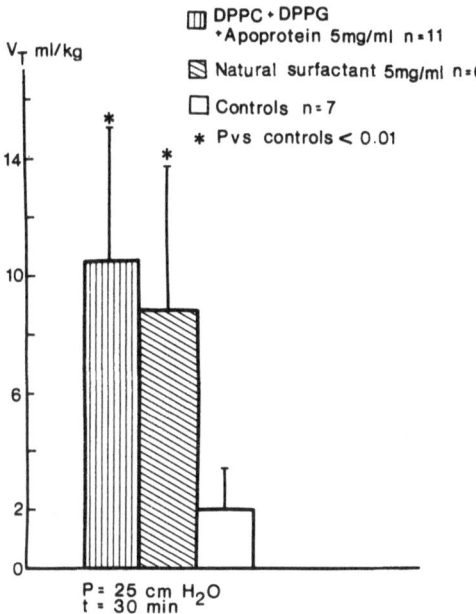

Figure 1 Tidal volumes in artifically ventilated immature newborn rabbits (day 27 of gestation), treated at birth with a mixture of DPPC, dipalmitoylphosphatidylglycerol, and apoprotein (75:25:5, w/w/w) or with natural porcine surfactant, and in littermate controls. Both surfactant preparations were administered via a tracheal cannula, at phospholipid concentration 5 mg/ml (dose volume 2 ml/kg). The recordings were obtained after 30 min of ventilation. Both groups of surfactant-treated animals have significantly larger tidal volumes than controls. The difference between the two groups of treated animals is not statistically significant. From Suzuki[35], reprinted with permission

CONCLUDING REMARKS

Despite promising results reported by many investigators (Table 1), the value of natural surfactant substitutes needs to be confirmed in randomized clinical trials. It would be of considerable interest if these studies could include evaluation of protein leakage, with particular attention paid to the possibility that variations in clinical response could reflect accumulation of surfactant inhibitors in the airspaces. Additional research work is also required to analyse the possible correlations between molecular organization ('dry' vs. 'wet' surfactant, unilamellar vs. multilamellar liposomes, etc.), surface properties (adsorption, spreading, minimal surface tension during surface compression, dynamic respreadability, etc.), and *in vivo* activity of surfactant substitutes. In particular, the role of apoproteins, indicated by the experimental data summarized above, should be considered in future studies of surfactant preparations for clinical use.

ACKNOWLEDGEMENTS

This work was supported by The Swedish Medical Research Council (Project No. 3351), The Swedish National Association against Heart and Chest Diseases, The 'Expressen' Prenatal Research Foundation, The Research Funds of the Karolinska Institute, Allmänna Barnbördshusets Minnesfond, and Stiftelsen Samariten.

References

1. Robertson, B. (1980). Surfactant substitution. Experimental models and clinical applications. *Lung*, **158**, 57–68
2. Jobe, A., Ikegami, M., Glatz, T., Yoshida, T., Diakomanolis, E. and Padbury, Y. (1981). Duration and characteristics of treatment of premature lambs with natural surfactant. *J. Clin. Invest.*, **67**, 370–5
3. Nilsson, R., Grossmann, G., Berggren, P. and Robertson, B. (1981). Surfactant treatment in experimental hyaline membrane disease. *Eur. J. Respir. Dis.*, **62**, 441–9
4. Ikegami, M., Jobe, A. and Glatz, T. (1981). Surface activity following natural surfactant treatment in premature lambs. *J. Appl. Physiol.*, **51**, 306–12
5. Jacobs, H., Jobe, A., Ikegami, M., Glatz, T., Jones, S. J. and Barajas, L. (1982). Premature lambs rescued from respiratory failure with natural surfactant: clinical and biophysical correlates. *Pediatr. Res.*, **16**, 424–9
6. Morley, C., Robertson, B., Lachmann, B., Nilsson, R., Bangham, A., Grossmann, G. and Miller, N. (1980). Artificial surfactant and natural surfactant. Comparative study of the effects on premature rabbit lungs. *Arch. Dis. Child.*, **55**, 758–65
7. Ikegami, M., Jobe, A., Jacobs, H. and Lam, R. (1984). A protein from the airways of premature lambs that inhibits surfactant function. *J. Appl. Physiol.*, **57**, 1134–42
8. Ikegami, M., Jobe, A., Jacobs, H. and Jones, S. J. (1981). Sequential treatments of premature lambs with an artificial surfactant and natural surfactant. *J. Clin. Invest.*, **68**, 491–6
9. Jobe, A., Ikegami, M., Jacobs, H., Jones, S. and Conaway, D. (1983). Permeabil-

ity of premature lamb lungs to protein and the effect of surfactant on that permeability. *J. Appl. Physiol.*, **55**, 169–76

10. Ikegami, M., Jacobs, H. and Jobe, A. (1983). Surfactant function in the respiratory distress syndrome. *J. Pediatr.*, **102**, 443–7

11. Fujiwara, T., Maeta, H., Chida, S., Morita, T., Watabe, Y. and Abe, T. (1980). Artificial surfactant therapy in hyaline-membrane disease. *Lancet*, **1**, 55–9

12. Kobayashi, T., Kataoka, H., Murakami, S. and Haruki, S. (1981). A case of idiopathic respiratory distress syndrome treated by newly developed surfactant (Surfactant CK). *J. Jpn. Med. Soc. Biol. Interface*, **12**, 1–6

13. Hallman, M., Merritt, T.A., Schneider, H., Epstein, B. L., Mannino, F., Edwards, D. K. and Gluck, L. (1983). Isolation of human surfactant from amniotic fluid and a pilot study of its efficacy in respiratory distress syndrome. *Pediatrics*, **71**, 473–82

14. Smyth, J. A., Metcalfe, I. L., Duffty, P., Possmayer, F., Bryan, M. H. and Enhorning, G. (1983). Hyaline membrane disease treated with bovine surfactant. *Pediatrics*, **71**, 913–17

15. Nohara, K., Muramatsu, K. and Oda, T. (1983). Six cases of RDS treated with Surfactant CK. *J. Jpn. Med. Soc. Biol. Interface*, **14**, 61–6

16. Berggren, P., Curstedt, T., Grossmann, G., Herin, P., Mortensson, W., Nilsson, R., Noack, G. and Robertson, B. (1984). Gynnsam effekt av surfaktantbehandling vid IRDS. *Läkartidningen*, **81**, 4180–2

17. Tanaka, Y., Takei, T., Kanazawa, Y., Kiuchi, A. and Fujiwara, T. (1982). Reconstitution of lung surfactant by adjusting chemical composition. *J. Jpn. Med. Soc. Biol. Interface*, **13**, 43–50

18. Robillard, E., Alarie, Y., Dagenais-Perusse, P., Baril, E. and Builbeault, A. (1964). Microaerosol administration of synthetic beta-gamma-dipalmitoyl-L-alpha-lecithin in the respiratory distress syndrome: a preliminary report. *Can. Med. Assoc. J.*, **90**, 55–7

19. Chu, J., Clements, J. A., Cotton, E., Klaus, M. H., Sweet, A. Y. and Tooley, W. H. (1967). Neonatal pulmonary ischemia. Part I. Clinical and physiological study. *Pediatrics*, **40**, 709–82

20. Ivey, H., Roth, S. and Kattwinkel, J. (1977) Nebulization of sonicated phospholipids (PL) for treatment of respiratory distress syndrome (RDS) of infancy. *Pediatr. Res.*, **11**, 573

21. Morley, C. J., Bangham, A. D., Miller, N. and Davis, J. A. (1981). Dry artificial lung surfactant and its effect on very premature babies. *Lancet*, **1**, 64–8

22. Friedman, Z. and Doody, M. (1982). Artificial surfactant (AS): A therapeutic trial in infants with hyaline membrane disease (HMD). *Pediatr. Res.* **16**, 287A

23. Wilkinson, A. R., Jeffery, J. A. and Jenkins, P. A. (1982). Controlled trials of dry surfactant in preterm infants. *Arch. Dis. Child.*, **57**, 802

24. Pettenazzo, A., Granati, B., Rossi, E., Carnielli, V., Baritussio, A., Jori, G. and Rubaltelli, F. F. (1983). Surfactant replacement with a synthetic suspension of phospholipids in the treatment of RDS. Presented at the *International Symposium on the Surfactant System of the Lung*, Rome, 2–4 March 1983. Abstract Book, p. 26

25. Milner, A. D., Vyas, H. and Hopkin, I. E. (1983). Effects of artificial surfactant on lung function and blood gases in idiopathic respiratory distress syndrome. *Arch. Dis. Child.*, **58**, 458–60

26. Morley, C. J., Greenough, A., Miller, N., Bangham, A., Wood, S., Hill, C. and Davies, R. J. (1984). Cambridge artificial surfactant trial. In von Wichert, P. (ed.). *Current Concepts in Surfactant Research. Prog. Respir. Res.*, Vol. 18, pp. 274–8. (Basel: Karger)

27. Halliday, H., McClure, G., Reid, M. McC., Lappin, T. R. J., Meban, C. and Thomas, P. S. (1984). Controlled trial of artificial surfactant to prevent respiratory

distress syndrome. *Lancet*, **1,** 476–8

28. Morley, C. J., Bangham, A. D., Johnson, P., Thorburg, G. D. and Jenkin, G. (1978). Physical and physiological properties of dry lung surfactant. *Nature*, **271,** 162–3

29. Egan, E. A., Notter, R. H., Kwong, M. S. and Shapiro, D. L. (1983). Natural and artificial surfactant replacement in premature lambs. *J. Appl. Physiol.*, **55,** 875–83

30. Kobayashi, T., Grossmann, G., Robertson, B. and Ueda, T. (1984). Effects of artificial and natural surfactant supplementation in immature newborn rabbits. *J. Jpn. Med. Soc. Biol. Interface*, **15,** 53–9

31. Jacobs, H., Jobe, A., Ikegami, M. and Conaway, D. (1983). The significance of reutilization of surfactant phosphatidylcholine. *J. Biol. Chem.*, **258,** 4156–65

32. King, R. J. (1984). The apolipoproteins of pulmonary surfactant. In von Wichert, P. (ed.). *Current Concepts in Surfactant Research. Prog. Respir. Res.*, Vol. 18, pp. 68–82. (Basel: Karger)

33. Benson, B. J., Williams, M. C., Hawgood, S. and Sargeant, T. (1984). Role of lung surfactant-specific proteins in surfactant structure and function. In von Wichert, P. (ed.) *Current Concepts in Surfactant Research. Prog. Respir. Res.*, Vol. 18, pp. 83–92 (Basel: Karger)

34. Suzuki, Y. (1982). Effect of protein, cholesterol, and phosphatidylglycerol on the surface activity of the lipid-protein complex reconstituted from pig pulmonary surfactant. *J. Lipid. Res.*, **23,** 62–9

35. Suzuki, Y. (1985). The role of apoproteins and phosphatidylglycerol in artificial surfactant. In Cosmi, E. V. (ed.). *Controversies in Perinatal Medicine.* (Ithaka, NY: Perinatology Press: in press)

46

Surfactant replacement studies in Belfast

H. L. Halliday, G. McClure, M. McC. Reid and C. Meban

INTRODUCTION

The respiratory distress syndrome affects over half of all babies born at less than 34 weeks gestation and accounts for at least 1500 deaths each year in the UK[1]. Following Pattle's discovery of surfactant Avery and Mead in 1959 suggested that its deficiency was the cause of RDS[2]. From 1964 many clinicians have tried to treat or prevent RDS by administering artificial surfactant to newborn babies. The results have generally been disappointing except perhaps for those of Morley et al.[3] which are presented in chapter 44 of this volume.

In the hope of developing an improved artificial surfactant we mixed dipalmitoylphosphatidylcholine (DPPC) with high-density lipoprotein (HDL) in a 10 : 1 ratio and showed that this was very effective at lowering surface tension and was rapidly adsorbed in vitro[4]. We undertook a randomized, controlled study to test this surfactant in 100 babies of less than 34 weeks gestation who were born in the Royal Maternity Hospital, Belfast.

PATIENTS AND METHODS

This study has already been reported in full elsewhere[5]. A dose of 30 mg of DPPC and 3 mg HDL in suspension was administered in a volume of 5 ml to half of a group of preterm babies born at Royal Maternity Hospital, Belfast between January 1982 and March 1983. Babies were excluded from the study if an antenatal L/S ratio was ≥ 2.0 (nine babies), significant congenital anomaly (six babies) or failure of a neonatologist or surfactant to be ready at birth (30 babies). The babies enrolled were randomly allocated to control and treatment groups. All babies were intubated by a consultant neonatologist and 51 control babies had a period of manual ventilation and 49 treated babies were given 5 ml of the DPPC/HDL suspension via an endotracheal tube before manual ventilation. Where possible gastric aspirate was obtained before surfactant was given to measure L/S ratio. Subsequent outcome and management of the babies was by a consultant neonatologist who was unaware of the treatment given at birth. Guidelines for the management, including those indications for assisted ventilation, have already been published[6].

RESULTS

The study and control groups were of similar birth weight and gestational age (Table 1). L/S ratio was measured in 78 babies (39 in each group) and there were no differences in mean levels. The treated group, however, had more immature L/S ratios prior to treatment ($\chi^2 = 4.45$, $p < 0.05$). There was less RDS in the control group (49% vs 67%) but this was not statistically significant (NS). The excess of RDS in the treated group was due to mild or moderate forms of the disease (oxygen concentration < 60%). There were no differences in mortality between the groups.

Table 1 Study groups and outcome

	Treated (n = 49)	Control (n = 51)
Birth weight (g)	1485±420	1590±425
Gestation (weeks)	30.3±2.4	31.0±2.13
SGA <10th centile	5 (10%)	8 (16%)
Male : female	23:26	25:26
Mean L/S ratio	1.74±0.59	1.94±0.63
L/S <2.0	29/39*	20/39
RDS	33 (67%)	25 (49%)
Mild	13 (26%)	8 (16%)
Moderate	9 (18%)	5 (10%)
Severe	11 (22%)	12 (23%)
Deaths in hospital	9 (18%)	9 (18%)
Neonatal deaths <28 days	6 (12%)	6 (12%)
Severe RDS		
L/S ratio <2.0	7/29 (24%)	9/20 (45%)
≥2.0	1/10 (10%)	0/19 —

* p <0.05
L/S ratio = lecithin/sphingomyelin ratio
Mean ± SD

Fewer babies with immature L/S ratios developed severe RDS in the treated group compared with controls (24% vs 45%, NS). The neonatal mortality rate in the babies < 30 weeks was lower in the treated group than control (12% vs 36%, NS). There were no differences in need for assisted ventilation or complications between the groups.

CONCLUSIONS FROM FIRST STUDY

Our suspension of DPPC/HDL did not prevent RDS in the babies studied. The reasons for this may be many:

1. perhaps the surfactant which is effective *in vitro* is not effective *in vivo*. We intend in the near future to test the surfactant in rabbits;
2. perhaps we used too low a dose and that 100 mg rather than 30 mg would be more appropriate;
3. some researchers have suggested that repeated doses of surfactant are necessary and this may be another reason for our failure.

It would certainly appear that any improvement likely to occur after surfactant replacement will most likely be seen in babies of 25–29 weeks gestation. Our treated babies who were subsequently proven to have had mature lungs at birth were not improved by surfactant administration and may indeed have suffered detrimental effects.

Table 2 Follow-up study

	Treated	*Control*	*Others*
Number	49	51	39
Died in hospital	9 (18%)	9 (18%)	8 (20%)
Died at home	1	1	0
Survived to follow-up	39	41	31
Age now >18 months	22	23	25
Examined in study	19 (86%)	21 (91%)	23 (92%)
Birth weight (g)	1530±390	1635±415	1610±360
Gestation (weeks)	30.7±2.1	31.3±1.6	31.1±1.8
Male : female	12:7	12:9	16:7
Obstetric risk score*	5.0±2.9	5.0±2.2	5.0±2.5
Hospital admissions			
Babies	6 (32%)	12 (57%)	11 (48%)
Admissions	13	20	15
Colds/year	2.3±2.0	2.5±2.2	3.0±1.9
Respiratory infections/year	1.3±2.0	0.9±1.2	2.2±1.5
Antibiotic courses/year	1.3±1.9	1.4±1.2	1.5±1.3
Wheezing	7 (37%)	4 (19%)	8 (30%)
Skin rashes	1 (5%)	6 (29%)	3 (13%)
Food intolerance	3 (16%)	1 (5%)	4 (12%)
Age at sitting (months)†	6.6±1.2	6.8±1.0	7.1±1.9
Age at walking (months)†	12.8±1.9	12.7±1.6	13.1±4.2
Developmental quotient (DQ)‡	95±9	96±10	93±19

* Jones *et al.* (1979)[7]
† Corrected for preterm
‡ Denver developmental screening test
Mean ± SD

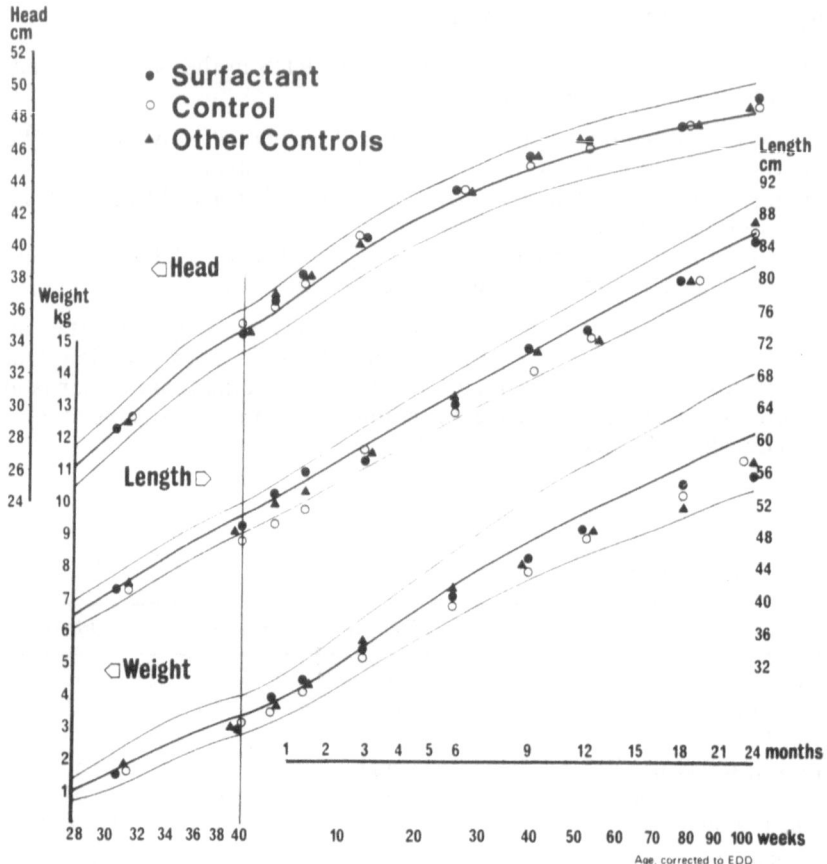

Figure 1   Growth chart showing weight, length and head circumference for the three groups of babies during the first 2 years of life

FOLLOW-UP STUDY

The survivors from our first randomized study plus the 39 babies (others) who were excluded because of mature antenatal L/S ratio and unavailability of surfactant or neonatologist have been followed up to 18 months of age (Table 2). Ninety per cent of the babies who are now over 18 months have been seen and assessed by a consultant neonatologist. The parents have been questioned about hospital admissions, colds, respiratory infections and courses of antibiotics. In addition we looked for signs of allergy, namely wheezing, skin rashes and food intolerance, and performed a Denver developmental screening assessment. There were no significant differences between the groups as regards any of these measurements. We also plotted growth throughout the first 2 years of life and found that the three groups did not differ significantly (Figure 1).

OVERALL CONCLUSIONS

Although our HDL/DPPC suspension of surfactant did not work *in vivo* except perhaps for infants less than 29 weeks gestation it does not appear to have had any long-term adverse effects.

Perhaps RDS is not just a simple surfactant deficiency and other factors such as immature alveoli, delayed fluid clearance, capillary permeability and protein leak, central and peripheral hypoventilation and the presence of PDA all interact to cause respiratory failure in the very immature newborn.

Future studies with artificial surfactant should concentrate on babies of gestational ages 25–29 weeks and should be carried out in a randomized controlled fashion.

ACKNOWLEDGEMENT

Our thanks are due to Dr Terry Lappin of the Department of Haematology, the Queen's University, Belfast, who prepared the high-density lipoprotein by ultracentrifugation of human serum.

References

1. Roberton, N. R. C. (1982). Advances in respiratory distress syndrome. *Br. Med. J.*, **284**, 917–18
2. Avery, M. E. and Mead, J. (1959). Surface properties in relation to atelectasis and hyaline membrane disease. *Am. J. Dis. Child.*, **97**, 517–23
3. Morley, C. J., Bangham, A. D., Miller, N. and Davis, J. A. (1981). Dry artificial lung surfactant and its effect on very premature babies. *Lancet*, **1**, 64–8
4. Meban, C. (1981). Effect of lipids and other substances on the adsorption of dipalmitoylphosphatidycholine. *Pediatr. Res.*, **15**, 1029–31
5. Halliday, H. L., McClure, G., Reid, M. Mc. C. Lappin, T. R. J. Meban, C. and Thomas, P. S. (1984). Controlled trial of artificial surfactant to prevent respiratory distress syndrome. *Lancet*, **1**, 476–8
6. Halliday, H. L., McClure, B. G. and Reid, M. McC. (1981). Respiratory problems. In: *Handbook of Neonatal Intensive Care*, pp. 102–16. (London: Baillière Tindall)
7. Jones, P. K., Halliday, H. L. and Jones, S. L. (1979). Prediction of neonatal death or a need for interhospital transfer by perinatal risk characteristics of mother. *Med. Care*, **17**, 796–806

Section 12
Perinatal Training

47

Higher training in fetal medicine in Britain

C. R. Whitfield

In the United Kingdom, although there has been considerable evolution of special interest work within the broad field of fetal medicine (for example in obstetric ultrasound, genetic and prepregnancy counselling, intrapartum care and fetal monitoring), no special training posts have been established and no training requirements have been recommended, so that obstetricians wishing to obtain further training in these areas must seek relevant experience and de-. velop special skills on a haphazard basis; as a consequence, they have usually been self-taught. Also, unlike subspecialization in the USA, there has as yet been no development towards a recognized subspecialty of fetal medicine (termed maternal–fetal medicine in the USA).

Recognizing that it has become impossible for the individual obstetrician/ gynaecologist to master in depth all, or even most, areas of his specialty, and aware that this process will continue and almost certainly accelerate, in 1980 the Royal College of Obstetricians and Gynaecologists (RCOG) formed a Working Party to consider, and make recommendations on, developments in further specialization within the field of obstetrics and gynaecology, including training implications. In its report (submitted at the end of 1982) the Working Party recommended the establishment of several subspecialties including fetal medicine (and also gynaecological oncology, reproductive medicine and gynaecological urology).

The RCOG Working Party recommended that there should be fewer *subspecialists*, defined as those who, having undertaken appropriate additional higher training, are recognized to have developed special expertise in fetal medicine and to devote at least half their working time to it, than *special interest consultants*, defined as those who, with or without a shorter period of special training, have developed their special interests, expertise and skills in the subspecialty or in part of it. The Working Party estimated that the national target for subspecialists in fetal medicine, achievable over a period of 10–15 years, might be 47 (for a total population of 56 million); and it proposed that every neonatal intensive care unit should be matched by, and work closely with, a subspecialist-led fetal medicine team.

For full subspecialist training in fetal medicine there would be a 3-year training programme, normally beginning after the trainee has passed the examination for Membership of the Royal College (MRCOG), i.e. usually at least 5½ years after graduation including 3½ years in obstetrics and gynaecology plus a required pre-MRCOG elective training year outside the specialty. Subspecialist training would therefore be mostly (or wholly) in the senior registrar grade. Flexibility will be essential and, in planning the content of training programmes to be approved in advance by the RCOG, account would be taken of relevant pre-MRCOG elective experience, although this would not be counted as part of the programme itself. There would be theoretical, clinical and research components, and the clinical training must include neonatal experience, ultrasound and at least 18 months of supervised intensive training in fetal medicine with increasing responsibility and a busy caseload of high-risk pregnancies. It was recommended, and has been agreed by the RCOG, that at least 1 year of subspecialty higher training would count towards the 3 years of general higher training required for specialist accreditation in obstetrics and gynaecology.

Appropriate arrangements, including training posts and attachments, are also required to enable more obstetrician/gynaecologists in training, and also established consultants, to obtain short periods of intensive training in fetal medicine as a whole or, probably more often, in a part of it, for example prepregnancy counselling, ultrasound and amniocentesis, maternal medicine, intensive intrapartum care, perinatal audit and epidemiology.

Appropriately trained clinical assistants and associate specialists, part-time or full-time, would have an important supporting role for fetal medicine teams, e.g. in obstetric ultrasound. The Working Party believed strongly that this could provide useful and expanding opportunities for married women doctors who might wish to develop and use special skills without the heavy commitment to full consultant training. It was nevertheless hoped that some of these doctors might continue training in obstetrics and gynaecology as far as the MRCOG examination.

The RCOG accepted all its Working Party's recommendations and, as a first step towards implementation, has established a Subspecialty Board to advise on, regulate and stimulate developments towards training in the four proposed subspecialties at both full subspecialist and special interest levels. It is encouraging that, in advance of the Subspecialty Board being established, a number of subspecialist and special-interest posts in fetal medicine – both in university departments and with the National Health Service – have developed *de facto*, and that for an increasing number of advertised posts special expertise in fetal medicine is required or at least preferred.

48

Perinatal training in Germany

F. Kubli

The West German contribution to the Workshop on Perinatal Training is limited by the simple fact that in contrast to the situation in the USA, and to what is planned in the UK, there is no subspecialty training for perinatal medicine in our country. There are probably several reasons for this being so. One of these is demonstrated by the fact that in West Germany obstetrics is highly decentralized and the number of departments with an annual rate of more than 2000 deliveries is exceedingly small. Thus, if there really is a need for a 'high-risk obstetrician', it is difficult to conceive the material basis for such positions. However we do have a specified postgraduate schedule for doctors who wish to specialize in obstetrics and gynaecology. This accords with EEC regulations and lasts a minimum of 5 years. Some of the requirements include.

1. conduct of at least 350 deliveries;
2. basic practice in operative obstetrics, i.e.
     15 caesarean sections
     10 vaginal operative deliveries
     100 episiotomies or tears
     10 manual removals of placenta;
3. knowledge of modern perinatal diagnostic procedures including ultrasound;
4. practical knowledge in resuscitation of the newborn.

A theoretical examination ('Board') has been introduced in recent years covering both obstetrics/perinatology and gynaecology. There seems to be little uniformity in the realization of this examination throughout the country.

'Special training' consisting of short-term courses and a sort of 'licence' issued by the local experts finally is needed in order to have ultrasound examinations paid by the various insurance bodies.

Overall, the quality of postgraduate training for obstetrics and gynaecology may be acceptable and some efforts are being made to improve its level, but there is no formal subspecialty training whatsoever, and there are few signs on the horizon which could indicate a change.

49

Training in perinatal pediatrics

D. Harvey

Neonatal medicine is now a recognized subspecialty of pediatrics. It is usually called perinatal pediatrics to emphasize the interest that a neonatal pediatrician must take in the fetus and the co-operation with obstetricians which is so essential

CO-ORDINATION OF PEDIATRIC TRAINING IN EUROPE

National and international organizations have been laying down training programmes. In the countries of the European Community (EC), this has been stimulated by the principle in the Treaty of Rome which allows free movement of workers, including doctors, from one member nation to another. The body concerned with the training of hospital doctors is the European Association of Specialist Doctors (known as UEMS from its title in French) and the monospecialty section for pediatrics is known as CESP, again from its French name. These organizations have gathered information from all the countries in the EC, about undergraduate and postgraduate training programmes. A directive of the EC has laid down that the minimum training period for pediatrics should be 4 years; in fact, several countries have programmes as long as 7 years.

PEDIATRIC TRAINING IN IRELAND AND GREAT BRITAIN

The body concerned with general medical and pediatric training is the Joint Committee on Higher Medical Training (JCHMT) which has a Specialist Advisory Committee (SAC) in pediatrics. The JCHMT is composed of representatives of a number of bodies including the four Royal Colleges of Physicians (one in Ireland, two in Scotland, and one in England). The Pediatric SAC has representatives from the British Paediatric Association.

The JCHMT will accredit doctors in a medical specialty or subspecialty. This was started in order to conform with the EC's plans for free movement of doctors. However, the JCHMT has been anxious to avoid any suggestion that accreditation should become a strait-jacket for doctors who wish to undertake an unusual and individual training programme. Flexible arrangements are permissible, and accreditation is not necessary for a consultant appointment; indeed, any consultant who is appointed will be accredited without any further formality.

The committees have had a recommended training programme in pediatrics for several years. They have now set out programmes for subspecialties. It was recognized that there should be a training programme for those intending to become full-time perinatal pediatricians, and a different plan for those with only a special interest in neonatal medicine.

SUBSPECIALTIES

There has been a lot of discussion about the advantages and disadvantages of subspecialization. Some have even cynically labelled the recent changes as superspecialization. It has certainly become a part of modern medicine, and newborn babies will be helped by pediatricians who specialize in their care.

The problem is that only university and regional centres will be able to sustain appointments for such subspecialists. For this reason it has been agreed that there should be training programmes for the full-time subspecialist and also for the general pediatrician outside a major centre who is expected to spend a large part of his time in a particular area of the care of children. We must therefore train doctors who are general pediatricians with a special interest in a subspecialty. For the newborn, there are therefore training programmes in general pediatrics alone, perinatal pediatrics, and general pediatrics with a special interest in neonatal medicine.

GENERAL PEDIATRICS

Any doctor in Ireland and the United Kingdom spends 1 year, as a house officer after qualification, before being put on the medical register. After that the doctor would expect to spend another 7 years before accreditation.

Three of these years are spent in general professional training. This basic period of training allows a doctor to change course and take up another specialty if he wishes. During the 3 years a pediatrician must spend at least 6 months as a resident house physician in a children's unit. Neonatal experience is essential as a part of a total of 2 years spent in the inpatient and outpatient care of ill children.

During these 3 years it is usual to obtain a higher qualification; in the case of pediatrics this is the membership of one of the Royal Colleges of Physicians (MRCP). Although this is a difficult examination, it is not meant as a qualification at the end of training, but shows that the doctor is suitable to undertake further training in order to become a specialist. There is no examination at the end of training and before accreditation.

After general professional training there is the final period of up to 4 years in higher specialist training. For the person intending to be a general pediatrician, experience in the care of the newborn is of course included in the obligatory experience. All the posts for higher specialist training have been inspected and approved for training.

PERINATAL PEDIATRICS

This is taken as a separate and additional accreditation to general pediatrics, because it is believed that the perinatal pediatrician should have sound training in the problems of older children. It is of course possible that a doctor specializing in the problems of newborn babies might want to switch to another part of pediatrics later in his career; in addition, many perinatal pediatricians wish to follow up the babies who have been in their care to be certain that they have not been impaired by their neonatal illnesses. The doctor wishing to undertake this subspecialty must therefore expect to spend at least 5 and probably 6 years in higher professional training.

The general professional training includes 6 months in each of pediatrics, obstetrics, and neonatal pediatrics. The higher specialist training must include 2 years in a referral neonatal intensive care unit as well the assessment and care of handicapped children. It is recommended that some time should be spent in research, particularly in such subjects as perinatal physiology or pharmacology.

PEDIATRICS WITH A SPECIAL INTEREST IN NEONATAL MEDICINE

Many pediatricians concerned with the care of ill newborn babies do not work in major centres, but in district general hospitals serving a total population of about 200 000 people. They will need to organize the care of preterm babies who need short-term ventilation, but cannot spend all their time in neonatal medicine. Since they will also be general pediatricians, a training programme has been devised for them.

In the general professional training at least 6 months in neonatology is required and a further 6 months in obstetrics is recommended. During the 4 years of higher specialist training, between 12 and 18 months of work in a neonatal unit is essential and it is hoped that some experience in research will be obtained.

CONCLUSION

An attempt has now been made to provide structured training for those hoping to take up perinatal pediatrics. It is important that the recommendations should be treated flexibly, and that there should be adequate training for those hoping to work full-time in the subspecialty and for those either having a special interest in it, or who intend to be general pediatricians and may therefore occasionally have to cover the neonatal service. It is encouraging to see so many young pediatricians taking up the challenge of neonatal care.

USEFUL DOCUMENTS

Two helpful booklets on the Irish and British training programmes can be obtained from the JCMHT Office at the Royal College of Physicians, St Andrew's Place, Regent's Park, London NW1 4LE, United Kingdom. They outline briefly the Committee's responsibilities and provide a handbook of the training programmes.

50

Subspecialization of neonatologists

E. L. Grauel and D. Gmyrek

In our country, the German Democratic Republic, there are now approximately 15 different subspecialities throughout the various fields of medicine. Each programme for such special education is developed by the respective medical society and has to be authorized by the Academy for Postgraduate Education of the Ministry of Health. The general purposes of all these subspecializations are:

1. to provide the physician with special knowledge and skills in the field of subspecialization,
2. to develop his ability to co-operate with other specialists in the complex management of his patients, and
3. to develop his ability to introduce new knowledge into medical practice.

The subspecialist should remain fully competent in his or her own basic speciality.

One of the youngest fields of subspecialization is neonatology. Neonatology is defined as a subspecialization of pediatrics with a lot of interdisciplinary facets. The most important co-operation is doubtless that with the obstetrician; but in addition there are various other strong interrelations, among others in the fields of anaesthesiology, pediatric surgery, pediatric neurosurgery, ophthalmology, orthopaedics, pediatric neuropsychiatry, human genetics, X-ray diagnostics, laboratory medicine, social medicine, medical engineering and the basic sciences of medicine.

The subspecialist should be able to do high-quality work in the basic care of healthy newborns as well as in the specialized and intensive care of premature and sick neonates. He should be able to discuss perinatal problems with the obstetrician and other specialists and to provide qualified metaphylactic care for infants who have had problems during the newborn period.

The subspecialization follows a programme which specifies different fields of knowledge and skills in

1. The basic sciences, especially in biochemistry, physiology, anatomy-embryology, pre- and postnatal development and their possible disturbances and abnormalities.
2. Clinical topics, such as classification of newborns; postnatal adaptation; cardiorespiratory system; gastrointestinal system; genitourinary system; central nervous system; infections; blood diseases; metabolic diseases; diseases of the eyes; diseases of ENT; diseases of the skin.
3. The technical problems of monitoring and therapy, especially of artificial respiration.
4. Diagnostics including ultrasonography.
5. Social and legal medicine concerning the rights of mother and child.

The preconditions for taking up this kind of postgraduate education are acknowledgement as a pediatrician and the successful defence of the doctoral thesis A.

To become a pediatrician one has to have a 4-year training in pediatrics after 2 years of preclinical, 3 years of clinical studies at a medical faculty, defence of a medical diploma dissertation and 1 year of clinical practice, for which surgery (4 months), internal medicine (4 months) and pediatrics (6 weeks) are compulsory.

After the preclinical year the student has to pass a major examination (physicum); two others are to be passed, one after the fifth year (state examination) and another one after the sixth year (interdisciplinary colloquium). Before acknowledgement as a pediatrician he is examined before the district board of pediatricians. Pediatric training includes at least 6 months in neonatology.

The doctoral thesis A is the second of three possible academic graduations in our country (Dipl. med., Dr. med., Dr. sc. med.). With such a dissertation the applicant has to prove his ability to do scientific work.

The subspecialization

Six months of basic care of healthy newborns and work in the delivery room. Six months of special care for premature and sick newborns. Twelve months intensive care in one – or even better – in two different neonatal centres. During this time the applicant is obliged to work with a metaphylactic service for high-risk newborns for several hours a week.

Since the majority of pediatricians, as well as neonatologists, are women there are different regulations if the training has to be interrupted (in case of child birth or family problems). This also holds true for the basic training in pediatrics. To get both qualifications in part-time work needs exceptional regulations, but is possible in principle.

The subspecialization ends with an examination taken before a special board.

According to the organization of our perinatal care, with about 20 grade III centres and about another 30 grade II centres, we estimate the needed number of specialized neonatologists to be about 200 at least and maximally 350 for the years to come. Basic care in the majority of obstetrical departments should be delivered by regular pediatricians, whose training includes neonatology. We hope that in this way we may provide our public health system with a sufficient number of highly qualified physicians for the care of newborn infants.

ADDENDUM

Legal regulations for specialization in pediatrics and subspecialization in neonatology:

1. Anordnung über die Weiterbildung der Ärzte und Zahnärzte – Facharzt/ Fachzahnarzt – v. 11.8.1978. *Gesetzbl. d. DDR*, T. I, **25,** 286–90.
2. Anweisung zur Facharzt-/Fachzahnarzt-Ordnung v. 11.8.1978. Verfügungen und Mitteilungen d. Ministeriums f. Gesundheitswesen Nr. 7/1978, S. 53.
3. Dittmer, A. and Schneeweiss, B. (1980). Comment of the Central Special Commission Pediatrics on the Program of Further Professional Education 'Specialist for Pediatrics'. *Kinderärztl. Prax.* **48,** 664–7.
4. Anordnung über die weiterführende Spezialisierung v. Fachärzten und Fachzahnärzten/Subspezialisierungsordnung v. 13.6.1983, *Gesetzbl. d. DDR*, T. I, **18,** 185–8.
5. Anweisung Nr. 1 z. Subspezialisierungsordnung v. 13.6.1983. Verfügungen und Mitteilungen d. Ministeriums f. Gesundheitswesen, Nr. 6/1983, 45–6.

51

Training of neonatologists in the USA

L. J. Butterfield

The American Medical Association House of Delegates adopted a historic policy on 'Centralized Community or Regionalized Perinatal Care' in 1971. Soon after, a National Committee on Perinatal Health was organized by the March of Dimes Birth Defects Foundation (MODBDF) with representation from the American Medical Association (AMA), the American Academy of Pediatrics (AAP), the American Academy of Family Physicians (AAFP) and the American College of Obstetricians and Gynecologists (ACOG). In 1976 the MODBDF published a monograph by the Committee, 'Toward improving the outcome of pregnancy', which set down broad guidelines for a systems approach to regional perinatal care.

Personnel was a key component in the definition of the levels of care of perinatal services. Select pediatricians and obstetricians had been focusing on high-risk maternal and high-risk newborn care for many years.

In the 1960s the premature infant centres in the USA began a gradual transformation to perinatal centres and several children's hospitals in the USA opened newborn centres. These centres were staffed by the precedents of perinatologists and neonatologists, although their training was quite varied in content.

The American Board of Pediatrics established the sub-board of neonatal–perinatal medicine in 1974 and held the first examination in 1975. With approximately 125 trainees graduating from 175 programmes each year, and a base of pediatricians who had specialized in neonatal–perinatal medicine, 1346 neonatologists had been certified by 1984.

There has been increasing concern that there are too few academic positions to absorb the 125 graduates per year, and that the excess number of subspecialists in neonatal–perinatal medicine would disrupt the established lines of referral and organization of regional perinatal care.

In 1984 a movement to certify training programmes took place. As a result

of the review process 84 programmes have been certified to train neonatologists.

That constriction of the output of neonatologists, and a forthcoming policy
statement on manpower by the AAP Committee on Fetus and Newborn,
should bring the neonatology manpower issue into some perspective and control.

As the American public pressures Congress for cost containment measures,
the number of centres caring for sick newborns and the number of neonatologists working in the perinatal system will be more carefully scrutinized than
in the past.

Section 13
Unexplained
Mature Stillbirth

52

Incidence of stillbirths in singletons and twins: national Swedish data – a preliminary report

H. Rydhström

It is well known that twins have a higher perinatal mortality than singletons. Less known is the fact that twins delivered preterm have a lower mortality than singletons delivered at the same gestational age. From the 38th gestational week on, the mortality of singletons continues to decrease while that of twins does not (Rydhström, to be published).

MATERIAL

All term twin stillbirths in Sweden 1973–81 were identified by using data from the National Board of Health and Welfare, and medical records from 107 twins were studied.

RESULTS

In 10 cases it was the first twin who died, in 71 cases it was the second, and in 13 cases both twins died. Eighty-four of the twins were subjected to a post-mortem. Lethal malformations were found in three cases. In the rest of the cases no obvious fetal reason for outcome of pregnancy was found. The mean weight ($m \pm 1$ SD) of the dead twins was 1990 ± 750 g. Nine of 107 had a weight of less than 1000 g.

CONCLUSIONS

One possible way to reduce the number of stillbirths would be to intensify sur-veillance with non-stress CTG, at least when symphysis–fundus height measurements and/or ultrasound indicate intrauterine growth-retardation of one or both twins. Another way to reduce the number of twin stillbirths could be to induce labour, for example, in the 37th–38th week of pregnancy. This,

however, will not save those twins dying *in utero* before term. In our material
we think that about half of the twin stillbirths actually succumbed before term.

EDITOR'S COMMENT

Dr Rydhström's manuscript is only a summary of his Congress presentation.
He and his co-authors will be publishing the full study when there has been sufficient time to consider not only twin stillbirths but the total twin perinatal
mortality in Sweden during the past 10 years.

53

Clinical characteristics of unexpected intrauterine death

J. Falck Larsen and B. Bødker

Stillbrith has always been a tragedy, and with a decreasing stillbirth rate, it is becoming even more difficult for either the mother or the obstetrician to accept an intrauterine death.

The obstetrician looks desperately for explanations in these cases – or for symptoms that might have been ignored – in order to reduce the incidence of stillbirth. Furthermore, it seems easier for the mother to cope with the situation if she can understand why she lost her baby.

Herlev University Hospital was opened in 1976. It is a regional hospital with a catchment area of approximately 200 000 inhabitants and has 1600 unselected deliveries per year. Only cases of rhesus incompatibility and diabetes mellitus are referred to another university hospital

Table 1 Perinatal deaths (gestational age ≥28 weeks), Herlev Hospital, November 1976–June 1984, 11 040 births

	Ante-partum	Intra-partum	Early neonatal	Total
≥1000 g	32 (2)*	2 (2)	11 (6)	45 (10)†
<1000 g	3	—	1 (1)	4 (1)
Total	35 (2)	2 (2)	12 (7)	49 (11)

In parentheses: included cases of lethal malformations
* Stillbirth rate 3.1 per 1000
† Perinatal mortality 4.1 per 1000
PM if malformations are excluded: 3.2 per 1000

Table 1 shows the 49 perinatal deaths that have occurred in the 11 040 pregnancies we have had in the department. Seventy-one per cent of the perinatal
deaths occurred before the onset of labour. The number of lethal malformations is indicated in parentheses.

Electronic monitoring was used routinely in all deliveries with infants
without known lethal malformations. No intrapartum death occurred during
the approximately 11 000 monitored deliveries. However, one infant died a
few minutes after delivery by emergency caesarean section because of a total
abruptio placentae. We feel that an intrapartum death rate of 1 : 11 000 monitored deliveries is strong circumstantial evidence for the statement that electronic monitoring can reduce – or eliminate – intrapartum death.

The perinatal mortality (≥ 1000 g) was 4.1 per 1000, and if lethal malformations were excluded 3.2 per 1000. The stillbirth rate was 3.1 per 1000. We
tried to analyse the causes of fetal death before the onset of labour. In all cases
a post mortem examination was performed and the clinical history was carefully reviewed.

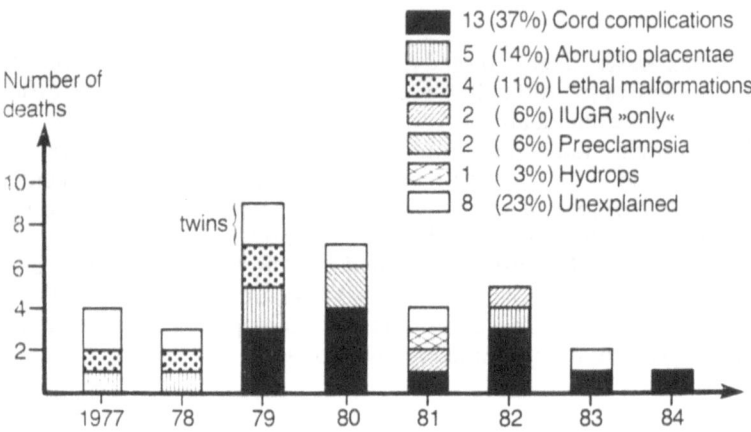

Figure 1   Antenatal deaths among 11 040 births, November 1976–June 1984 at the
Herlev University Hospital, Copenhagen, Denmark

Figure 1 shows the individual cases. In cases of cord complications we felt
that we have a good explanation for the intrauterine death. The following
complications have been recorded: True knots (2), tight coiling (4), torsion or
stricture (3), length less than 30 cm (2), thrombosis (2), and compression (prolapse) (1). However, we must admit that we often see a liveborn infant with a
true knot on the umbilical cord or coiling of the cord. Therefore, some of these
fetal deaths may belong to the 'unexplained' cases.

Much more certain is the diagnosis of abruptio placentae, when we have
clinical signs of increased uterine tonus, haemorrhage, and evidence of placental haematoma. Abruptio placentae was probably the case in 14%, which is in

accordance with the findings in the Scottish Perinatal Survey[1] and another Danish study from Odense university[2].

In nine of our 35 cases of intrauterine death before onset of labour the fetus was light for dates. However, in three of these cases the birth weight was very close to the 10th centile, and in four other cases the fetuses had lethal malformations. Thus, only in two cases was the death caused by 'chronic placental insufficiency'. This is in contrast to the Scottish Perinatal Study[1], in which intrauterine growth retardation (IUGR) was found in 63% of the cases with low birth weight and no other complication.

The most interesting group is that of unexplained intrauterine death. This occurred in five cases with a birth weight of 2500 g or more – or in about 10% of the total number of perinatal deaths.

We have tried to analyse if hormone assays or counting of fetal movements could have predicted or prevented the intrauterine deaths. We have used oestriol (E_3) and human placental lactogen hormone (hPL) for screening of the function of the fetoplacental unit until about 1 year ago, so we have hormone assays in most of the cases. Abnormal hormone values were found in eight cases. Very low E_3 values were measured in two cases of neural tube defects. In one case of cord complication we found a sharp decrease in E_3 but the values were within the normal reference area, and no fetal heart action could be detected at the next examination. This infant was born with the umbilical cord coiled tight around the legs and neck.

Significant falls in E_3 were observed in both cases of IUGR. The patients were contacted as soon as the results of the assays were known but the fetal deaths occurred before the mothers came to the hospital.

E_3 assays did not offer much help in the 'unexplained' cases. However, in one case the E_3 value was very low. Ultrasound examinations gave suspicion of malformation, but it could not be conformed when the infant was born dead at 30 weeks gestation. The placenta appeared to be normal.

Neither did hPL give any warning except in one case of unexplained death. The hPL dropped below the lower limit and the patient was immediately contacted, but the fetus was dead when the mother arrived at the hospital.

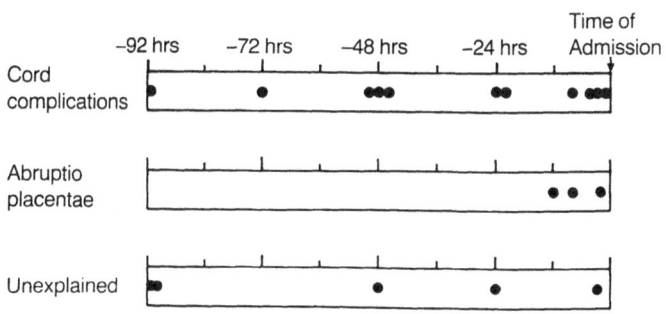

Figure 2 Interval between last registered fetal movements and admission to hospital in 19 cases of unexpected intrauterine death

We have analysed the interval between the last time fetal movements were registered by the mother and admission (Figure 2). We found that in cases of abruptio placentae this interval was very short. In cases of cord complications the interval varied from few minutes to several days. No certain pattern could be found in the cases of unexplained death.

One randomized trial indicated that counting of fetal movements may reduce antenatal death[3]. However, the cases of unexplained death often occur in low-risk pregnancies, and Grant and Mohide[4] calculated that a randomized trial on low-risk cases would need 15 000 women in each arm of the trial. The value of this method has still to be evaluated.

SUMMARY AND CONCLUSIONS

1. Intrapartum death of normal infants can be avoided by careful monitoring.
2. Cord complications may be the cause in one-third of the cases.
3. Antepartum death because of placental insufficency can be reduced.
4. Hormone assays may be useful in risk cases, but immediate action with supplementary methods is necessary if the fetal death is to be avoided.
5. Counting of fetal movements may reduce intrauterine death, but more studies are necessary to prove the value of this.
6. One-fifth of antepartum deaths are unexplained and more research is needed to find the causes for these.

References

1. McIlwaine, G. M., Dunn, F., Howat, R. C. L., Smalls, M., Wyllie, M. M. and Mac-Naughton, M. C. (1984). The Scottish Perinatal Mortality Survey. University of Glasgow, Departments of Social Paediatrics and Obstetric Research Unit, and Department of Obstetrics and Gynaecology, Glasgow, Scotland.
2. Poulsen, H. K., Ipsen, L., Andreasen, E. and Kristoffersen, K. (1982). Perinatal mortalitet. *Ugeskr. Laeg.*, **144**, 3505–7
3. Neldam, S. (1983). Fetal movements as an indicator of fetal well-being. *Dan. Med. Bull.*, **30**, 274–8
4. Grant, A. and Mohide, P. (1982). Screening and Diagnostic Tests in Antenatal Care. In Enkin, M. and Chalmers, I. (eds.) *Effectiveness and Satisfaction in Antenatal Care*. pp. 33–42. (London. Spastics International Medical Publications/ William Heinemann Medical Books)

54

Unexplained mature stillbirth: review of clinical and laboratory data

H. P. van Geijn, J. T. J. Brons, J. I. Puyenbroek and N. F. Th. Arts

INTRODUCTION

This paper reports on the incidence of unexplained mature stillbirth in the Academic Hospital of the Vrije Universiteit between 1980 and 1984, and gives a description of the cases identified during this period.

Table 1 Details of four unexplained mature stillbirths

	A	B	C	D
Grav./par.	1/1	1/1	1/1	3/2
Age (years)	23	31	28	40
Pregnancy control	Midwife	Midwife	Obstetrician	Obstetrician
Antenatal visits	12	9	20	15
Gestational age (wks)	38 1/7	37 6/7	39 0/7	40 4/7
Sex infant	Female	Male	Female	Female
Birthweight (g)	2750	3040	2890	3190
Percentile	25–50	25–50	25–50	25–50

Between January 1980 and June 1984, 4188 women delivered in our obstetrical department. Thirteen infants had died before birth following the 37th week of pregnancy (3.1 per 1000). For nine of these infants an obvious explanation for the occurrence of intrauterine demise was available: five abruptio placentae, two severe preeclampsia with intrauterine growth retardation, one bleeding from vasa previa, one prolonged rupture of membranes. For four cases (1 per 1000), however, a clear explanation for the near-term occurrence of fetal death could not be found, and they were classified as unexplained since they had the following characteristics: gestational age at birth 37–42 weeks, maternal diastolic blood pressure during pregnancy ≤ 85 mmHg, intact membranes upon arrival and no vaginal bleeding, no medication during pregnancy except iron supplementation, birth weight of the infant between the 25th and 75th percentile, absence of fetal congenital anomalies. Table 1 summarizes data on these four cases regarding gravidity, parity, maternal age at delivery, pregnancy control, number of antenatal visits, gestational age at delivery and infant's sex and birth weight. A short description of each case is given.

CASES

Patient A

This is her first pregnancy. Her age is 23 years. There is no history of disease. She does not smoke. The course of pregnancy is uneventful: diastolic blood pressure 60–70 mmHg, weight gain 10 kg, normal fundal growth, no glucosuria or proteinuria. Laboratory findings at 32 weeks of gestation are normal: Hb 7.4 mmol/l, creatinine 44 µmol/l, uric acid 190 µmol/l. At 38 weeks of gestation fetal movements are absent and following the diagnosis of stillbirth, labour is induced. A macerated female infant is born, birth weight 2750 g (25th–50th percentile). At post mortem, congenital anomalies are not found, nor are signs of a intrauterine infection. The only abnormal finding is absence of one umbilical artery. Follow-up examinations (diabetes mellitus, SLE, fetomaternal transfusions, infections) do not give deviating results.

Patient B

Her age is 31 years, she is healthy and does not smoke. It is her first pregnancy. Diastolic blood pressure during pregnancy varies between 60 and 70 mmHg. Weight gain is 10 kg. Fundal growth is normal. Glucosuria and proteinuria are absent. Serum levels at 32 weeks of gestation: Hb 7.9 mmol/l, creatinine 35 µmol/l, uric acid 350 µmol/l. At 37 weeks, fetal heart tones are absent. Polyhydramnios is observed on ultrasound examination. Because of the stillbirth, labour is induced and a macerated male fetus is born, birth weight 3040 g (25th–50th percentile). The pathologist finds no congenital abnormalities nor signs of a chorioamnionitis. Placental weight is 750 g. There are no signs of a fetomaternal transfusion. This pregnancy is followed by two missed abortions and D/C at 12 weeks of gestation. Oral glucose tolerance is normal. Hysterography shows a normally shaped uterus. Cell cultures of both parents demonstrate normal chromosomes.

Patient C

Her age is 28 years and it is her first pregnancy. She has a history of repeated cystitis. She smokes 15–20 cigarettes per day. Diastolic blood pressure during pregnancy varies between 50 and 70 mmHg. Weight gain is 5 kg. Fundal growth is normal. Glucosuria is absent. At 33 weeks of gestation she is admitted to the hospital for social problems (emotional stress) and low oestriol levels in 24-hour urine collections (see Figure 1). During hospitalization oestriol levels increase, protein excretion is present in variable concentrations

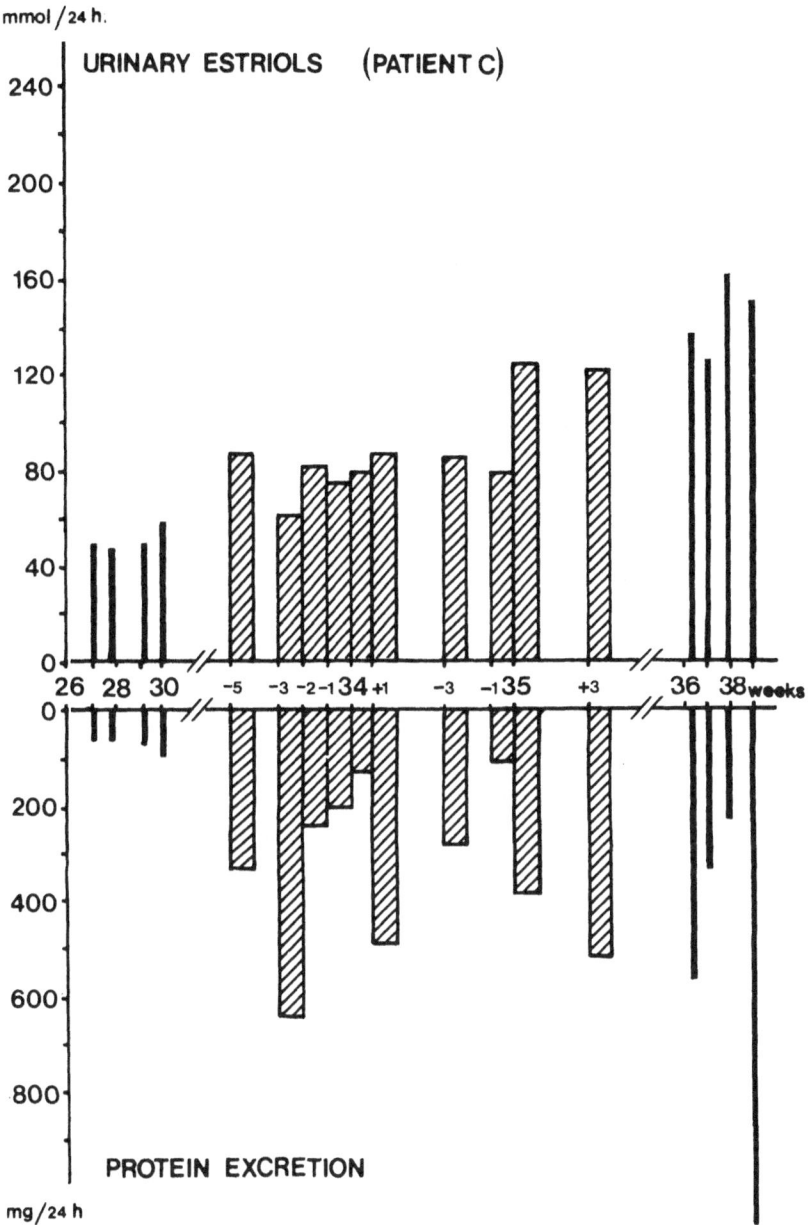

Figure 1 Patient C: maternal oestriol and protein excretion in 24-hour urine samples

with a maximum of 1070 mg/24 hours (see Figure 1). Haemoglobin levels increase towards the end of pregnancy to 8.4 mmol/l. Creatinine levels during pregnancy are 55–62 µmol/l, uric acid levels 180–280 µmol/l. At 39 weeks during a morning visit to the antenatal clinics fetal heart tones appear absent, while fetal movements have been felt the evening before. Labour is induced and a stillborn female infant is delivered, birthweight 2890 g (25–50 percentile). The placenta weighs 800 g and is normal on examination. The pathologist finds signs of a congested circulatory failure. Congenital anomalies are not found.

Patient D

Her age is 40 years. This is her third pregnancy. The first pregnancy resulted in 1962 in the birth of a daughter, birth weight 2250 g, at 34 weeks of gestation. The second pregnancy ended in a miscarriage at 8 weeks. During the current pregnancy blood pressure varies between 65 and 85 mmHg. Weight gain is 9.3 kg. Fundal growth is normal. Glucosuria is absent. At 35 weeks of gestation she is admitted to the hospital for low back pain. During hospitalization blood pressure is normal and frequent collections of 24-hour urine give normal oestriol values. Towards the end of pregnancy haemoglobin, creatinine, and particularly uric acid levels increase (see Figure 2). Two days before fetal death, for the first time an elevated protein excretion of 490 mg/h is noted. Following the diagnosis of stillbirth, labour is induced and at 40⁴/₇ week a female infant is delivered, birth weight 3190 g (25th–50th percentile). Congenital abnormalities are absent. Placenta weight is 610 g. The placenta has no infarctions and there are no signs of a chorioamnionitis.

COMMENTS

Four cases of 'unexplained' mature stillbirth have been described. According to the initial criteria – normal maternal blood pressure, intact membranes at moment of stillbirth, no vaginal bleeding, no maternal medication, normal birth weight of the infant, no fetal congenital anomalies – all four pregnancies should be regarded as uneventful. However, on closer inspection of the clinical and laboratory data, all four pregnancies reveal some abnormality:

   A: one umbilical artery;
   B: polyhydramnios;
   C: elevated haemoglobin, proteinuria;
   D: increased creatinine and uric acid levels, proteinuria.

Although these abnormal findings certainly cannot serve as an easy explanation for each fetal death and a clear cause–effect relationship between these findings and the final bad outcome of pregnancy is lacking, they point to an underlying problem in each case possibly related to the occurrence of fetal death. In case A the presence of one umbilical artery on pathological examination raises the suspicion of other congenital anomalies, possibly undetected due to maceration of the infant's organs. The presence of a polyhydramnios in case B and the course of the next two pregnancies indicate a diminished obstetric performance, for which at present no cause can be found, but which may become apparent in future. The course of pregnancy in cases C and D certainly has not been uneventful and both patients show signs of a reduced

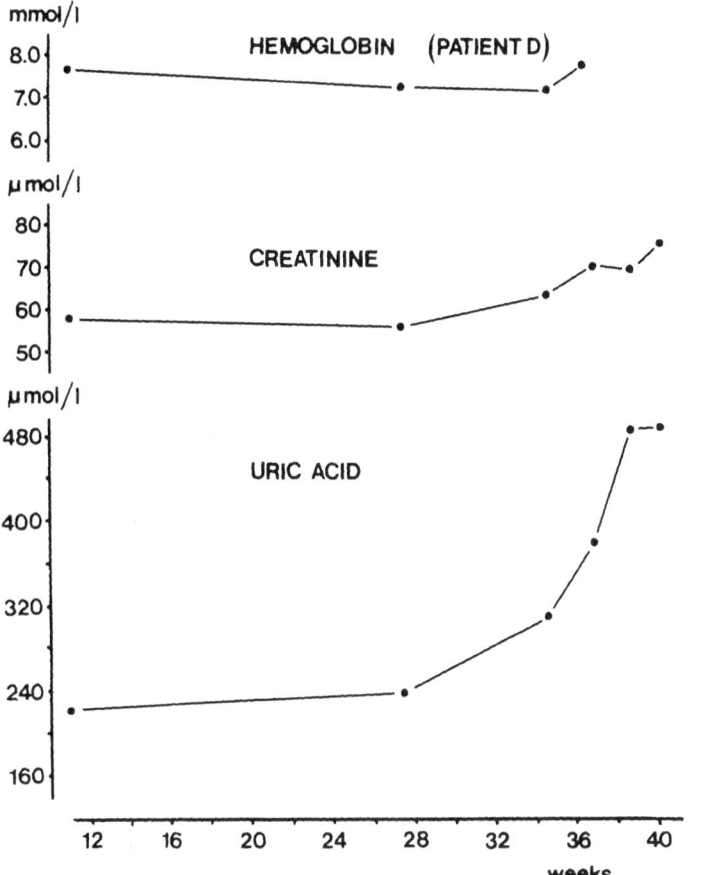

Figure 2 Patient D: maternal serum haemoglobin, creatinine and uric acid levels during pregnancy

maternal plasma volume. Both are suspect for some form of pre-eclampsia and fetal death might even have been prevented by intensive monitoring, e.g. by daily antepartum cardiotocography. All four cases can be considered as 'unexplained' only because all possible available information is lacking. In the population studied – all deliveries at our hospital during the past 4 years – a mature stillbirth following a fully normal pregnancy was not found, which raises doubt if a fully unexplained stillbirth, similar to the so-called sudden infant death syndrome (SIDS) does exist during intrauterine life.

EXAMINATION SCHEME FOLLOWING UNEXPLAINED STILLBIRTH

After an unexplained stillbirth the following scheme is recommended. A complete anamnesis of the mother's history and complaints should be repeated.

After the diagnosis of fetal death, a systematic ultrasound examination should follow, since this is the only opportunity to collect data that will be lost afterwards, e.g. concerning the amount of amniotic fluid, cord entanglements, trans-sonic spaces behind the placenta, fetal stomach and bladder filling, etc. Laboratory investigations should include maternal haemoglobin levels, an evaluation of the blood coagulation system, renal and liver functions, a test to rule out fetomaternal transfusion (Kleihauer–Bethke), search for irregular antibodies and infections (Torch, listeriosis, lues), glucose tolerance testing, lupus erythematosus and determination of the infant's chromosomes. A post mortem of the infant should be performed by a pathologist trained in fetal and neonatal problems. The placenta should be examined macroscopically and microscopically. Following birth of the infant a full-bladder ultrasound examination of the maternal female organs is recommended to detect or rule out uterine anomalies. Since an infant with an appropriate birth weight has been born, and in general each following pregnancy by itself has a better outcome, the prognosis for future offspring should be regarded as good.

55

Pathological investigations

J. S. Wigglesworth

Pathological investigation in a case of stillbirth at term represents merely one example of the sorting process involved in performance of the perinatal autopsy. Although I have published more extensive details elsewhere[1], the whole process can be summarized as shown in Figure 1. It is important for the pathologist to be provided with full clinical information. Diagnosis can often only be made on the basis of non-histopathological investigation (microbiology, haematology, cytogenetics, biochemistry) and there will not be a second opportunity to collect the necessary specimens. Photography and radiography are valuable adjuncts to histopathological study.

The investigation has two aims: firstly, to diagnose any specific condition or significant lesion that may be present and secondly, if no specific diagnosis is possible, to construct a profile of events leading to death. The combination of microbiology and histopathology may establish a diagnosis of β-haemolytic streptococcal infection in one case, while organ weights, indices of maturity and signs of acute and chronic stress in another case may indicate an acute anoxic death following a prolonged period of growth retardation, but without revealing a specific cause.

The process of examination in an infant born dead unexpectedly near term can be depicted in the form of an algorithm as shown in Figure 2. Some of the main pointers which will lead to particular lines of investigation being followed include the recognition of hydrops, of fetal growth retardation and of maceration. Limitation in the clinical database means that the pathologist has to make maximum use of all information that can be obtained. A considerable number of major diagnoses are possible even in the mature, normally grown, non-hydropic stillborn infant, and it may be necessary to put subsidiary questions to the clinicians at any time during the investigations (e.g. as to what infection screen studies were performed on the mother or cord blood). This underlines the necessity for close liaison between pathologist, obstetrician and

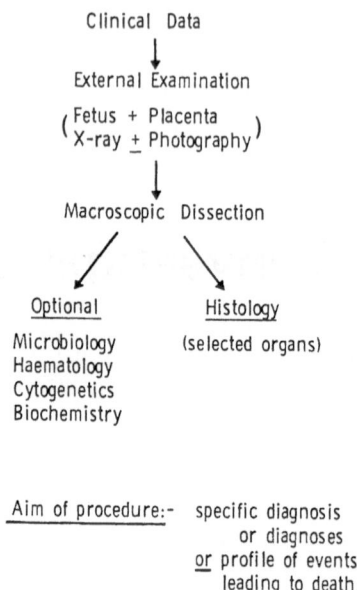

Figure 1 Procedure for perinatal post mortem examination

Table 1 Procedure if consent for post mortem dissection not obtained

---

External examination of fetus
Surface cultures (e.g. ear)
Photography
X-ray
? Other imaging procedures
Cord blood studies (Hb, group, etc.)
Dissection ⎤
Cultures   ⎬ of placenta
Histology ⎦

---

pediatrician in order to achieve accurate diagnosis as an aid to provision of informed explanation and advice to the parents.

In those cases where permission for a formal autopsy is not obtained, it may still be feasible to carry out a range of useful investigations as indicated in Table 1. It is possible to make quite sophisticated diagnoses by such means without causing distress to parents whose sincerely held beliefs may forbid post mortem dissection. In addition to photography and radiography the modern imaging techniques such as real-time ultrasound may allow recognition, or exclusion, of cardiac or renal anomalies or a range of intracranial

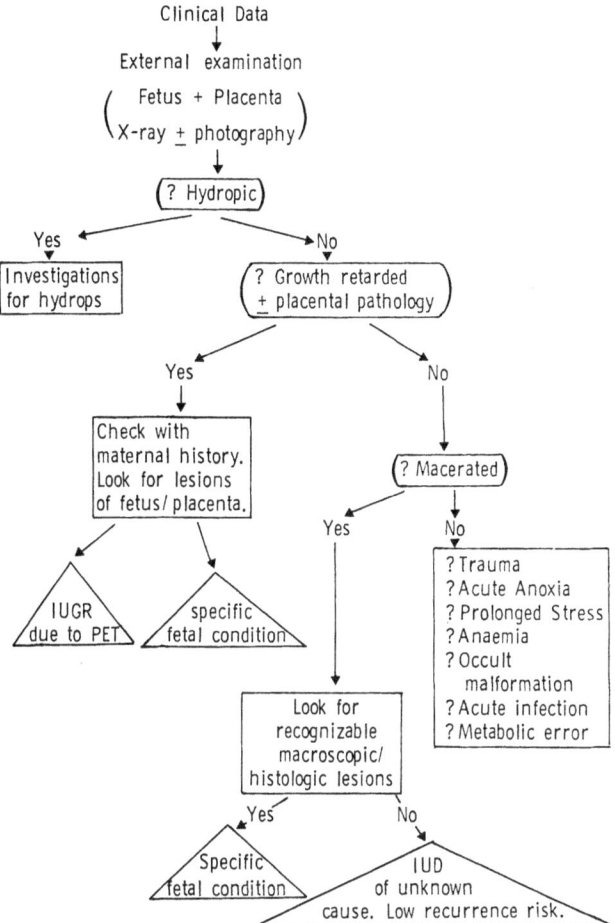

Figure 2 Post mortem examination in cases of unexplained late fetal death

lesions. Cord blood studies for haematological, microbiological or cytogenetic investigations will usually be considered acceptable, and the placenta provides a mass of tissue which can be assessed by histopathological techniques.

Reference

1. Wigglesworth, J. S. (1984). *Perinatal Pathology*. (Philadelphia: W. B. Saunders)

Chairman's summary

R. Derom

INTRODUCTION

A large number of cases will remain where, after consideration of the clinical and autopsy findings, no basis for foetal death can be recognized.

Morison[1]

In some instances careful autopsy examination fails to disclose pathological lesions. This is especially true of deaths occurring before the onset of labor...

Potter and Craig[2]

The macerated stillborn fetus has been a neglected topic in perinatal pathology.

Wigglesworth[3]

Unexplained late fetal death is a challenge to obstetricians and perinatal pathologists. Its importance cannot be overemphasized because, with the reduction in the number of deaths associated with labour and diminishing early neonatal mortality, its relative share in perinatal mortality is increasing.

Major causes of antepartum fetal death and their relative incidence in 249 cases investigated in Belfast by Morison[1] and 511 cases investigated in Chicago by Potter and Adair[4] and Potter and Dieckman[5] are listed in Table 1. There is good agreement, at least concerning the major categories of cause of death. Notice that in roughly one out of two cases there is no evidence available about the cause of death. Notice also the differences in the incidences of accidents to the umbilical cord and premature placental detachment.

The careful analyses of consecutive series of hospital records by Falck Larsen (chapter 53 of this volume) and van Geijn *et al.* (chapter 54 of this volume) and of national figures of single and twin pregnancies by Rydhström[6], show that definite progress has been made in recent decades regarding the aetiology of late antepartum fetal death. One is still left with a number

Table 1 Causes of antepartum stillbirth and incidence per hundred cases*

Cause	Belfast (up to 1952)	Chicago (1931–46)
Congenital anomalies	6	7
Infection: non-specific	1	1
Syphilis	3	1
Erythroblastosis fetalis	7	5
Diabetic or prediabetic mother	2	—
Miscellaneous	—	1
Extrinsic anoxia		
Accidents to cord	1 ⎫	8 ⎫
Haemorrhage: placenta praevia	1 ⎪	3 ⎪
Haemorrhage: cause uncertain	23 ⎬ 27	— ⎬ 32
Abruptio placentae	— ⎪	15 ⎪
Miscellaneous	2 ⎭	6 ⎭
Not ascertained		
No evidence available	54	53

* Modified from Morison[1]

of unexplained cases, but the incidence is much less than the 50% found in Belfast and Chicago during the 1930s and 1940s. I am convinced that the more we learn about the physiology and pathology of pregnancy, the smaller will be the number of fetal deaths for which no direct or indirect cause can be found. van Geijn and his colleagues (chapter 54) even doubt if a mature stillbirth can occur in an otherwise fully normal pregnancy.

Excellent guidelines for the pathological investigation in cases of stillbirth are given by Wigglesworth[7]. Flow charts describe the different steps leading to one or more specific diagnoses, or to the recognition of a profile of events leading to death. Very useful is his list of investigations which can be performed where permission for a formal autopsy is not obtained.

In addition to the contributions made by the participants in the workshop I would like to raise three points, two of which I have had the opportunity of discussing recently with Naeye.

UMBILICAL CORD: ACCIDENTS AND ABNORMALITIES

Whether or not accidents to the umbilical cord are responsible for otherwise unexplained fetal death is still a controversial subject. The large difference in incidence of umbilical cord-related antenatal fetal death in Morison's (1%) and Potter's (8%) series illustrates differences of opinion between leaders in the field of perinatal pathology (see Table 1). Looking into the charts of cases in which such accidents are deemed the cause of death is mostly a frustrating exercise. Detailed description of entanglement of the cord is generally lacking except in the mostly well-documented but very exceptional instances of intertwining of the cords in monoamniotic twins.

What is the evidence that, in a particular case, an accident to the cord may be responsible for antepartum fetal death? A number of abnormalities of the cord have been listed, e.g. true knots, tight wrapping around the infant's head, neck, rump or extremity, strangulation and venous thrombosis.

However, one should be very careful in establishing a causal relationship between the abnormality and the fetal death. It is known, for instance, that strangulation of the umbilical cord can occur after fetal death and is, therefore, a consequence and not a cause of it. Clear-cut criteria should be agreed on by the experts; these would be helpful to the clinicians who are frequently in doubt with regard to the relationship between varieties of positioning of the cord and antepartum fetal death.

A single umbilical artery, as found in one of the cases presented in chapter 54 of this volume by van Geijn et al., may also be related to late fetal death. In the US Collaborative Perinatal Project stillbirths were six times more frequent in such cases as compared to cases in which the vascular structure of the cord was normal.

BACTERIAL INFECTION

Chorioamnionitis has been recognized as an important cause of late fetal death. According to Naeye and Tafari[6] 'it is the most frequent cause of preterm birth and fetal and neonatal death wherever it has been studied'. Histology of the extraplacental membranes, plate of the placenta, and umbilical cord should be performed in all cases of stillbirth in order to recognize the disorder. Some years ago the infectious origin of chorioamnionitis had been doubted because in many instances it was not possible to isolate the bacterial agent. With improved bacteriological techniques the aetiological agent can now be cultured. In a recent study[7] bacteria were recovered from 26/31 placentas showing chorioamnionitis, whereas 25/30 placentas without chorioamnionitis were sterile. One should always perform anaerobic cultures because in approximately one-third of cases only a single such organism could be isolated.

The incidence of fatal amniotic fluid bacterial infections increases markedly at the end of pregnancy[6]. Reliable figures on the role of infection in late fetal death are not available, at least in Europe. Certainly this is one area in which more research is needed, preferably on a multicentric scale because the number of cases in most units is small.

MATERNAL BLOOD VOLUME

The marked increase in maternal blood volume during pregnancy has been recognized as a major factor in fetal growth and well-being. It is also known that low pregnancy weight gain is associated with lower blood volume expansion and with an increased incidence of antepartum fetal death.

The evidence linking low maternal blood volume and fetal demise is one of the recent contributions to the physiopathology of pregnancy. Analysing the data from the US Collaborative Perinatal Project Naeye[6] pointed out that only about one-third of the excessive fetal/neonatal mortality associated with low pregnancy weight gain was associated with acetonuria, so there must be additional causes of the deaths. There is strong indirect evidence that low maternal blood volume is another major contributor to this mortality.

Clinicians rarely have the opportunity of determining blood volume, but a correlation can be made by assessing maternal haemoglobin values and oedema of hands and face[7,8]. In the third trimester of pregnancy absence of oedema and high haemoglobin values or haematocrit reflect smaller expansion of blood volume with less haemodilution. In van Geijn's paper (chapter 54) case C, in which the haemoglobin levels increase towards the end of pregnancy, illustrates this point.

The message could be to look carefully at weight gain, oedema and haemoglobin levels during the third trimester of pregnancy in order to screen for cases in which the risk of late fetal death is increased.

References

1. Morison, J. E. (1970). *Foetal and Neonatal Pathology*, 3d edn. (London: Butterworths)
2. Potter, E. L. and Craig, J. M. (1976). *Pathology of the Fetus and the Infant*. (Chicago: Year Book Medical Publishers)
3. Wigglesworth, J. S. (1984). *Perinatal Pathology*. (Philadelphia: Saunders)
4. Potter, E. L. and Adair, F. L. (1943). Clinical-pathological study of the infant and fetal mortality for a ten-year period at the Chicago Lying-in Hospital. *Am. J. Obstet. Gynecol.*, **45**, 1054–65
5. Potter, E. L. and Dieckman, W. J. (1948). Fetal and infant mortality for the Chicago Lying-in Hospital, 1941–46. *Am. J. Obstet. Gynecol.*, **56**, 593–7
6. Naeye, R. L. and Tafari, N. (1984). *Risk Factors in Pregnancy and Diseases of the Fetus and Newborn*. (Baltimore: Williams & Wilkins)
7. Pankuch, G. A., Appelbaum, P. C., Lorenz, R. P. *et al.* (1983). Placental microbiology in the diagnosis of chorio-amnionitis. *Abstracts of the American Society of Microbiology*, p. 319
8. Naeye, R. L. (1979). Weight gain and the outcome of pregnancy. *Am. J. Obstet. Gynecol.*, **135**, 3–9

Index

337